Essential Revision Notes in Surgery for Medical Students

TEL: 01803 656700

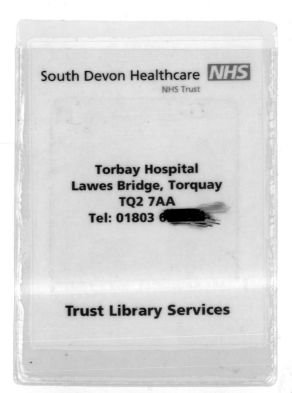
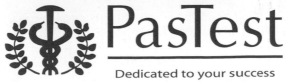

PasTest
Dedicated to your success

Essential Revision Notes in Surgery for Medical Students

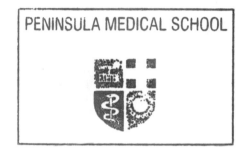

PENINSULA MEDICAL SCHOOL

Edited by
Irfan Halim MBBS MRCS MSc

Specialist Registrar in General Surgery

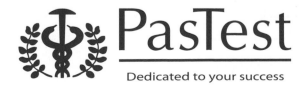

PasTest

Dedicated to your success

First published 2008

ISBN: 1 905635 39 7

978 1 905635 33 9

A catalogue record for this book is available from the British Library.

The information contained within this book was obtained by the author from reliable sources. However, while every effort has been made to ensure its accuracy, no responsibility for loss, damage or injury occasioned to any person acting or refraining from action as a result of information contained herein can be accepted by the publishers or author.

PasTest Revision Books and Intensive Courses

PasTest has been established in the field of postgraduate medical education since 1972, providing revision books and intensive study courses for doctors preparing for their professional examinations.

Books and courses are available for the following specialties:

MRCGP, MRCP Parts 1 and 2, MRCPCH Parts 1 and 2, MRCS, MRCOG Parts 1 and 2, DRCOG, DCH, FRCA, PLAB Parts 1 and 2, Dentistry.

For further details contact:

PasTest, Freepost, Knutsford, Cheshire WA16 7BR

Tel: 01565 752000   **Fax: 01565 650264**
www.pastest.co.uk   **enquiries@pastest.co.uk**

Text prepared by Saxon Graphics Ltd, Derby

Printed and bound in the UK by Cambridge University Press, Cambridge, UK

Contents

Contents

Contributors

Barnaby Garner Chappell BSc MBBS MRCS MSc (Urol)
Specialist Registrar in Urology, Department of Urology, Guy's Hospital, London
Urology

Rajib Das MBBS, BMedSci, MRCS
Clinical fellow, Breast and General Surgery, Department of Breast and General Surgery, St. George's Hospital, London
Abdominal Surgery

Gilles D Dreyfus
Professor of Cardiothoracic Surgery, Royal Brompton and Harefield NHS Trust, London
Cardiac Surgery, Thoracic Surgery

Ibraheim El-Daly MBBS
Foundation Year 1 in General Surgery, Kings College Hospital, London
Abdominal Surgery, Head, Neck, Neurosurgery and Orthopaedics

Amir Halim BMBS
Foundation Year 1 in Vascular Surgery, Derriford Hospital, Plymouth
Principles of Surgery

Irfan Halim MBBS MSc MRCS
Specialist Registrar in General Surgery, St. George's Hospital, London
Principles of Surgery, Abdominal and Breast Surgery

Ahmed Farhan Haq MB BCh BAO MSc MRCS
Research in Surgery, St. Mary's Hospital, London
Vascular Surgery

Karim Jamal BSc (Hons) MBBS
ST1 in Surgery, Kingston Hospital, London
Urology

Shelain Patel MBBS BSc MRCS
Senior House Officer, Trauma and Orthopaedics, Kingston Hospital NHS Trust, London
Plastic Surgery

Shahzad Raja
Details to come
Cardiac and Thoracic Surgery, Surgical Pathology

Nirooshun Rajendran BSc MRCS
Clinical Surgical Research Fellow, St. George's Hospital, London
Abdominal Surgery

Seyed MM Ameli Renani MBBS BSc (Hons)
Foundation Year 1 in Vascular Surgery, Department of Vascular Surgery, St. George's Hospital, London
Abdominal Surgery

Saima Saeed MBBS, MRCP
Clinical Fellow in Cardiothoracic Intensive Care, Cardiothoracic Intensive Care Unit, St. George's Hospital, London
Peri-operative Care and Anaesthetics

Naveed Shaikh MRCS (Eng)
Specialist Registrar in Trauma and Orthopaedics, St. George's Hospital, London
Orthopaedics and Trauma Surgery

Akash Sharma BSc (Hons) MBBS
Foundation Year 1 in Plastic Surgery, Department of Plastic Surgery, St. George's Hospital, London
Introduction to Surgery

Editor's Preface

There are many textbooks of surgery aimed at the undergraduate level in the bookstores today. Each one has particular aims with strengths and weaknesses. This textbook aims to provide exactly what the title says; a revision guide to the essential topics in surgery for students. It should be noted that it is not intended to replace the undergraduate surgical textbook from which students should learn concepts for clinical practice. The revision format makes it ideal to cover large volumes of essential and commonly occurring topics in both clinical practice and examinations. It also allows the book to be used as a quick reference text for future recap.

Essential Revision Notes in Surgery for Medical Students makes an ideal complement to the existing Medicine title by Philip Kalra. It has been written in the style of the existing Revision Notes series for post-graduate MRCS examinations. Particular highlights of this textbook in addition to standard surgical revision include a section on peri-operative care and an extended section on Pathology. Both of these topics are often omitted from formal undergraduate teaching programs as distinct subjects and often lose their value as they become incorporated into the newer "problem-based learning" modules. Students will find these sections extremely helpful in both medicine and surgery revision.

This book could not have been completed without the support of particular individuals who have helped me see this project through from start to finish. I would like to thank all the contributing chapter authors for making this book possible, Cathy Dickens from PasTest for all her support in making this project happen, Sarah Price and Fiona Power for looking over and proofing the text, and my family for all their support in all my endeavours. I would also like to thank a few particular trainers and mentors who have been exceptional in supporting me in my career and have helped me develop as a surgeon, in particular, Ahsan Zaidi, Rene Chang, Femi Olagbaiye, David Melville, Ciaran Healy, Shamim Khan, Ali Tavakkolizadeh, and my programme director Peter Leopold.

This book is dedicated to my little baby girl Zara, my wife Saila, and my parents for all their support, always.

Essential Revision Notes in Surgery for Medical Students is designed as a revision aid for medical undergraduates. It aims to accompany the clinical medical syllabus and has been developed by individuals with a particular interest in teaching surgery at the undergraduate level. The authors themselves range from Foundation Year doctor to Consultants and Professor, representing every main specialty within surgery. The junior doctors have been involved from a variety of medical schools to allow an adequate representation of the medical teaching syllabus from around the UK.

About this book

Medical training has changed considerably over the last decade with less emphasis on rote learning and a shift towards problem-based and systems-based learning. Post-graduate training has also considerably changed with the advent of the MMC and Foundation programmes. This has led to an overall shortened training period within a working week with fewer hours (EWTD). The pressures and challenges to adequately train the medical student and junior doctor are increasing by the day. This book aims to ease the burden of medical undergraduates by condensing a wealth of essential information required for clinical practice and passing undergraduate exams. .

There are many surgical textbooks of varying quality out in the markets today. This particular title is not a replacement for a proper surgical textbook. It is intended to complement a baseline knowledge derived from a combination of clinical learning and experience. Many of the sections are presented in bullet-point format with other sections requiring more explanation for "less digestible" topics. Diagrams and pictures are kept to a minimum and this is intentional in producing the essential revision notes format.

Particular highlights of this book in addition to the standard surgical core topics include a section on Peri-operative care and a section on Pathology. Both of these essential topics are often neglected from revision or core textbooks as they are assumed to be integrated into the relevant system of study. It is hoped that the student will be able to recap on these added sections as he or she feels necessary and that it will aid revision in general.

Essential Revision Notes in Surgery for Students:

- Helps you focus your revision
- Takes a succinct but detailed look at each specialty
- Draws on a wealth of knowledge from a list of experienced authors
- Incorporates figures and images to illustrate revision notes

This title incorporates a number of features designed to make your reading of the book as fruitful as possible.

Editor's Note

At the start of each chapter you will find a brief overview of the chapter subject broken down into specialisation where appropriate. General advice is also given on how to focus on revision topics that are commonly covered in medical final exams.

Revision Aids

Throughout the book we have highlighted sections that give the reader succinct lists to aid revision.

Essential Notes

As you read through each chapter, you will see pertinent points highlighted as 'Essential Notes'. Each of our subject-specific authors has used this feature to highlight certain key learning notes you should remember.

Notes on revision

Above all, it is important to be prepared. Leave yourself enough time to study and develop a true understanding of the subjects on which you are examined. Know where and when your examinations will be held and leave plenty of time to get there.

When you begin revising, you will soon discover what study techniques work best for you. Here are a few general tips to get you started:

Planning your revision

- Do not be too selective in your revision. It is dangerous to anticipate ('spot') specific questions and revise only those topics. Just because a particular topic appeared in an examination one year does not mean that it will not be examined in the following year.

- Aim to do equally well in all of your subjects. It is not a good tactic to attempt to do very well in some subjects and to neglect others.
- Make a realistic estimate of how much time you will be able to spend on concentrated revision. Make a timetable for your revision and try to keep to it This will help you to be more organised in your revision. During revision of one subject you will worry less about how much or how little revision you have done in another subject. Also, if you keep to your revision timetable, you will be able to enjoy your relaxation time without feeling guilty that you are not revising.
- In planning your revision timetable, allow some spare time for unexpected problems; for example, illness, or relationship problems.
- Allow some time immediately before the examinations to practise answering questions from previous examinations. It is a fallacy to assume that if you know a subject well you will automatically be able to write well about it.
- *Do not let the construction and constant alteration of revision schedules become a substitute for revision itself!*

Revision

- At the beginning of your revision of a subject, scan through the section of your notes that you wish to revise to get an overview. Then split the subject area into smaller sections, and tackle these in turn.
- Read through your notes actively, thinking about what they mean. If you refer to text books at this stage, integrate the information from them into your notes.
- Make a set of skeleton notes using the main headings and sub-headings of the material. Use flow diagrams, annotated illustrations or lists of topics. For lists which that have to be learnt 'by heart', try making a mnemonic, that is, a word in which the letters, or sentence in which the first letters of the words, trigger your thoughts to items on the list. For example, Richard Of York Gave Battle In Vain, for the colours of the spectrum in their correct order, Red, Orange, Yellow, Green, Blue, Indigo, Violet.
- Using your skeleton notes alone, test yourself to see how much you can recall.
- Look at questions from past examination papers, and check how you would answer them. Do not write out answers in full, but do make a written plan of what you would

include, and in what order. Remember that many examination questions will require the synthesis or comparison of material from more than one lecture, so to be fully prepared for an examination you should not learn lecture notes 'by heart', but you should understand and be prepared to apply the material which that you have been taught.

- Remember that during revision the general principles of private study apply. Familiar and reasonably comfortable surroundings aid concentration. There is an optimum time for concentrated study; too short a time interrupts your concentration, and after too long a time your ability to concentrate will decline.
- Immediately before the examinations, try to establish a routine with sufficient sleep and relaxation. There is little point in being full of facts but mentally or physically exhausted as you enter the examination.

The sections 'Planning your revision' and 'Revision' above are courtesy of the Study Skills sections of www.liverpool.ac.uk.

Notes on the exam

Common things are common and these will be concentrated on in the MB exam. Think carefully

if you find yourself answering a question by describing a rare disease – is there a more common condition you should be concentrating on?

- In general brevity is good – even in essays the examiner will have a mental tick list of important points and if these appear in your text you will generally do well.
- Read the newspapers – examiners do. They may light upon an item of topical medical news to discuss in an oral exam.
- When faced with an image that you do not recognise, describe it to yourself – many conditions in medicine have descriptive similes attached and describing the image may trigger the right memory.
- Knowledge learnt in one subject will overlap with other subjects, making the load of learning easier than it may first appear.
- In a multi-part question the subject (eg a disease) will usually be the same throughout.
- In oral examinations you dig your own holes – if you mention a rare and interesting condition that is relevant to the discussion then expect to be questioned about it.

Principles of surgery

CONTENTS

1.1.1 Learning surgery

Your first exposure to surgery and to seeing patients being cut open on the operating table will usually occur in your first clinical year. Your experiences of surgery may be varied, depending on your surgical firm, and the teaching quality can range anywhere from excellent to an unacceptable waste of time. Often this diversity in teaching can motivate or dishearten you about a genuinely exciting subject. This section aims to provide advice on how you can maximise your clinical learning experience in surgery.

My personal advice on learning surgery is to start early, even before joining a surgical firm. Some points that you should follow routinely include:

- Speak to students already on the firm before joining
- Establish a rapport with the surgical team you are joining
- Get a good surgical textbook for theory and one for examinations. Read them at least once properly and then as needed. My personal recommendations are:
  - Theory – *Lecture Notes in General Surgery* by Ellis et al
  - Examination – *Introduction to Symptoms and Signs of Surgical Disease* by Browse et al
- Attend all the teaching offered regularly
- Use free time to explore clinical experience (theatres, clinics, clerking)
- Stick to good teachers and spend time with them regularly
- Try to clerk and present as many patients as possible
- Have doctors demonstrate clinical signs and examination techniques to you
- Have doctors observe the way you examine and present patients
- Scrub in to as many cases as possible
- Try to observe patients and cases from other surgical firms with permission
- Learn relevant procedures and skills from day 1
- Do not be put off if doctors are too busy to teach you. Use self-directed learning here
- Read further about clinical cases encountered during the day
- Never be disheartened by doctors who treat you in an unacceptable manner. This is common in surgery and actually means nothing to you in the long run. Do not let them take you off your path to learning surgery. Be good and proper as a student

It is not difficult to follow the above points if these are built into a routine. They will not always apply, but their aim is to make your surgical experience fulfilling and your exams much easier. For those of you pursuing surgery in the future, you will be building upon these skills. For those of you pursuing other specialties, this may be the last opportunity for you to explore and learn surgery and become comfortable with assessing surgical patients.

Surgery is fun. Surgery is challenging. Surgery requires an engaged mind with a skilled hand. Learn it, apply it, teach it!

1.1.2 Diagnosing surgical patients

Diagnosing patients involves:

- History
- Examination
- Investigation

Every patient being seen for the first time should have a history taken and an examination performed as the minimum in diagnosing conditions. The only exception to this rule not being followed is in the acute state where a critically ill patient may require resuscitation and stabilisation first before reverting to the thorough clinical history and detailed examination when appropriate.

There is no good substitute for taking a thorough history when seeing patients for the first time. Regardless of your own level of surgical expertise, it is best to start taking full histories to obtain as much information as possible. Later on, as the student or junior doctor becomes more experienced, a focused and targeted history can be a more efficient means of assessment. This is required during busy times such as in the outpatient clinics and emergency departments.

Although this book is intended as purely a revision guide to surgery, no apology is made for recapping the very important history-taking section below, which is vital in any patient being assessed.

History taking follows a standard approach anywhere in the world and comprises the following:

- Introduction
- Presenting complaint
- History of the presenting complaint
- Past medical/surgical history
- Medications and allergies
- Family history
- Social history
- Systems review

Relevant sections such as immunisations, obstetric history and developmental milestones may be added as required, depending on the patient.

One of the commonest presenting symptoms in surgery as well as medicine is that of pain. In general surgery, abdominal pain is part of most disease processes in combination with other symptoms. The SOCRATES approach to ascertaining a history in patients presenting with abdominal pain allows for an easy and thorough assessment. This method is covered further in Chapter 4 and can also be applied to other common presenting complaints.

If you find it difficult to take histories, it is probably best to learn it via a combination of books, videos and personal observations of more senior doctors. Most importantly, though, is the self-directed practice of history taking with patients one-on-one. There is no substitute for this and it should be done with as many patients as possible. Once the full history is mastered, you should aim to make this more efficient by taking it in less time, or taking a more focused approach. Presenting histories is also equally important as this often alerts you to what you are doing right and what you are missing out. Many medical students of mine have taken a near-perfect history and presented it to me, often forgetting a single key question in the presenting complaint (eg forgetting to ask about dysuria or last menstrual period in a young woman with abdominal pain). Another great thing about taking and presenting histories is that it can be done before having learnt any examinations.

1.1.3 Surgical examinations
Surgical examinations are slightly different from the standard medical examinations applied in a general clerking, although the same principles apply, such as inspect, palpate, percuss and auscultate. Different conditions are focused upon in examination settings. Also, different examination algorithms exist for assessing particular surgical conditions and these must be learnt in order to complete any patient's surgical assessment.

Examples of surgical examinations include:

- Abdominal examination
- Vascular – arterial examination (usually lower limbs and systemic)
- Vascular – venous examination (lower limbs)
- Lump examination
- Ulcer examination
- Breast examination
- Neck/thyroid examination
- Hernia/groin-lump examination
- Scrotal examination
- Joint examination

Genuine effort should be made to learn these examinations as they are easy to learn and perform as well as appearing in every surgical exam! These are best learnt from surgical outpatient clinic settings as well as from emergency patients admitted on-take and elective surgical patients awaiting a surgical procedure (eg a patient awaiting a thyroidectomy with a palpable goitre).

Some chapters of this book cover an outline of the relevant surgical examinations as a revision tool, but this is not the book's main focus. There are many excellent textbooks to read in conjunction with practising and performing examinations under supervision. It is the supervision by and feedback from different doctors that will enhance your diagnostic skills, by learning how to pick up signs and combine the clinical assessment with a history. Demonstration of normal signs in addition to key signs is needed to learn them properly. How can you be expected to recognise an abnormal breath or heart sound if you don't yet know what a normal one sounds like?

1.2 SURGICAL METHODOLOGY

1.2.1 Incisions
Recognition and identification of surgical incisions is a key element of inspection in a clinical examination. The organ being operated on dictates the incision choice, in addition to other factors listed below:

- Site – depends on which organ is being operated on
- Size – access to the organ dictates size of incision
- Orientation – follow Langer's line to allow for better healing and cosmesis
- Surrounding tissues – healthy and non-infected tissues
- Anatomy of site – underlying structures that may need avoiding (eg nerves and arteries)
- Cosmesis – hidden scar (eg inframammary scar for breast implants)

With the advent of laparoscopic surgery, large incisions are now disappearing and nowadays scars as small as 5–12 mm are located in various sites around the abdomen. The combination of sites of these incisions can give a clue to the laparoscopic operation performed, although it is beyond the scope of undergraduate and early postgraduate teaching to learn these.

The most common incisions are shown and listed below, along with potential organs that may have been operated on through them (Figure 1.1, Table 1.1).

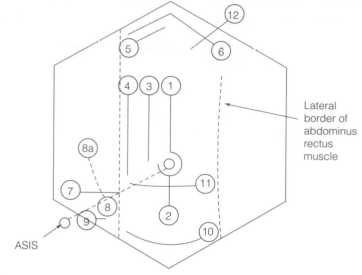

(1)   Mid-line incision through linea alba
(2)   Sub-umbilical incision
(3)   Para-median incision
(4)   Para-rectal 'Battle's' incision
(5)   Kocher's incision
(6)   Double Kocher's (rooftop) incision
(7)   Transverse muscle-cutting incision
(8)   McBurney's/Gridiron incision
(8a) Rutherford Morrison incision
(9)   Lanz incision
(10) Pfannenstiel incision
(11) Transverse incision
(12) Thoraco-abdominal incision

Figure 1.1: Common abdominal incisions

Table 1.1 Common incisions

Organ	Approach	Organ	Approach
Oesophagus	Cervical	Colon	Midline
Upper thoracic	Right 4/5 postero-lateral thoracotomy		Right paramedian
Mid thoracic	Right 5/6/7 postero-lateral thoracotomy		Right transverse
Lower thoracic	Right 5/6/7 postero-lateral thoracotomy		Rutherford–Morrison
	Left 6/7 postero-lateral thoracotomy		Gridiron
	Left thoracoabdominal	Appendix	Gridiron
Abdominal	Left thoracoabdominal		Lanz
	Rooftop		Midline
	Upper midline		Left paramedian
Stomach	Left thoracoabdominal		Left transverse
	Rooftop	Rectum	Midline
	Upper midline		Left paramedian
Liver	Right thoracoabdominal		Left transverse
Biliary tree	Rooftop		Perineal
	Upper midline	Uterus, ovaries	Midline
	Right paramedian		Pfannenstiel
	Kocher	Aorta	Midline
	Transverse		Transverse
Pancreas	Rooftop	Iliac vessels	Midline
Duodenum	Upper midline		Transverse
	Right paramedian		Rutherford–Morrison
	Kocher	Bladder	Lower midline
	Transverse		Pfannenstiel
Small	Midline	Kidney	Midline
intestine	Paramedian	Adrenal	Kocher
	Transverse	glands	12th rib incision

1.2.2 Sutures

Sutures are used in surgery to appose tissue edges that have been cut, as well as to tie off structures and provide secure ligation. Sutures may be found attached to needles or on their own as 'ties'.

Many different materials can be used to suture and there is much commercial competition between differing suture brands. At the undergraduate level, a basic understanding and classification of sutures is provided here with examples.

- Sutures may be absorbable or non-absorbable
- Sutures may be synthetic or natural
- Sutures may be monofilament or braided

Absorbable sutures are used for tissues that heal quickly, such as bowel anastomosis, skin suturing, ligation of vessels and mesentery and stoma creation. These sutures are understood to provide initial strength to achieve their purpose and then to degrade and dissolve over time by natural processes within the human body. Examples include Vicryl, Monocryl, Dexon, PDS and catgut (no longer used).

Non-absorbable sutures are used for tissues that heal slowly. They retain strength for a longer period of time to allow greater healing to occur (eg abdominal wall closure). They also cause less tissue reaction compared with absorbable sutures so they have some cosmetic advantage (exception is silk, which causes an inflammatory reaction). Examples include steel wire (sternotomy closure), nylon, silk, Prolene and PTFE. Although it is often assumed that non-absorbable sutures do not absorb within the body as their title suggests, this is not often the case and almost all suture materials (except steel) lose their strength and absorb over time. The main difference is the length of time which may elapse before a non-absorbable suture is dissolved (months to many years) as compared to an absorbable suture (weeks to months).

Synthetic sutures include Dexon, Vicryl, PDS, nylon, Prolene and PTFE.

Natural sutures include catgut and silk.

Monofilament sutures have a single filament and are easier to pass through tissues. They do not have braids in them in which infection can reside so they are less of an infection source. Disadvantages include the fact that they are slippery and difficult to knot due to the stiffness. Knots may not hold as securely because of this and lead to inadequate closures.

Braided sutures have multiple filaments running through them. Examples include Dexon, Vicryl, silk and nylon. They have the advantage of providing a more secure closure. They can cause more of a tissue reaction than monofilaments and also harbour bacteria between the braids, leading to infections.

1.2.3 Drains

Drains are used in various parts of the body to drain and collect air or fluids that can accumulate in compartments around the body. Some indications for usage of drains include but are not limited to:

- Wound drain (eg post-thyroidectomy or mastectomy)
- Abscess cavity drainage (eg corrugated drain)
- Abdominal drainage for ascites or post-operatively to check for blood, bile, urine, or anastomotic leakage
- Chest drain for air, effusion, blood, or rarely chyle
- Ventricular drains (eg external ventricular drains following subarachnoid haemorrhage)

Drains come in many forms and varieties. Drains are best classified into:

- Open or closed drains
  - **Open drains** allow drainage into dressings or a stoma bag through gravity or natural flow. Often, just making an incision into a superficial collection creates an open drain which can then be dressed appropriately. This is more often used in heavily infected cases or where a natural fistula has already formed. A corrugated drain is an example of an open drain.
  - **Closed drains** allow drainage of substances into a bag or bottle. As this is a closed system, infections are less likely to develop. A Robinson's drain is an example of a closed drain.
- Suction or non-suction drains
  - **Suction drains** help to collapse down wound cavities and drain them. If vacuum is applied, this can also help wound healing. Examples include Redivac drains, sump drains with suction and Vac dressings. Never apply a suction drain in a brain ventricle.
  - **Non-suction drains** are usually used in the brain ventricles or abdominal cavities post-operatively or for chest drains generally. They allow for natural collection of fluids, air, or other content as necessary within the body cavity.

1.2.4 Attending operations

It is a privilege as a student to be allowed to scrub in and assist a surgical procedure. This allows you to appreciate the anatomy and pathology of the surgical procedure and to feel part of the team involved in caring for a surgical patient.

Scrubbing-in

Always ask permission of the most senior surgeon if you can scrub up in the procedure to observe. If allowed to, make sure you learn the appropriate technique for scrubbing up from the theatre sister or surgeon. Once this has been learned properly and practised a few times, it should become a natural act provided it has been practised regularly as well. Try to wear a mask at all times with visor protection. This is to ensure that no bodily fluids get splashed onto your eyes and into your mouth. This is extremely common in surgery and following these simple measures can save a lot of unnecessary distress. The standard rule for hand washing is to scrub up for 5 minutes for the first scrub of the day and for 3 minutes between subsequent cases. The closed gloving technique is preferred over the open one, although it is best to learn both for comparison and personal choice.

Scrub brushes should not be used as they promote bacteria on the skin and also irritate the skin's surface. They can be used if necessary on the fingertips and nails, but they should not be used on skin. An appropriate glove size should also be checked prior to scrubbing up to allow for smooth assisting. Try to double-glove as much as possible to ensure universal precautions are carried out in every patient regardless of who they are and the nature of their operation. The human immunodeficiency virus (HIV) and hepatitis status of most surgical patients is not known and there is no point risking your life and career over something that could have been avoided. This advice is no different from asking all drivers to wear seatbelts whilst driving regardless of where and when they drive. If the law didn't insist on it, would all drivers neglect the seatbelt?

Assisting

Assisting in an operation can be exciting as it allows you access to view the operation upfront. It can also be boring, tiring and may not give you the view and angle you wanted to see the operation from. In certain cases, it is not always ideal to scrub up to get the best view and remaining unscrubbed also allows you freedom of movement within the case. Always follow the lead of the senior surgeon and do not ever risk the life and well-being of the patient by interfering or not following orders. You may often have to provide retraction for long periods of time in a particular stance and this can get painful for anyone. If there is a particular discomfort, it is best to ask politely for a break to readjust at the right moment in a surgical case. This allows you to carry on doing your job well and does not put the patient at any risk.

The operating room

When you are in the operating room you should notice that there are many things in this new environment that you haven't encountered before. Firstly, the people around the operating room have particular, defined job roles and you should introduce yourself to them so that they know how to help you and how you may be able to help them. Always try to assist them in any way possible, including the transferring of patients. They will, in return, teach you how to scrub and assist

in cases, and teach you about the operating room environment. In other moments when you are not assisting or learning, it is advisable to introduce yourself to the anaesthetist as well, who can teach you a lot. Many skills such as cannulation, intubation, central venous pressure (CVP) and arterial line insertion, lumbar puncture (LP)/spinal and ventilation can be learnt in a short time. Topics such as physiology and pharmacology can also be applied really well during the anaesthetic course and it is an asset to learn from these doctors as well. Rules include:

- Do not touch anything unless you know what you are doing
- Stay off the green sterile field unless you are scrubbed and sterile
- Always wear a mask as a student, even if not assisting
- Be polite to everyone and introduce yourself to make your own life easier
- Help out at all times
- Use every free moment to learn in the operating room, ask questions appropriately, take a surgical textbook to read on the side, read through patient notes and learn from anaesthetists
- Thank everyone for taking the time to accommodate you and for teaching you

Post-operative care

As a junior doctor, it is good practice to see the patient in the recovery room as they wake up. Many vital signs can be monitored here and on occasion a patient who may have to go back to the operating theatre can be recognised by following good clinical judgement (eg excess bleeding from a drain site in the recovery room, or blood-soaked dressings). After recovery, it is also advisable to see the patient on the ward at the end of an operating list or between cases if possible. This allows you to see the patient recovering and to speak to them about what happened during surgery. This helps in building rapport through communication and often allows you to speak to any family members at the same time so that any concerns are alleviated. If you get into this practice as a student, it becomes part of your good clinical practice and routine and makes you feel part of the surgical team. Students often spend more time with patients talking to them than the doctors looking after them. If a rapport has been established pre-operatively, the patient may expect to see the student after surgery as a friendly face who cares about their well-being.

1.3 PERI-OPERATIVE SURGICAL CARE

1.3.1 Preparing for surgery

When preparing for surgery, many things need to be considered in advance. It is surprising to see how often most of these things can go wrong. The following need consideration and addressing well before undertaking surgery on any patient:

- Ensuring appropriate indication for surgery
- Ensuring that the patient wishes to go ahead with surgery
- Ensuring appropriate setting and facilities (eg ITU, laparoscopic unit, anaesthetists with special skills)
- Full clerking of patient and identification of any special needs, medications or investigations
- Liaising with anaesthetists, theatre staff and the consultant/registrar about the cases
- Ordering and submitting the theatre list with appropriate case load and mix
- Ordering any special equipment well in advance of surgery
- Ensuring all investigations are adequate and results acted upon in the week before surgery
- Ensuring all patients have a bed on the wards or are admitted pre-operatively
- Ensuring that all patient's have been consented and marked appropriately (if necessary)
- Ensuring that all the patient's notes and scans are available well in advance (few days) of the operation
- Ensuring that any special adjuncts have been addressed on the day (ITU bed, surgical equipment, blood products, etc)
- Making sure that an appropriate time has elapsed since the patient last ate or drank
- Ensuring that the anaesthetist and theatres are aware of the patient's location (ward)

Although these points seem like a long list of chores, they often become second nature to the junior doctor once they are established on a surgical firm. For those who are still finding their way, there is never any harm in reverting back to the above checklist.

1.3.2 Informed consent

Informed consent should be sought before undertaking any investigation, treatment, screening, or research on a patient. All patients have a right to information about their condition and any options for further investigation and management plans. They also have the right to refuse any investigation or treatment offered to them at any time, even after a consent form has been signed. Acting against a patient's wishes can be regarded as assault. Most informed consent applies to competent patients who can:

- Understand the information given to them
- Retain the information
- Contemplate the information

It is good practice to ask if patients have understood the information and if they have any further questions of their own before proceeding.

Different laws apply for patients deemed incompetent and for children:

- For children under 16 years – parents should consent to treatment. If a child is deemed competent and understands the risks and benefits of treatment, they can consent to treatment even if their parents refuse. The converse is also true if a competent child refuses treatment, but the parents wish for it, then treatment may be given. A court order can be obtained in life-threatening cases where both child and parent refuse treatment.
- For incompetent adults (including temporary and transient incompetence) – the doctrine of necessity applies, where a physician can act in the patient's best interests.

Informed consent can be implied or acquired. Informed consent is implied in situations where there are no major complications resulting from it. A good example is when a doctor cannulates a patient or takes blood from them; no consent form is signed for the procedure or investigation. Any situation in which a major complication can arise should ideally have a signed consent form. This happens to be a grey area in most hospitals for intermediate ward procedures such as CVP line insertions, chest drains and LPs, which all have well-defined major complications listed. They are often treated as no different from any other ward procedure provided the appropriate precautions are taken and the procedure is discussed with the patient in the usual manner.

Informed consent in all other situations should include:

- Details of the clinical condition, including prognosis
- Management options
- Explanation of any proposed procedures
- Risks, benefits, side-effects and complications which may arise from it
  - Common (>1%) and serious complications and risks should be discussed
- The doctor responsible for their treatment
- An opportunity for the patient and family members to ask any questions

Normally, the consent forms provided these days in most hospitals have sections laid out which comply with the above points (except the last one) and can easily be gone through in a stepwise approach. Remember that patients may change their minds at any stage, even after signing the consent form. Consent should ideally be obtained by the doctor performing the procedure although it can be delegated to an appropriate team member of sufficient seniority and knowledge.

1.3.3 Communication

Communication is regarded as the most important part of any aspect of patient care. It is extensively taught and examined nowadays in the medical school curriculum. It is very briefly recapped in this section and the following skills should be learnt well as part of learning in surgery. They are only included here to remind you of the skills necessary and are not expanded upon any further in this book.

- Informed consent
- Explaining common procedures for a lay person to understand (eg gastroscopy, hernia repair, magnetic resonance imaging (MRI) scan)
- Breaking bad news (eg post- or peri-operative death)
- Dealing with angry patients (eg cancelling their operation due to lack of beds or overbooked lists)
- Communicating with foreign-language-speaking patients (eg use of translators, family, etc)

1.3.4 Post-operative review

The first post-operative review of a patient should ideally be done in the recovery area of theatres as the patient is waking up from anaesthesia. In reality, time pressures and other cases may prevent a surgeon from seeing a patient in recovery for review. It is good clinical practice to see all post-operative patients after the operating list has finished on the same evening. A quick ward round can be done to assess the patients for any potential problems as well as communicate with the patient as to the progress made by the surgical procedure. Analgesics and antibiotics can be given as well as permission to eat and drink as appropriate. Blood tests can also be ordered for the next morning during this round.

During the subsequent daily ward rounds it is important to monitor the surgical patient carefully to ensure that they are on the path to recovery from their surgical procedure. The aims of the ward round are to:

- Identify and address any problems reported by the patient or nursing staff
- Check routine observations:
  - Temperature
  - Heart rate
  - Blood pressure
  - Respiratory rate
  - O_2 saturations
  - Blood glucose (diabetics)
  - Fluid balance
    - Input
    - Output
  - Nutritional status ladder
    - Sips of water

  - 30 ml/60 ml/90 ml per hour of water
  - Clear free fluids
  - Free fluids (anything liquid)
  - Soft light diet
  - Light diet
  - Full diet
- Check analgesic control
- Examine the patient
  - Cardiorespiratory
  - Abdomen
  - Wound
  - Calves for deep vein thrombosis (DVT)
- Inspect the wound and drains
  - Note future date for suture removal
  - Drains (eg nasogastric tube, catheter, cavity drains, lines)
- Check blood and imaging results and compare with previous results
- Communicate findings
  - To patient (and relatives)
  - To own team
  - To nurses and other allied health professionals (eg physiotherapist, dietitian)
- Document findings
  - Clear legible and accurate notes

1.3.5 Post-operative complications

Post-operative complications occur frequently. They may be easily categorised by timing or by cause:

- Timing
  - Immediate (within 24 hours of surgery)
  - Early (occur up to 30 days for outpatients or during the inpatient stay)
  - Late (post-discharge or more than 30 days post-op)
- Cause
  - General complications of surgery (haemorrhage, infection, DVT)
  - Specific operative complication (eg anastomotic leak)
  - Complications as a result of patient co-morbidities (eg cardiac failure)

The commonest causes of post-operative complications in general are found in Section 3.3. I would highly recommend reading that section to familiarise yourself with a description of the commonest post-operative complications.

Complications should also be learnt which are specific to the procedure being performed (eg common bile duct injury during laparoscopic cholecystectomy). Although this is a post-graduate topic, some knowledge is tested in the written exams as well as in OSCEs.

The goal of a junior doctor in the post-operative period is to recognise complications early and prevent their progress by initiating appropriate management.

REFERENCES

Burnand K, Thomas W, Black J, Browse N. 2005. *Browse's Introduction to the Symptoms and Signs of Surgical Disease.* London: Hodder Arnold.

Ellis H, Calne R Y. 2002. *Lecture Notes on General Surgery*, 10th revised edition. Oxford: Blackwell Science.

Surgical pathology

CONTENTS

Surgical pathology

2.1 SURGICAL WOUND HEALING

Advances in pathology have resulted in better understanding of the basic mechanisms of wound healing. A detailed knowledge of these mechanisms allows surgeons to influence healing as well as anticipate and prevent problems of infection and incomplete or excessive repair. Despite marked improvements in wound care, poor healing, infection and excessive scarring continue to be leading causes of disability and death after surgical procedures.

2.1.1 Types of healing
Wound healing is conventionally divided into healing by first intention or by second intention.

- **Healing by first intention (primary)** occurs when tissue is cleanly incised and re-approximated and repair occurs without complication.
- **Healing by second intention (secondary)** occurs in open wounds through formation of granulation tissue and eventual coverage of the defect by spontaneous migration of epithelial cells. This type of healing is most commonly seen in infected wounds and burns. Primary healing is simpler and requires less time and material than secondary healing.
- These two forms may be combined in **delayed primary closure**, when a wound is allowed to heal open for about 5 days and is then closed as if primarily. Such wounds are less likely to become infected than if closed immediately.

2.1.2 Process of wound healing
The process of wound healing and repair is complex and involves signalling processes that include growth factors, complement, classic inflammatory mediators and metabolic signals such as hypoxia and accumulated lactate. For easy understanding, the complex process of wound healing can be described as a stepwise process involving:

- Coagulation and inflammation
- Fibroplasia and matrix deposition
- Angiogenesis
- Epithelialisation
- Collagen maturation
- Wound contraction

Coagulation and inflammation
Immediately after injury, inflammatory cells – particularly neutrophil macrophages – are attracted into the wound by the coagulation products and complement components. Activated platelets also release insulin-like growth factor 1 (IGF-1), transforming growth factor alpha (TGFα) and beta (TGFβ) and platelet-derived growth factor (PDGF), which further attract leucocytes and fibroblasts into the wound. Receptors for integrin molecules on the cell membranes of leucocytes are expressed by damaged endothelial cells in response to a signal cascade involving complement product C5a, tumour necrosis factor alpha (TNFα), interleukins 1 and 8 (IL-1 and IL-8). This enables circulating leucocytes to adhere to the endothelium and then migrate into the injured tissue. The inflammatory mediators released by leucocytes cause blood vessels to constrict initially in aid of haemostasis, and later dilate, becoming so porous that blood plasma and leucocytes can move freely into the area. At the same time lactate accumulation

secondary to hypoxia and increased lactate production by stimulated macrophages stimulates angiogenesis and collagen deposition. By the third or fourth day the reparative cells – macrophages and fibroblasts – are arranged in a characteristic spatial relationship.

Fibroplasia and matrix deposition

Replication of fibroblasts (fibroplasia) is stimulated by several growth factors released by platelets, macrophages and fibroblasts. Dividing fibroblasts are seen mainly near the wound edge, where they are exposed to the growth environment and to an oxygen tension of approximately 10 mmHg in normally healing wounds. These newly replicated fibroblasts secrete the collagen and proteoglycans of the connective tissue matrix that hold wound edges together.

Angiogenesis

Formation of new blood vessels (angiogenesis), an essential feature of repair, becomes visible about 4 days after injury but begins 2 or 3 days earlier when new capillaries sprout out of pre-existing venules and grow towards the injury in response to chemoattractants released by platelets and macrophages.

Epithelialisation

Epithelial cells also undergo replication in response to growth factors. Replication commences in epithelium a few cells away from the wound edge. The new cells migrate over the cells at the edge and into the unhealed area, perhaps attracted by a growth factor or cytokine, and anchor on the first unepithelialised place, forming a new wound edge.

Collagen maturation and contraction

Collagen maturation and lysis occur side by side. Collagenases released by fibroblasts and leucocytes ensure the lytic process. Collagen maturation and controlled lysis determine wound strength and durability. Finally, both open and closed wounds tend to contract if not subjected to a superior distorting force. The phenomenon is best seen in surface wounds, which, in areas of loose skin, may close 90% or more by contraction alone. Fibroblasts provide the motive force for contraction. Fibroblasts attach to collagen and each other and pull the collagen network together when the cell membranes shorten as the fibroblasts migrate. The fibres are then fixed in the packed positions by a variety of cross-linking mechanisms. Healing of wounds stops once the stimulants such as local hypoxia and lactic acidosis disappear.

2.1.3 Abnormalities of wound healing

Abnormalities of wound healing can be grouped under three categories.

1 **Formation of contractures**
- Contraction in the size of a wound is an important part of the normal healing process. An exaggeration of this process is called a contracture and results in deformities of the wound and the surrounding tissues. Contractures are particularly prone to develop on the palms, the soles, and the anterior aspect of the thorax. Contractures are commonly seen after serious burns and can compromise the movement of joints.

2 **Deficient scar formation**
- Inadequate formation of granulation tissue or assembly of a scar can lead to two types of complications: wound dehiscence and ulceration. **Dehiscence** or rupture of a wound is most common after abdominal surgery and is due to increased abdominal pressure. This mechanical stress on the abdominal wound can be generated by vomiting, coughing, or ileus. Wounds can **ulcerate** because of inadequate vascularisation during healing. For example, lower extremity wounds in individuals with atherosclerotic peripheral vascular disease typically ulcerate. Non-healing wounds also form in areas devoid of sensation. These **neuropathic ulcers** are occasionally seen in patients with diabetic peripheral neuropathy.

3 **Excessive formation of the repair components**
- Excessive formation of the components of the repair process can also complicate wound healing. Aberrations of growth may occur even in what may begin initially as normal wound healing. The accumulation of excessive amounts of collagen may give rise to a raised scar known as a **hypertrophic scar**; if the scar tissue grows beyond the boundaries of the original wound and does not regress, it is called a **keloid**. Keloid formation appears to be an individual predisposition, and for unknown reasons this aberration is somewhat more common in African-Americans. The mechanisms of keloid formation are still unknown. Another deviation in wound healing is the formation of excessive amounts of granulation tissue, which protrudes above the level of the surrounding skin and blocks re-epithelialisation. This has been called **exuberant granulation** or proud flesh. Excessive granulation must be removed by cautery or surgical excision to permit restoration of the continuity of the epithelium. Finally (fortunately rarely), incisional scars or traumatic injuries may be followed by exuberant proliferation of fibroblasts and other connective tissue elements that may, in fact, recur after excision. These are called **desmoids**, or aggressive fibromatoses. These lie in the interface between benign proliferations and malignant (though low-grade) tumours.

2.1.4 Factors affecting wound healing

Wound healing is affected by both local and general factors (Box 2.1).

Local factors that influence healing include the following:

- **Infection:** the single most important cause of delay in healing because it results in persistent tissue injury and inflammation.
- **Mechanical factors** (such as early motion of wounds): can delay healing, by compressing blood vessels and separating the edges of the wound.
- **Foreign bodies** (such as unnecessary sutures or fragments of steel, glass, or even bone): constitute impediments to healing.
- **Size, location, and type of wound:** influence healing. Wounds in highly vascularised areas, such as the face, heal faster than those in poorly vascularised ones, such as the foot. Small incisional injuries heal faster and with less scar formation than large excisional wounds or wounds caused by blunt trauma.

General or systemic factors that affect healing include the following:

- **Impaired perfusion and oxygenation:** the most frequent causes of healing failure. Oxygen is required for successful inflammation, angiogenesis, epithelialisation and matrix deposition. Collagen deposition in human wounds is proportionate to wound oxygen tension ($PaO2$). Human healing is profoundly influenced by local blood supply, vasoconstriction and all other factors that govern perfusion and blood oxygenation.
- **Cardiopulmonary diseases:** influence wound healing, but vasoconstriction due to sympathetic nervous system activity is the principal source of clinical problems. Prevention or resolution of problems can be achieved by minimising sympathetic activity by correcting blood volume deficits, alleviating pain and avoiding hypothermia.
- **Drugs:** impaired healing is common in patients taking anti-inflammatory corticosteroids, immunosuppressants, or cancer chemotherapeutic agents and whose inflammatory responses are blunted. Open wounds suffer more than primarily healing ones. The administration of these agents after inflammation has been established is less detrimental. Healing impaired by inadequate inflammation, especially that due to corticosteroids, can be accelerated by vitamin A systemically or locally.
- **Excessive and inadequate inflammatory responses:** can also influence wound healing. Inflammation may also be excessive. A mild excess may produce a hypertrophic scar. Prolonged inflammation due to infection or foreign bodies is a common cause of excess scarring. A major excess (eg

in response to endotoxin) can excite inflammatory cells to produce cytolytic amounts of cytokines and large amounts of proteinases with the consequence of lysis of newly formed tissue. In Gram-negative wound infections or septic shock, granulation tissue may not develop or it may be lysed.

- **Malnutrition:** impairs healing, since healing depends on cell replication, specific organ function (liver, heart, lungs) and matrix synthesis. Weight loss and protein depletion have been shown experimentally to be risk factors for poor healing. Deficient healing is seen mainly in patients with acute malnutrition (ie in the weeks just before or after an injury or operation). Even a few days of starvation measurably impairs healing, and an equally short period of repletion can reverse the deficit. Wound complications increase in severe malnutrition.
- **Diabetes mellitus:** is associated with delayed healing, as a consequence of the microangiopathy that is a frequent feature of this disease.

Box 2.1: Factors affecting wound healing

General factors
- Infection
- Hypoxaemia and hypovolaemia (eg cardiorespiratory disease)
- Radiation injury
- Uraemia
- Diabetes mellitus
- Jaundice
- Drugs: cancer chemotherapy, immunosuppressants, steroids
- Advanced age
- Starvation (protein depletion)
- Severe trauma
- Inflammation
- Smoking

Local factors
- Tissue injury
- Poor blood supply
- Wound mobility
- Poor apposition of surrounding tissues (unreduced fracture, unclosed dead space)
- Infection
- Foreign bodies

Inflammation is the complex biological response of vascularised tissues to noxious stimuli, such as pathogens, physical trauma, or irritants (Box 2.2). It is a protective attempt by the organism to remove the injurious stimuli as well as to initiate the healing process for the tissue. Inflammation is not a synonym for infection. Infection is caused by a pathogen, while inflammation is the response of the organism to the pathogen.

Box 2.2: Causes of inflammation

- Thermal burns
- Chemical irritants
- Foreign bodies
- Frostbite
- Immune reactions due to hypersensitivity
- Infection by pathogens
- Ionising radiation
- Necrosis
- Physical injury, blunt or penetrating
- Toxins

2.2.1 Types of inflammation

Inflammation can be classified as either **acute** or **chronic**. The two types differ from each other as shown in Table 2.1 below.

- **Acute inflammation** is a short-term process that is characterised by the classic signs of inflammation – swelling, redness, pain, heat and loss of function – due to the infiltration of the tissues by plasma and leucocytes. It occurs as long as the injurious stimulus is present and ceases once the stimulus has been removed, broken down, or walled off by scarring (fibrosis).

- **Chronic inflammation** is a pathological condition characterised by concurrent active inflammation, tissue destruction and attempts at repair. Chronic inflammation is not characterised by the classic signs of acute inflammation. Instead, chronically inflamed tissue is characterised by the infiltration of mononuclear immune cells (monocytes, macrophages, lymphocytes and plasma cells), tissue destruction and attempts at healing, which include angiogenesis and fibrosis.

The inflammatory response consists of two main components, a vascular reaction and a cellular reaction.

Vascular events in acute inflammation

Acute inflammation is characterised by marked vascular changes:

- Vasodilation
- Increased permeability
- Slowing of blood flow

These are induced by the actions of various inflammatory mediators (Tables 2.2 and 2.3). Vasodilation occurs first at the arteriolar level, progressing to the capillary level, and brings about a net increase in the amount of blood present, causing the redness and heat of inflammation. Increased permeability of the vessels results in the movement of plasma into the tissues, with resultant stasis due to the increase in the concentration of the cells within blood – a condition characterised by enlarged vessels packed with cells. Stasis allows leucocytes to marginate along the endothelium, a process critical to their recruitment into the tissues. Normal flowing blood prevents this, as the shearing force along the periphery of the vessels moves cells in the blood into the middle of the vessel.

Table 2.1: Comparison between acute and chronic inflammation

Characteristic	Type of inflammation	
	Acute	Chronic
Causative agent	Pathogens, injured tissues	Persistent acute inflammation due to non-degradable pathogens, persistent foreign bodies, or autoimmune reactions
Major cells involved	Neutrophils	Mononuclear cells (monocytes, macrophages, lymphocytes, plasma cells), fibroblasts
Primary mediators	Vasoactive amines, eicosanoids	INF-γ and other cytokines, growth factors, reactive oxygen species, hydrolytic enzymes
Onset	Immediate	Delayed
Duration	Few days	Up to many months, or years
Outcomes	Healing, abscess formation, chronic inflammation	Tissue destruction, fibrosis

Table 2.2: Plasma-derived inflammatory mediators (PAR-1 = protease-activated receptor-1)

Inflammatory mediator	Source	Function(s)
Bradykinin	Kinin system	A vasoactive protein which is able to induce vasodilation, increase vascular permeability, cause smooth muscle contraction and induce pain
C3	Complement system	Cleaved to produce C3a and C3b. C3a stimulates histamine release by mast cells, thereby leading to vasodilation. C3b is able to bind to bacterial cell walls and act as an opsonin, which marks the invader as a target for phagocytosis
C5a	Complement system	Stimulates histamine release by mast cells, thereby producing vasodilatation. It is also able to act as a chemoattractant to direct cells via chemotaxis to the site of inflammation
Factor XII (Hageman factor)	Liver	A protein which circulates inactively, until activated by collagen, platelets, or exposed basement membranes via conformational change. When activated, it in turn is able to activate three plasma systems involved in inflammation: the kinin system, fibrinolysis system and coagulation system
Membrane attack complex	Complement system	A complex of the complement proteins C5b, C6, C7, C8, and multiple units of C9. The combination and activation of this range of complement proteins forms the membrane attack complex, which is able to insert into bacterial cell walls and causes cell lysis with ensuing cell death
Plasmin	Fibrinolysis system	Able to break down fibrin clots, cleave complement protein C3, and activate factor XII
Thrombin	Coagulation system	Cleaves the soluble plasma protein fibrinogen to produce insoluble fibrin, which aggregates to form a blood clot. Thrombin can also bind to cells via the PAR-1 receptor to trigger several other inflammatory responses, such as production of chemokines and nitric oxide

[a]Non-exhaustive list.

Table 2.3: Cell-derived inflammatory mediators (IFN-γ = interferon-γ; IL = interleukin; NK = natural killer; TNF = tumour necrosis factor)

Name	Type	Source	Description
Lysosomal enzymes	Enzymes	Granulocytes	Granulocytes have lysosomes that contain granules with a large variety of enzymes which perform a number of functions. Granules can be classified as either specific or azurophilic, depending upon the contents, and are able to break down a number of substances, some of which may be plasma-derived proteins, allowing these enzymes to act as inflammatory mediators
Histamine	Vasoactive amine	Mast cells, basophils, platelets	Stored in preformed granules, histamine is released in response to a number of stimuli. It causes arteriolar dilation and increased venous permeability
IFN-γ	Cytokine	T cells, NK cells	Antiviral, immunoregulatory, and anti-tumour properties. This interferon was originally called macrophage-activating factor, and is especially important in the maintenance of chronic inflammation
IL-8	Chemokine	Primarily macrophages	Activation and chemoattraction of neutrophils, with a weak effect on monocytes and eosinophils
Leukotriene B4	Eicosanoid	Leucocytes	Able to mediate leucocyte adhesion and activation, allowing them to bind to the endothelium and migrate across it. In neutrophils, it is also a potent chemoattractant, and is able to induce the formation of reactive oxygen species and the release of lysosome enzymes by these cells
Nitric oxide	Soluble gas	Macrophages, endothelial cells, some neurones	Potent vasodilator, relaxes smooth muscle, reduces platelet aggregation, aids in leucocyte recruitment, direct antimicrobial activity in high concentrations
Prostaglandins	Eicosanoid	Mast cells	A group of proteins which can cause vasodilation, fever and pain
TNF-α and IL-1	Cytokines	Primarily macrophages	Both affect a wide variety of cells to induce many similar inflammatory reactions: fever, production of cytokines, endothelial gene regulation, chemotaxis, leucocyte adherence, activation of fibroblasts. Responsible for the systemic effects of inflammation, such as loss of appetite and increased heart rate

[a]Non-exhaustive list.

Cellular events in acute inflammation

Neutrophils (and perhaps a few macrophages) are critically involved in the initiation and maintenance of inflammation. These cells must be able to get to the site of injury from their usual location in the blood, so mechanisms exist to recruit and direct leucocytes to the appropriate place. The process of leucocyte movement from the blood to the tissues through the blood vessels is known as **extravasation**.

The first step is the binding of the neutrophils to the endothelium of the blood vessels. The binding is due to molecules called **intercellular adhesion molecules (ICAMs)**, which are found on the surfaces of neutrophils and on endothelial cells in injured tissue. The binding occurs in two steps. In the first, adhesion molecules called **selectins** lightly tether the neutrophil to the endothelium, so that it begins rolling along the surface. In a second step, a much tighter binding occurs through the interaction of **ICAMs** on the endothelial cells with **integrins** on the neutrophil.

Once bound to the endothelium, neutrophils squeeze through gaps between adjacent endothelial cells into the interstitial fluid, a process called **diapedesis**. Once outside the blood vessel, a neutrophil is guided towards the injurious agent by various diffusing **chemotactic factors** (Tables 2.2 and 2.3).

Morphological patterns of inflammation

Specific patterns of acute and chronic inflammation are seen during particular situations that arise in the body, such as when inflammation occurs on an epithelial surface, or when pyogenic bacteria are involved.

- **Fibrinous inflammation:** Inflammation resulting in a large increase in vascular permeability allows larger molecules such as fibrinogen to pass the vascular barrier, and fibrin is formed and deposited in the extracellular space. If an appropriate procoagulant stimulus is present, a fibrinous exudate is deposited. This is commonly seen in serous cavities, where the conversion of fibrinous exudate into a scar can occur between serous membranes, limiting their function.
- **Granulomatous inflammation:** Inflammation characterised by the formation of granulomas. A granuloma is a group of epithelioid macrophages surrounded by a cuff of lymphocytes. Granulomatous inflammation is seen in diseases such as tuberculosis, leprosy and syphilis.
- **Purulent inflammation:** Inflammation characterised by the formation of a large amount of pus, which consists of neutrophils, dead cells and fluid. Infection by pyogenic bacteria such as staphylococci is characteristic of this kind of inflammation. A large, localised collection of pus enclosed by surrounding tissues forming a pyogenic membrane is called an abscess.
- **Serous inflammation:** Inflammation characterised by the copious effusion of non-viscous serous fluid, commonly produced by mesothelial cells of serous membranes. Pleural effusion seen in connective tissue disorders is an example of serous inflammation.
- **Ulcerative inflammation:** Inflammation of epithelial surface resulting in the necrotic loss of tissue from the surface, exposing lower layers. The subsequent excavation in the epithelium is known as an ulcer.

Outcome of inflammation

The final outcome of inflammation is modified by many variables, including the nature and intensity of the injury, the site and tissue affected, and the responsiveness of the host. In general, however, acute inflammation may have one of three outcomes:

- **Resolution:** Characterised by the complete restoration of the inflamed tissue back to a normal status. Inflammatory events such as vasodilation, chemical production and leucocyte infiltration cease, and damaged parenchymal cells regenerate. In situations where limited or short-lived inflammation has occurred this is usually the outcome.
- **Fibrosis:** Seen when large amounts of tissue destruction take place or when tissues unable to regenerate are damaged. Fibrous scarring occurs in these areas of damage, forming a scar composed primarily of collagen. The scar will not contain any specialised structures, such as parenchymal cells, so functional impairment may occur.
- **Chronic inflammation:** In acute inflammation, if the injurious agent persists then chronic inflammation will ensue. This process, marked by inflammation lasting many days, months or even years, may lead to the formation of a chronic wound. Chronic inflammation is characterised by the dominating presence of macrophages in the injured tissue. These cells are powerful defensive agents of the body, but the mediators they release (including reactive oxygen species) are injurious to the organism's own tissues as well as to invading agents. Consequently, chronic inflammation is almost always accompanied by tissue destruction.

2.2.2 Surgical infections

A surgical infection is an infection that (1) occurs in an operated site or (2) is unlikely to respond to non-surgical treatment (it usually must be excised or drained), and occupies an unvascularised space in tissue. Common examples are appendicitis, empyema, gas gangrene and most abscesses.

This section deals with surgical infections in the following divisions:

- Pathogenesis
- Spread of infection
- Diagnosis
- Treatment
- Complications

Pathogenesis of surgical infections

Three features are common to surgical infections:

1 An infectious agent
2 A susceptible host
3 A closed, unperfused space

The infectious agent

A variety of organisms are capable of causing surgical infections. *Staphylococcus aureus* is the most common pathogen in wound infections and around foreign bodies. Among the other aerobic organisms, streptococci may invade even minor breaks in the skin and spread through connective tissue planes and lymphatics. *Klebsiella* often invades the inner ear and enteric tissues as well as the lung. Enteric organisms, especially the Enterobacteriaceae and enterococci, are often found together with anaerobes. Among the anaerobes, *Clostridium* species are major pathogens in ischaemic tissue while *Bacteroides* species and *Peptostreptococcus* are also often present in surgical infections.

Opportunistic organisms such as *Pseudomonas* and *Serratia* are usually non-pathogenic surface contaminants but can become lethal invaders in critically ill or immunosuppressed patients. Some fungi (*Histoplasma*, *Coccidioides*) and yeasts (*Candida*), along with *Nocardia* and *Actinomyces*, cause abscesses and sinus tracts, and even animal parasites (amoebas and *Echinococcus*) may cause abscesses, especially in the liver. Destructive granulomas, such as tuberculosis, once required excision, but antibiotic therapy has now superseded surgery for this purpose in most cases. Other rare diseases such as cat-scratch fever, psittacosis, and tularaemia may cause suppurative lymphadenitis and require drainage or excision.

Identification of the pathogen by smear and culture remains a crucial step in treatment. It is extremely important that maximum information is provided to the microbiologist of peculiar circumstances associated with any given specimen, so that appropriate smears and cultures can be done; serious errors may otherwise occur.

The susceptible host

The outcome of any infection, either surgical or non-surgical, is determined by the ability of the microbe to infect, colonise and damage host tissues and the ability of host defence mechanisms to eradicate the infection. Host barriers to infection prevent microbes from entering the body and consist of innate and adaptive immune defences. Innate immune defence mechanisms exist before infection and respond rapidly to microbes. These mechanisms include physical barriers to infection, phagocytic cells and natural killer cells, and plasma proteins, including the complement system proteins and other mediators of inflammatory responses (cytokines, collectins, acute-phase reactants). Adaptive immune responses are stimulated by exposure to microbes and increase in magnitude, speed and effectiveness with successive exposures to microbes. Adaptive immunity is mediated by T and B lymphocytes and their products.

Surgical infections such as appendicitis and furuncles occur in patients whose only defect in immunity is a closed space in tissue. However, patients with suppressed immune systems are being seen with increasing frequency, and their problems have become a major surgical challenge. Diabetes, acquired immunodeficiency syndrome (AIDS), transplant immunosuppression and agammaglobulinaemia are some of the conditions associated with increased susceptibility to infection. Defects in leucocyte chemotaxis, phagocytosis and oxidative killing are possible mechanisms resulting in increased susceptibility to infection.

The closed space

Most surgical infections start in a susceptible, usually poorly vascularised place in tissue, such as a wound or a natural space. The common denominators are poor perfusion, local hypoxia, hypercapnia and acidosis. Some natural spaces with narrow outlets, such as those of the appendix, gallbladder, ureters and intestines, are especially prone to becoming obstructed and then infected.

The peritoneal and pleural cavities are potential spaces, and their surfaces slide over one another, thereby dispersing contaminating bacteria. However, foreign bodies, dead tissue and injuries interfere with this mechanism and predispose to infection. Fibrin inhibits the clearing of bacteria. It polymerises around bacteria, trapping them. This encourages abscess formation but at the same time prevents dangerous spread of infection.

Foreign bodies may have spaces in which bacteria can reside. Infarcted tissue is markedly susceptible to infection. Thrombosed veins, for example, rarely become infected unless intravenous catheters enter them and act as entry points for bacteria.

Spread of surgical infections

Surgical infections usually originate as a single focus and become dangerous by spreading and releasing toxins. Spreading occurs by several mechanisms.

Spread of infection via the bloodstream

Surgical infections can spread via the bloodstream. Empyema and endocarditis caused by intravenously injected contaminated drugs are now common. Brain abscesses resulting from infections elsewhere in the body (especially the face) occur in infants and diabetics. Liver abscesses may complicate appendicitis and inflammatory bowel disease, sometimes as a result of suppurative phlebitis of the portal vein (pylephlebitis).

Spread of infection via the lymphatic system

Lymphangitis produces red streaks in the skin and travels proximally along major lymph vessels. However, it may also occur in hidden places such as the retroperitoneum in puerperal sepsis.

Necrotising infections

Necrotising infections tend to spread along anatomically defined paths. Necrotising fasciitis spreads along poorly perfused fascial and subcutaneous planes. The toxins cause thrombosis even of large vessels ahead of the necrotic area, thus creating more ischaemic and vulnerable tissue.

Abscesses

If not promptly drained, abscesses enlarge, killing more tissue in the process. Leucocytes contribute to necrosis by releasing lysosomal enzymes during phagocytosis. Natural boundaries can be breached, eg intestinal cutaneous fistulas may form, or blood vessel walls may be penetrated.

Phlegmons and superficial infections

Phlegmons contain little pus but much oedema. They spread along fat planes and by contiguous necrosis, combining features of both abscesses and necrotising infections. Retroperitoneal peripancreatic inflammation or infection is typical. Superficial infections may spread along skin not only by contiguous necrosis but also by metastasis.

Diagnosis of surgical infections

Diagnosis of surgical infections involves the following steps.

Physical examination

Physical examination is the easiest way to locate a surgical infection. When infection is suspected but cannot be found initially, repeated examination will often reveal subtle warmth, erythema, induration, tenderness, or splinting due to a developing abscess. Failure to repeat the physical examination is the most common reason for delayed diagnosis and therapy.

Laboratory findings

- **General findings:** Laboratory data are of limited value. Leucocytosis may give way to leucopaenia when the infection is severe. Acidosis is helpful in diagnosis, and signs of disseminated intravascular coagulation are useful as well. Otherwise unexplained respiratory, hepatic, renal and gastric (ie stress ulcers) failure is strong evidence for sepsis.
- **Cultures:** Positive cultures help to differentiate systemic inflammatory response syndrome (SIRS) from sepsis even though 50% of cases of sepsis are culture-negative. If infection is suspected, cultures of blood, sputum and urine are collected routinely initially, especially in hospitalised patients, given the high frequency of nosocomial pneumonia and urinary tract infections. Other fluids, such as cerebrospinal fluid, pleural and joint effusions, and ascites can be aspirated and cultured based on signs or symptoms that specifically indicate these sites as potential sources of infection. In general, pus from abscesses should be cultured, unless the causative organism is known. In rapidly advancing cases, two separate blood cultures should be taken within 15 minutes. In less urgent situations, cultures should be taken over a 24-hour period, and up to six should be taken if the patient has a cardiac or joint prosthesis or vascular shunt. False-negative blood culture results occur in about 20% of cases. False-positive results are difficult to define, since skin commensals (even some diphtheroids and *Staphylococcus epidermidis*), regarded as contaminants in the past, have proved occasionally to be true pathogens. Arterial blood cultures may be necessary to detect fungal endocarditis.

Imaging studies

Radiological examination is frequently helpful, particularly for the diagnosis of pulmonary infections. Whenever infection is close to bone, radiological examination is indicated to detect early signs of osteomyelitis, which might require more aggressive surgical or antibiotic therapy. Computed tomography (CT) scanning is useful for detecting abscesses in solid organs. CT scanning and ultrasonography are particularly useful in locating occult infection. Numerous radionuclide scans have been tested, all with fair results. The best radionuclides for labelling leucocytes are gallium (^{67}Ga) and indium (^{111}In).

Source of infection

An early diagnosis of sepsis is usually based on a combination of suspicion and inconclusive evidence, because the results of blood cultures are often unavailable during this stage. An important initial step is to identify the source. Once identified, any septic focus amenable to surgical therapy should be excised or drained.

Treatment of surgical infections

Incision and drainage
Abscesses must be opened, and bacteria, necrotic tissue and toxins drained to the outside. The pressure and the number of bacteria in the infected space are lowered due to incision and drainage. This inhibits the spread of toxins and bacteria. An abscess with systemic manifestations is a surgical emergency.

Fluctuation is a reliable but late sign of a subcutaneous abscess. Abscesses in the parotid or perianal area may never become fluctuant, and if the surgeon waits for this sign, serious sepsis may result. Drainage creates an open wound, but the tissue will heal by secondary intention with remarkably little scarring. Deep abscesses difficult to drain surgically may be drained by a catheter placed percutaneously under guidance by CT scanning or ultrasonography.

It may appear that a patient with sepsis cannot withstand operation. In fact, operation to drain an abscess may be the most important of all therapeutic measures. There is no substitute for obliteration of the focus of infection when it is surgically accessible.

Excision
Some surgical infections can be excised (eg an infected appendix or gallbladder). In these cases, drainage may not be necessary, and the patient is cured on the operating table. Clostridial myositis may require amputation of the infected limb. The success of such operations is greatly facilitated by intensive specific antimicrobial therapy.

Enhancement of vascularity
Just as infections due to vascular ischaemia are cured by restoring arterial patency, chronic infections in poorly vascularised areas, as in osteoradionecrosis, can be cured by transplanting a functioning vascular bed (eg a musculocutaneous flap or omental transposition) into the affected area.

Antibiotics
Antibiotics are not necessary for simple surgical infections that respond to incision and drainage alone – furuncles and uncomplicated wound infections. Infections likely to spread or persist require antibiotic therapy, best chosen on the basis of sensitivity tests. In 'toxic' infections, including septic shock, antibiotics must be started promptly and empirically and the regimen modified later according to the results of blood cultures. The choice of drugs must take into account the organisms most often cultured from similar infections in previous patients, the results of Gram-stained smears and specific characteristics of the patient.

Nutritional support
In malnourished, septic, or severely injured patients, the ability to avoid or recover from infection is often enhanced by aggressive nutritional therapy. Specific measurable effects include improved immunocompetency and blunting or reversal of catabolism.

Complications of surgical infections

Fistulas and sinus tracts
A fistula is an abnormal connection or passageway between two epithelium-lined organs or vessels that normally do not connect. A sinus is a chronically infected tract such as a passage between an abscess and the skin. Fistulas and sinus tracts often result when abdominal abscesses contiguous to bowel open to the skin.

Suppressed wound healing
Suppressed wound healing is a consequence of infection. The mechanism is probably stimulation by bacteria of cytokines, which in turn stimulates proteolysis, especially collagenase production.

Immunosuppression and superinfection
Immunosuppression is a common consequence of injury, which includes surgery, trauma, shock, or infection or sepsis. Superinfection occurs when immunosuppression provides an opportunity for invasion by opportunistic, often antibiotic-resistant, organisms.

Bacteraemia
The term bacteraemia is defined as the presence of bacteria in blood. The significance of bacteraemia is variable. It occurs during dental work, and in instrumentation of the gastrointestinal tract or infected urinary tract. In most cases it is transient, rapidly cleared and harmless. However, patients with damaged heart valves, cardiac, vascular, or orthopaedic prostheses, or impaired immunity are at increased risk and should receive an appropriate prophylactic antibiotic regimen.

Organ dysfunction
Uncontrolled infection leads to clinical deterioration, manifested as dysfunction of the brain (delirium), lungs (hypoxia), heart and blood vessels (shock and oedema), kidneys (oliguria), intestines (ileus), liver (hyperbilirubinaemia), and the haematological (coagulopathy, anaemia) and immunological systems (immunosuppression). This syndrome is referred to as multiple organ dysfunction syndrome (MODS). The risks of

organ failure in general are directly proportionate to the duration and severity of infection and inversely proportionate to the age and underlying health of the patient. It is frequently difficult or impossible to determine whether the cause of organ dysfunction in critically ill patients is severe infection or inflammation.

2.2.3 Infection control measures

Patients can acquire infection in hospital (nosocomial infection) through contact with personnel or from a non-sterile environment, or infection may develop from bacteria harboured by the patient before operation. Microorganisms are transmitted in hospitals by several routes, and the same microorganism may be transmitted by more than one route. There are five main routes of transmission: contact, droplet, airborne, common vehicle and vector-borne. Infection control measures include the following:

Universal precautions

Traditionally, patients with infection were individually isolated. In 1985 – partly in response to the human immunodeficiency virus (HIV) epidemic – a more general kind of isolation called 'universal precautions' was substituted. In this system, any procedure involving close contact with any patient – and especially those involving contact with blood – is performed by hospital personnel wearing gloves and other protective devices. As blood is the single most important source of HIV and other blood-borne pathogens (eg hepatitis B virus), the concept of universal precautions emphasises:

1   Prevention of needlestick injuries
2   The use of traditional barriers such as gloves and gowns
3   The use of masks and eye coverings to prevent mucous membrane exposure during procedures
4   The use of individual ventilation devices when the need for resuscitation is predictable

The Centres for Disease Control and Prevention (CDC) recommends that universal precautions apply to blood, semen and vaginal secretions; to amniotic, cerebrospinal, pericardial, peritoneal, pleural and synovial fluids; and to other body fluids contaminated with blood. Universal precautions are not recommended for faeces, nasal secretions, sputum, sweat, tears, urine, or vomitus unless they contain visible blood. The need for hand washing is not diminished by this system.

Precautions to be adopted by hospital personnel

- Most nosocomial acquired bacteria are transmitted through human contact. In order to minimise transmission in hospital, rules made for behaviour, dress and hygiene should be obeyed.

- Unwashed hands are by far the most frequent source of nosocomial infections such as pneumonia, intravenous catheter-related sepsis and wound infection. Routine hand washing should be a matter of reflex conditioning. In today's atmosphere, failure to wash one's hands between patient contacts in a hospital is essentially an unethical act.

Precautions to be adopted in operating theatres

- Any breach in sterility noted by any member of the operating team should be corrected immediately.
- Members of the team should not operate if they have cutaneous infections or upper respiratory or viral infections that may cause sneezing or coughing.
- Scrub suits should be worn only in the operating room and not in other areas of the hospital. If they must be worn outside the operating room, they should be changed before re-entering.
- Physicians and nurses should always wash their hands between patients. Careful hand washing should follow all contact with infected patients. For pre-operative preparation, hands and forearms up to the elbows should be scrubbed for 2–5 minutes with any approved agent if the surgeon has not scrubbed earlier in the same operating list. Shorter scrubs are allowable between operations.
- Traffic and talking in the operating room should be minimised.
- Though many parts of the operating environment are sterile, the operative field is not – it is merely as sterile as it can be made. Attempts to achieve a level of sterility beyond normal standards have not led to further reductions in wound infection rates. This reflects the fact that bacteria are also present in the patient, and immune variables are also important determinants of infection not affected by more aggressive attempts to achieve sterility.
- Many special and expensive techniques have been devised to minimise bacterial contamination in the operating room. Ultraviolet light, laminar flow ventilation and elaborate architectural and ventilation schemes have been advocated, but none has proved more effective than common sense and good surgical discipline.
- The only completely reliable methods for sterilisation of surgical instruments and supplies are steam under pressure (autoclaving), dry heat and ethylene oxide gas. Saturated steam, at 2 atmosphere pressure and a temperature of 120°C destroys all vegetative bacteria and most resistant dry spores in 13 minutes, but exposure of surgical instrument packs should usually be extended to 30 minutes to allow heat and moisture to penetrate to the centre of the package. Shorter times are allowable for unwrapped instruments with the vacuum-cycle.

Safe dry-heat sterilisation for instruments requires 4 hours at 160°C.

- Gaseous ethylene oxide destroys bacteria, viruses, fungi and various spores. It is used for heat-sensitive materials, including telescopic instruments, plastic and rubber goods, sharp and delicate instruments, electrical cords and sealed ampoules. It damages certain plastics and pharmaceuticals. The technique requires a special pressurised-gas autoclave, with 12% ethylene oxide and 88% freon-12 at 55°C, 8 PSI pressure above atmospheric pressure. Most items must be aerated, in sterile packages on the shelf for 24–48 hours before use in order to rid them of the dissolved gas. Implanted plastics should be stored for 7 days before use. Ethylene oxide is toxic and represents a safety hazard unless it is used according to strict regulations.
- Miscellaneous sterilisation procedures include soaking in antiseptics such as 2% glutaraldehyde to remove viruses from instruments with lenses. Total sterilisation by this method requires 10 hours.
- Chemical antiseptics are often used to clean operating room surfaces and instruments that need not be totally sterile.
- Other disinfectant solutions include synthetic phenolics, polybrominated salicylanilides, iodophors, alcohols, other glutaraldehyde preparations, and 6% stabilised hydrogen peroxide. These agents maintain high potency in the presence of organic matter and usually leave effective residual antibacterial activity on surfaces. They are also used to clean anaesthetic equipment that cannot be sterilised.
- Prepackaged instruments and supplies can be sterilised with gamma radiation by manufacturers.
- Synthetic fabrics have now proved to be superior barriers to bacteria and less costly than the traditional cotton. They can be used in gowns and drapes.
- Commensal bacteria on the patient's skin are a common cause of infection. Pre-operative showers or baths with antiseptic soap reduce the infection rate in clean wounds by 50%.
- Shaving of the operative field hours prior to incision is associated with a 50% increase in wound infection rates and should not be done.
- The skin to be included in the operative field should be cleansed with antiseptic. Non-irritating agents such as benzalkonium salts should be used in or around the nose or eyes. For other skin areas, the iodophors (eg povidone-iodine) and chlorhexidine are used most commonly.

2.2.4 Antibiotics

An antibiotic is a chemical compound produced by a microbe that inhibits or abolishes the growth of microorganisms, such as bacteria, fungi, or protozoans. The first antibiotic compounds used in modern medicine were produced and isolated from living organisms, for example the penicillin class produced by fungi in the genus *Penicillium*, or streptomycin from bacteria of the genus *Streptomyces*.

Mechanism of action of antibiotics

Antibiotics active against bacteria are bacteriostatic or bacteriocidal; that is, they either inhibit growth of susceptible organisms or destroy them. On the basis of their mechanism of action, antibiotics are classified as:

1 Those that affect bacterial cell-wall biosynthesis, causing loss of viability and often cell lysis (penicillins and cephalosporins, bacitracin, cycloserine, vancomycin)
2 Those that act directly on the cell membrane, affecting its barrier function and leading to leakage of intracellular components (polymyxin)
3 Those that interfere with protein biosynthesis (chloramphenicol, tetracyclines, erythromycin, spectinomycin, streptomycin, gentamicin)
4 Those that affect nucleic acid biosynthesis (rifampicin, novobiocin, quinolones)
5 Those that block specific steps in intermediary metabolism (sulphonamides, trimethoprim)

Antibiotics active against fungi are fungistatic or fungicidal. Their mechanisms of action include:

1 Interaction with the cell membrane, leading to leakage of cytoplasmic components (amphotericin, nystatin)
2 Interference with the synthesis of membrane components (ketoconazole, fluconazole)
3 Interference with nucleic acid synthesis (5-fluorocytosine)
4 Interference with microtubule assembly (griseofulvin)

For an antibiotic to be effective, it must first reach the target site of action on or in the microbial cell. It must also reach the body site at which the infective microorganism resides in sufficient concentration, and remain there long enough to exert its effect. The concentration in the body must remain below that which is toxic to the human cells. The effectiveness of an antibiotic also depends on the severity of the infection and the immune system of the body, being significantly reduced when the immune system is impaired. Complete killing or lysis of the microorganism may be required to achieve a successful outcome.

Routes of administration of antibiotics

Antibiotics can be given by injection, orally or topically. When given orally, they must be absorbed into the body and transported by the blood and extracellular fluids to the site of the infecting organisms. When they are administered topically, such absorption is rarely possible, and the antibiotics then exert their effect only against those organisms present at the site of application.

Selection of appropriate antibiotic

For optimal treatment of an infectious process, a suitable antimicrobial agent must be administered as early as possible. This involves a series of decisions:

1 The judgement, on the basis of clinical impression, that a microbial infection probably exists
2 Formulation of a differential diagnosis and possible microbial pathogens
3 Procurement of specimens likely to provide a microbiological diagnosis
4 Selection of the drug most likely to be effective against the suspected organisms ('empiric therapy')

5 Observation of the clinical response to the prescribed antimicrobial and laboratory identification of a putative microbial pathogen
6 Continuation of the empiric regimen or a switch to pathogen-directed therapy

When an aetiological pathogen has been isolated from a specimen, it is often possible to select the drug of choice on the basis of current clinical experience. Such a listing of drug choices is given in Table 2.4. Given the rising rates of multidrug-resistant bacteria and geographic differences in antibiogram data (tables setting forth the antibiotic sensitivities of pathogens), laboratory tests for antimicrobial drug susceptibility are necessary, particularly if the isolated organism is of a type that often exhibits drug resistance, eg enteric Gram-negative rods.

Table 2.4: Drugs of choice for suspected and empiric regimens[a]

Suspected or proved aetiological agent		Drugs of first choice	Alternative drugs
Gram-negative cocci	*Moraxella catarrhalis*	Amoxicillin-clavulanic acid or TMP-SMZ[b] ceftriaxone, penicillin[f]	Cephalosporins,[c] erythromycin,[d] tetracycline,[e] cefixime, ciprofloxacin, spectinomycin,[c] ampicillin, chloramphenicol
	Gonococcus		
	Meningococcus		
Gram-positive cocci	*Streptococcus pneumoniae* (penicillin-susceptible)	Penicillin,[f] ceftriaxone + vancomycin (combination therapy may be indicated)	Erythromycin,[d] cephalosporin,[g] vancomycin
	Streptococcus pneumoniae (penicillin-resistant)		
	Streptococcus, haemolytic, groups A, B, C, G	Penicillin[f]	Erythromycin,[d] cephalosporin,[g] vancomycin
	Viridans streptococci	Penicillin,[f] ±aminoglycosides[h]	Cephalosporin,[g] vancomycin
	Staphylococcus, methicillin-resistant	Vancomycin + gentamicin or rifampin (or both)	TMP-SMZ, ciprofloxacin
	Staphylococcus, non-penicillinase-producing	Penicillin	Cephalosporin, vancomycin
	Staphylococcus, penicillinase-producing	Penicillinase-resistant penicillin[i]	Vancomycin, cephalosporin[g]
	Enterococci	Ampicillin ± gentamicin	Vancomycin + gentamicin
Gram-negative rods	*Acinetobacter, Bacteroides, oropharyngeal strains*	Aminoglycoside[h] + imipenem, penicillin,[f] clindamycin	Minocycline, TMP-SMZ,[b] metronidazole, cephalosporinc, [g]
	Brucella	Tetracycline[e] + streptomycin	Tetracycline,[e] ciprofloxacin
	Campylobacter	Erythromycin[d]	Imipenem, newer cephalosporins[c]
	Enterobacter	TMP-SMZ,[b] aminoglycoside[h]	Ampicillin, TMP-SMZ[b]
	Escherichia coli (sepsis)	Aminoglycoside,[h] newer cephalosporins[c]	Ampicillin, cephalosporin[g]
	E. coli (first urinary infection)	Sulfonamide,[j] TMP-SMZ[b]	Ampicillin and chloramphenicol[b]

Table 2.4: *continued*

Suspected or proved aetiological agent	Drugs of first choice	Alternative drugs
Haemophilus (meningitis, respiratory infections)	Cephalosporins[c]	TMP-SMZ,[b] aminoglycoside[h]
Klebsiella	Cephalosporins[c]	TMP-SMZ
Legionella (pneumonia)	Macrolide + rifampin	Chloramphenicol
Pasteurella (Yersinia) (plague, tularaemia)	Streptomycin, tetracycline[e]	Cephalosporins,[c] aminoglycoside[h]
Proteus mirabilis	Ampicillin	Aminoglycoside[h]
Proteus vulgaris and other species	Newer cephalosporins[c]	Ceftazidime or cefoperazone + aminoglycoside; imipenem + aminoglycoside; aztreonam
Pseudomonas aeruginosa	Aminoglycoside[h] + antipseudomonal penicillin[k]	Chloramphenicol, tetracycline,[e] TMP-SMZ
Burkholderia pseudomallei (melioidosis)	Ceftazidime	Chloramphenicol + streptomycin
Burkholderia mallei (glanders)	Streptomycin + tetracycline[e]	TMP-SMZ,[b] ciprofloxacin, ampicillin, chloramphenicol
Salmonella	Ceftriaxone	TMP-SMZ[b]
Serratia, Providencia	Cephalosporins,[c] aminoglycoside[h]	Ampicillin, tetracycline,[e] ciprofloxacin, chloramphenicol
Shigella	TMP-SMZ[b]	
Stenotrophomonas maltophilia	TMP-SMZ[b]	
Vibrio (cholera, sepsis)	Tetracycline[e]	TMP-SMZ[b]
Gram-positive rods *Actinomyces*	Penicillin[f]	Tetracycline[e]
Bacillus (eg anthrax)	Penicillin[f]	Erythromycin[d]
Clostridium (eg gas gangrene, tetanus)	Penicillin[f]	Metronidazole, chloramphenicol, clindamycin
Corynebacterium diphtheriae	Erythromycin[d]	Penicillin[f]
Corynebacterium jeikeium	Vancomycin	Ciprofloxacin
Listeria	Ampicillin + aminoglycoside[h]	TMP-SMZ[b]
Acid–fast rods *Mycobacterium tuberculosis*	INH + rifampin + pyrazinamide + ethambutol	Other antituberculosis drugs
Mycobacterium leprae	Dapsone + rifampin, clofazimine	Ethionamide
Mycobacterium kansasii	INH + rifampin + ethambutol	Other antituberculosis drugs
Mycobacterium avium intracellulare	Ethambutol + rifampin + clarithromycin	Other antituberculosis drugs
Mycobacterium fortuitum chelonae	Amikacin + doxycycline	Cefoxitin, erythromycin, sulphonamide
Nocardia	Sulphonamide,[j] TMP-SMZ[b]	Minocycline

Table 2.4: *continued*

Suspected or proved aetiological agent		Drugs of first choice	Alternative drugs
Spirochaetes	*Borrelia* (Lyme disease, relapsing fever)	Tetracycline,[e] ceftriaxone	Penicillin,[f] erythromycin[d]
	Leptospira	Penicillin[f]	Tetracycline[e]
	Treponema (syphilis, yaws, etc)	Penicillin[f]	Erythromycin,[d] tetracycline[e]
Mycoplasmas		Macrolide or tetracycline[e]	
Chlamydiae	*C. psittaci*	Tetracyline[e]	Chloramphenicol
	C. trachomatis (urethritis or pelvic inflammatory disease)	Doxycycline or erythromicin[d]	Ofloxacin or azithromycin
	C. pneumoniae	Tetracycline[e]	Erythromycin[d]
Rickettsiae		Tetracycline[e]	Chloramphenicol

[a]Pathogen-directed therapy should utilise antibiogram data from clinical microbiology laboratory.
[b]TMP-SMZ is a mixture of 1 part trimethoprim and 5 parts sulfamethoxazole.
[c]Cephalosporins include cefotaxime, cefuroxime, ceftriaxone, ceftazidime, ceftizoxime.
[d]Erythromycin estolate is best absorbed orally but carries the highest risk of hepatitis; erythromycin stearate and erythromycin ethylsuccinate are also available.
[e]All tetracyclines have similar activity against microorganisms. Dosage is determined by rates of absorption and excretion of various preparations.
[f]Penicillin G is preferred for parenteral injection; penicillin V for oral administration – to be used only in treating infections due to highly sensitive organisms.
[g]Older cephalosporins are cephalothin, cefazolin, cephapirin, and cefoxitin for parenteral injection; cephalexin and cephradine can be given orally.
[h]Aminoglycosides – gentamicin, tobramycin, amikacin, netilmicin – should be chosen on the basis of local patterns of susceptibility.
[i]Parenteral nafcillin or oxacillin; oral dicloxacillin, cloxacillin, or oxacillin.
[j]Oral sulfasoxazole and trisulfapyrimidines are highly soluble in urine; parenteral sodium sulfadiazine can be injected intravenously in treating severely ill patients.
[k]Antipseudomonal penicillins: ticarcillin, carbenicillin, mezlocillin, azlocillin, piperacillin.
[l]First choice for previously untreated urinary tract infection is a highly soluble sulphonamide or TMP-SMZ.

Duration of antibiotic therapy

The duration of drug therapy depends on the nature of the infection and the severity of the clinical presentation. Treatment of acute uncomplicated infections should be continued until the patient has been afebrile and clinically well for at least 72 hours. Infections at certain sites (eg endocarditis, septic arthritis, osteomyelitis) require more prolonged therapy. In evaluating the patient's clinical response, the possibility of adverse reactions to drugs must be considered (Table 2.5). Such reactions can mimic continuing activity of the infectious process by causing fever, skin rashes, central nervous system disturbances and changes in blood and urine. In the case of many drugs, it is desirable to assess hepatic and renal function at intervals. Adverse events may require dose reduction or drug discontinuation.

Table 2.5: Common antibiotic-induced adverse reactions

Drug	Reaction
Aminoglycosides	Nephrotoxicity, ototoxicity
Cephalosporins	Diarrhoea or colitis, hypersensitivity reactions
Clindamycin	Diarrhoea or colitis, morbilliform skin eruption
Fluoroquinolones	Gastrointestinal intolerance, central nervous system abnormalities
Macrolides, azolides	Gastrointestinal intolerance
Metronidazole	Gastrointestinal intolerance, neurological toxicity
Penicillins	Hypersensitivity reactions
Tetracyclines	Gastrointestinal intolerance, candidal vaginitis
Trimethoprim-sulfamethoxazole	Gastrointestinal intolerance, hypersensitivity reactions
Vancomycin	Hypersensitivity reactions (red-neck or red-man syndrome)

Combination therapy

Indications

Occasionally combinations of antibiotics are used. Possible reasons for employing two or more antibiotics simultaneously instead of a single drug are as follows:

1 The necessity for prompt treatment in a severely ill patient suspected of having a serious microbial infection. A good guess about the most probable two or three pathogens is made, and drugs are empirically targeted to those organisms. Before such treatment is started, it is essential that adequate specimens are obtained for identifying the aetiological agent in the laboratory.
2 The presence of mixed infections, particularly those following massive trauma. Each drug is aimed at an important pathogenic microorganism likely to cause bacteraemia.
3 The need to delay the emergence of antimicrobial resistance to one drug in chronic infections by the use of a second or third non-cross-reacting drug. Treatment of active tuberculosis is a good example.
4 To achieve bactericidal synergism. Synergism is usually defined as more rapid and complete bactericidal action from a combination of antibiotics (usually a cell-wall-active agent, ie a β-lactam or vancomycin, plus an aminoglycoside) than could be achieved by either antibiotic alone. Unfortunately, such synergism is unpredictable, and a given drug pair may be synergistic for only a single microbial strain.

Disadvantages

The following disadvantages of using antibiotics in combinations must always be considered:

1 The more drugs administered, the greater the chance for drug reactions to occur or for the patient to become sensitised to drugs.
2 Combined drug regimens may be unnecessarily expensive.
3 Antimicrobial combinations often accomplish no more than an effective single drug.
4 Empiric, broad-spectrum antimicrobial coverage may compromise the effort to establish a specific aetiological diagnosis.
5 On rare occasions, one drug can antagonise a second drug given simultaneously. Antagonism resulting in increased rates of illness and death has been observed mainly in bacterial meningitis when a bacteriostatic drug (eg tetracycline or chloramphenicol) was given with (or prior to) a bactericidal drug (eg penicillin or ampicillin). However, antagonism can usually be overcome by giving a larger dose of one of the drugs in the pair and is therefore an infrequent problem in clinical therapy.

Antibiotic resistance

Resistance to an antibiotic may be inherent in a particular bacterial species or may be acquired as a result of mutations or acquisition of genes from another organism that encode for antibiotic resistance. Mechanisms for resistance that are encoded by these genes are briefly described in Table 2.6. Resistance genes can be transmitted between two bacterial cells by transformation (uptake of naked DNA from another organism), transduction (infection by a bacteriophage), or conjugation (exchange of genetic material in the form of either plasmids, which are pieces of independently replicating extrachromosomal DNA, or transposons, which are movable pieces of chromosomal DNA). Plasmids and transposons can rapidly disseminate resistance genes.

Table 2.6: Common mechanisms of resistance to antibiotics	
Mechanism	Example
Decreased cell wall permeability	Loss of outer cell wall D2 porin in imipenem-resistant *Pseudomonas aeruginosa*
Enzymatic inactivation	Production of β-lactamases that inactivate penicillins in penicillin-resistant *Staphylococcus aureus, Haemophilus influenzae, Escherichia coli*
	Production of aminoglycoside-inactivating enzymes in gentamicin-resistant enterococci
Changes in target	Decreased affinity of penicillin-binding proteins for β-lactam antibiotics (eg in *Streptococcus pneumoniae* with reduced penicillin sensitivity)
	Decreased affinity of methylated ribosomal RNA target for macrolides, clindamycin and quinupristin in MLSB-resistant *S. aureus*[a]
	Decreased affinity of altered cell wall precursor for vancomycin (eg *Enterococcus faecium*)
	Decreased affinity of DNA gyrase for fluoroquinolones in fluoroquinolone-resistant *S. aureus*
Increased antibiotic efflux pump	Increased efflux of tetracycline, macrolides, clindamycin, or fluoroquinolones (eg *S. aureus*)
Bypass of antibiotic inhibition	Development of bacterial mutants that can subsist on products (eg thymidine) present in the environment, not just products synthesised within the bacteria (eg trimethoprim-sulfamethoxazole)

[a]MLSB = macrolide, lincoside, streptogramin B.

2.3 METABOLIC AND NEUROENDOCRINE RESPONSES TO TRAUMA AND SURGERY

The metabolic and neuroendocrine responses to trauma and surgery are important components of the stress reaction as they improve the individual organism's chances of surviving under adverse circumstances or when injured. Although the magnitude of the biological responses varies according to the severity of the injury and is determined by the extent of injuries, the number of organs involved, the suddenness of the event, and whether or not a body cavity has been entered or damaged, the nature of these responses to injury or surgery are similar (Table 2.7).

Table 2.7: Influence of extent of injury on biological responses to injury

Extent of injury	Biological responses
Minimal surgery: laparoscopy, thoracoscopy, inguinal hernia repair, no large incision into body cavity	Minimal and appropriate. Minor changes in the homeostatic thermostat
Major surgery and non-life-threatening injury: large incision into a body cavity or multisystem injury	Major changes that seem to be interrelated and coordinated. Homeostasis seems evident
Life-threatening injuries, operations, or illnesses	Biological chaos – dyshomeostasis. The individual is overwhelmed by the multiplicity of changes that should be protective but become self-destructive

2.3.1 Phases of biological response to trauma and surgery

Francis Moore was the first to describe the four phases in the response to trauma and surgery (Table 2.8).

- The first phase begins at the time of injury or, for an elective operation, during preparation, when the patient stops oral intake, becomes anxious about the experience and receives pre-operative medication. The injury phase normally lasts 2–5 days, depending on the magnitude of injury and the presence or absence of complications.
- In normal convalescence, the second phase – the 'turning point' – is a transient period marked physiologically by a turning off of the neuroendocrine response and clinically by the appearance of getting well.
- The third phase is characterised by gain in muscular strength, or positive nitrogen balance.
- The fourth phase is characterised by gain in weight and body fat; or positive caloric balance. These patterns seem to be specific to trauma and surgery and are not observed in medical patients with sepsis.

Table 2.8: Phases of the biological response to trauma and surgery

Phase	Description
1 Injury phase	Lasts 2–5 days or longer. Duration is related to the magnitude of injury and the presence or absence of complications
2 Turning point	The neuroendocrine response turns off. A transient period. May occur overnight or develop over 1 or 2 days
3 Anabolic phase	Gain in muscular strength. Phase of positive nitrogen balance. Lasts 3–12 weeks or longer
4 Late anabolism	Gain in weight and body fat. Phase of positive caloric balance. Lasts months to years

2.3.2 Afferent pathways

The neuroendocrine and metabolic responses to trauma and surgery are initiated by the neural and mediator signals to the central nervous system primarily by way of nociceptors, baroreceptors, chemoreceptors and from the wound. A variety of stimuli can trigger a biological response and reset the homeostatic thermostat (Box 2.3).

The wound or surgical incision site also functions as a somewhat independent organ, calling on the rest of the body for support. It establishes a high biological priority for itself and triggers many of the changes in metabolism and responses to injury. It not only provides afferent stimuli to the central nervous system but also provides efferent stimuli to the liver, the temperature control centre and elsewhere. The inflammatory mediators produced by cells in the wound (Box 2.4) provide the afferent and efferent signals. These mediators have an autocrine function, along with paracrine activity. When produced in larger amounts, there is also a remote endocrine function. Many of these wound mediators – particularly the cytokines – stimulate the hypothalamus–pituitary–adrenal (HPA) axis. More importantly, these inflammatory mediators play a central role in the healing of the wound itself.

2.3.3 Efferent pathways

Trauma and surgery result in a variety of neurohormonal alterations (Box 2.5), which are responsible for the acute phase response (Box 2.6) and have an impact on the eventual outcome. The magnitude of this neuroendocrine response is proportionate to the severity of injury or operation, to body fluid and blood loss, sequestration of fluid into the wound (so-called third-spacing), and other factors. A summary of these neuroendocrine alterations is provided below.

- Hypothalamic stimulation leads to antidiuretic hormone (ADH) release from the neurohypophysis, adrenaline (epinephrine) secretion from the adrenal medulla and noradrenaline (norepinephrine) release from sympathetic nerve endings. Corticotropin-releasing hormone (CRH) travels to the adenohypophysis, stimulating adrenocorticotropic hormone (ACTH) production.

- Although the normal or primary stimulus to ACTH secretion is CRH, with trauma and surgery ADH and angiotensin II from the kidneys also stimulate ACTH. ACTH acts on the adrenal cortex, producing cortisol release. Significant effects of cortisol relevant to recovery from trauma and surgery are restoration of blood volume after haemorrhage, inhibition of extrahepatic protein synthesis, potentiation of glucose production and inhibition of various immune responses. Angiotensin II and aldosterone also serve as direct stimulants for cortisol secretion with injury. The immunosuppressive and anti-inflammatory properties of the glucocorticoids are well known. It has been suggested that they prevent the normal responses to trauma from proceeding to a stage of producing tissue damage and threatening homeostasis.

- Catecholamine production and release from both the adrenal medulla (adrenaline and noradrenaline) and sympathetic nerve endings (only noradrenaline) increase with injury, anxiety and after administration of many anaesthetic agents. Catecholamines are the primary agents producing the hypermetabolism that accompanies burns and other injuries, along with many other effects. Circulating catecholamine levels correlate positively with the severity of injury, particularly when there is head injury.

- ADH secretion is stimulated by factors such as fear, pain, haemorrhage; decreased atrial, arterial and portal pressures; and certain drugs, including morphine, barbiturates and anaesthetic agents, leading to water conservation. Normally, the primary stimulus for ADH secretion is increased plasma osmolality. However, the primary stimulant after injury is decreased effective blood volume. Angiotensin II may also affect ADH release.

- Aldosterone secretion also increases greatly with injury. Normally, the renin-angiotensin system controls its production. Sympathetic system or local stimulation of the myoepithelial cells of the juxtaglomerular apparatus results in renin production. Renin circulates and cleaves an α1-globulin produced in the liver to form angiotensin I. Angiotensin-converting enzyme (ACE) converts angiotensin I to the active form, angiotensin II, in the lungs, kidneys, or blood. Angiotensin II, which has a very short half-life, is a potent general vasoconstrictor with direct chronotropic and inotropic effects on the heart. This agent also seems to have an endocrine effect, increasing vasopressin secretion and sympathetic and adrenal medullary activity. Angiotensin II is the major stimulus for aldosterone secretion from the zona glomerulosa of the adrenal cortex. ACTH, which has a minor role in stimulating aldosterone secretion in normal individuals, is more important after injury or operation. Aldosterone secretion, causing sodium conservation, occurs with injury regardless of whether renal blood flow, vascular volume and renin production are altered. Secretion can be lessened, however, if sodium intake and plasma volume are increased.

- Thyroid-stimulating hormone (TSH) levels remain the same or decrease somewhat after injury, as do the levels of thyroxine (T_4). However, reverse triiodothyronine (rT_3) levels increase, with T3 decreasing, indicating a shift of circulating thyroid hormone from an active to an inactive form. This has been called the euthyroid sick (or low T_3) syndrome.

- Glucagon secretion and circulating levels are increased following trauma or surgery. Insulin levels remain normal or increase slightly but do not respond proportionately to the hyperglycaemia that occurs with injury. Thus, a period of insulin resistance resembling diabetes mellitus is a consequence of injury. Cortisol, glucagon and the catecholamines have been called the counter-regulatory or catabolic hormones.

- The endogenous opioid system modulates noxious stimuli and the sympathetic response. Circulating levels of endorphin (opioid peptides) rise after operation for as long as 72 hours. They produce some analgesia and a calming effect, along with other receptor interactions. Beta-endorphins from the central nervous system may contribute to hyperglycaemia and glucose intolerance after injury. Alkaloid compounds similar to morphine and codeine are also produced in the central nervous system. These neurotransmitters help integrate the response to injury.

In addition to the neuroendocrine alterations, immune modulation is also a component of the biological response to trauma and surgery. The specific or cell-mediated immune system is suppressed after injury and there is a reduction in expression of the class II major histocompatibility complex molecule HLA-DR in monocytes and reduction also in the expression of soluble HLA-DR molecules. In addition, B cells become differentiated into plasma cells that produce antibodies to specific antigens.

The non-specific immune system is also activated after trauma and surgery. Polymorphonuclear leucocytes (PMNs) increase and are activated. PMN priming and activation may play a major role in remote organ damage after ischaemia and reperfusion and severe injury.

Box 2.3: Stimuli triggering biological response to trauma and surgery

- Anaesthetic agents
- Anxiety
- Blood and body fluid (extracellular fluid) loss
- Drugs
- Fear
- Immobilisation
- Infection
- Invasive sepsis
- Long bone and pelvic fractures
- Major burns
- Organ injury – spleen, liver, lung, bowel, heart
- Pain
- Prolonged starvation
- Shock
- Tissue injury
- Tissue necrosis

Box 2.4: Inflammatory mediators central to biological response to trauma and surgery

- Cytokines
- Platelet-activating factor (PAF)
- Complement
- Kinins and kallikreins
- Endorphins
- Neutrophils, superoxides, proteases
- Immune complexes
- Histamine
- Nitric oxide (NO_2), endothelium-derived relaxing factor (EDRF)
- Myocardial depressant factor (MDF)
- Adhesion molecules
- Coagulation cascades
- Serotonin

Box 2.5: Neurohormonal alterations in response to trauma and surgery

Hypothalamus (neural control)

- Adrenaline (epinephrine): secretion from adrenal medulla increased
- Arginine vasopressin, antidiuretic hormone (ADH): increased production in hypothalamus and release from posterior pituitary gland
- Corticotropin-releasing factor (CRF): stimulates release of adrenocorticotropin
- Luteinising hormone-releasing hormone (LHRH): no recognised role
- Noradrenaline (norepinephrine): secretion from sympathetic nerve endings increased
- Somatostatin [growth hormone (somatotropin)-releasing inhibitory factor; SRIF]: uncertain role
- Thyrotropin-releasing hormone (TRH): no recognised role

Endorphins (encephalins) and pituitary (neural and hormonal control)

- Alpha-melanocyte-stimulating hormone: unknown function
- Arginine vasopressin: increased
- Beta-lipotropin hormone: unknown
- Corticotropin: increased
- Follicle-stimulating hormone/luteinising hormone (FSH/LH): decreased
- Growth hormone (somatotropin): increased
- Prolactin: increased; function obscure
- Thyroid-stimulating hormone (TSH): no change or decrease

Adrenal gland cortex (hormonal control)

- Adrenal oestrogens and androgens: no change or decreased
- Aldosterone: increased
- Cortisol: increased

Adrenal medulla (autonomic control)

- Catecholamines: increased

Thyroid gland (hormonal control)

- Reverse triiodothyronine: increased
- Thyroxine: no change
- Triiodothyronine: decreased

Box 2.5: *continued*

Pancreas (autonomic, hormonal and substrate control)
- Glucagon: increased
- Insulin: less increase than hyperglycaemia would produce

Kidney (autonomic and local control)
- Erythropoietin produced
- Renin-angiotensin activation

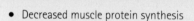

Box 2.6: Acute phase response to trauma and surgery

- Decreased muscle protein synthesis
- Hepatic gluconeogenesis
- Hepatic protein synthesis (acute phase reactants)
- Initial increased gut mucosal synthesis and export
- Kidney response
- Lung response (glutamine)
- Skeletal muscle proteolysis through the ubiquitin-proteasome pathway

2.3.4 Physiological effects

The physiological effects of the biological response to trauma and surgery can be summarised as:

1 Blood pressure and cardiac output maintenance by cardiovascular compensation and capillary refilling
2 Salt and water retention to maintain vascular and extracellular fluid volume
3 Increased metabolic rate (hypermetabolism)
4 Altered metabolism, with insulin resistance, hyperglycaemia, gluconeogenesis, excess catabolism and negative nitrogen balance, with release of intracellular components
5 Mobilisation of fats
6 Beginning of wound healing
7 Immunomodulation

2.3.5 Clinical effects

The clinical effects of the biological response to trauma and surgery are important as they can indicate whether the response is normal or complications are developing. During the injury phase, patients are quiet, lethargic and look ill. They are not interested in their surroundings or appearance. The patient's pulse increases modestly; temperature increases, with low grade fever of 37.7–38.3°C, oliguria tends to develop,

appetite decreases, the gastrointestinal tract and peristalsis are quiet and pain is present. A temperature elevation greater than 38.3°C suggests other problems such as atelectasis.

If the injury phase continues, weight loss, fatigue and weakness progress. The patient may have difficulty ambulating without help and eventually could be bedridden, with an altered sensorium, impaired ventilatory reserve and impaired ability to cough. Initially, body weight increases each day for 1–3 days as extracellular fluid and blood normally are sequestered in the injury site. After that time, daily body weight loss is equal to catabolism unless nutrition is provided.

If the patient is adequately resuscitated during the injury phase, the wound is adequately managed and complications avoided then the turning point is reached. This transitional phase may occur suddenly and dramatically overnight or may last 1–2 days or longer. This has also been called the corticoid withdrawal phase or the endorphin withdrawal phase and is characterised by shutting off of neuroendocrine stimulation. After a clean elective operation, the turning point is often clearly evident. Clinically during this phase the patient looks as if he or she is recovering, regains appetite and becomes interested in their surroundings. The patient becomes interested in personal grooming and wants to get up and move about. Pulse and temperature return to normal, and the patient has a sense of well-being.

The turning point is immediately followed by the anabolic phase, especially if the patient can take nourishment or is provided with parenteral nutrition. The patient at this time may begin to mobilise but feels weak and tired. Weakness is in good part due to the previous hypermetabolic catabolic response, loss of lean body mass and duration of bedrest. It is not unlike a febrile illness such as the flu, with loss of appetite, decreased oral intake and inactivity with bedrest. This has been called the period of ambition without fulfilment. Patients may feel great, feel like they are convalescing and believe they should be able to get out of bed and go home. Recovery of strength, positive nitrogen balance and restoration of muscle protein are slow procedures. If enteral or parenteral caloric intake during this period exceeds expenditure, some fat may be deposited as well.

The early anabolic phase overlaps with the final late anabolic phase, which is characterised by positive caloric and carbon balance. Fat stores are replaced. Although the fat gain may continue for months or years, some fat is restored earlier, along with protein. After nitrogen balance has been achieved, it becomes zero. Weight gain accelerates, but the extent of injury or surgery may dictate the amount of weight restored.

2.3.6 Strategies to minimise the biological response to trauma and surgery

The following strategies are adopted to minimise the biological response to trauma and surgery and expedite recovery.

- **Adequate resuscitation:** This is the first step towards recovery. Correcting volume loss, pain relief, repairing injured organs, supporting damaged organs, closing wounds and cleaning body cavities should stop the wounding and shorten the injury phase.
- **Effective surgery:** Careful surgical technique aimed at reducing the load of necrotic tissue and minimising the risk of post-injury or post-operative infection, either in the wound or elsewhere, ensures that the injury phase is curtailed. Debridement, irrigation, and cleaning and stopping continued pleural, peritoneal, bone, or muscle contamination are critical.
- **Minimally invasive surgical techniques:** Minimally invasive surgical procedures will decrease the response to stress and injury. In general, laparoscopic surgery reduces the stress response to injury compared with comparable procedures performed via an open approach.
- **Good anaesthesia:** Epidural or spinal anaesthesia and agents such as fentanyl and morphine decrease the response to injury by decreasing the cortisol, cAMP and glucose responses. Epidural analgesia also prevents the sensitisation of the spinal cord by pain. This effect may be enough to decrease morbidity. Thus, a combined neural and hormonal blockade inhibits the global stress response to operation. Epidural anaesthesia appears to attenuate the hormonal response to stress by blocking afferent pain stimuli that can still elicit a subconscious sympathetic response even in a patient under general anaesthesia.
- **Maintenance of temperature:** Clinical evidence suggests that even mild hypothermia during an operation is deleterious. Normothermia should be maintained during major surgery because it reduces the incidence of morbid cardiac events, reduces the incidence of surgical wound infection and shortens hospitalisation. Trauma patients should be rewarmed rapidly, because doing so improves survival.
- **Nutrition:** Nutritional support will decrease total protein loss. Early post-injury enteral feeding should be provided whenever possible, particularly if the patient will not be able to resume normal nutrition after 3–4 days or is severely hypermetabolic. Evidence is accumulating that additives such as glutamine, arginine, omega-3 fatty acids, branched-chain amino acids and antioxidants (vitamins C, A, and E and glutathione) may decrease the incidence of infection and provide immune enhancement.

- **Hormonal manipulations:** Evidence is also accumulating that hormonal manipulations with the anabolic hormones such as exogenous insulin, growth hormone and insulin-like growth hormone may have some positive effects in reducing protein loss, preserving body composition, increasing strength and decreasing complications such as infection. However, these agents are not recommended as yet for general use in injured and operated patients.

2.4 DISORDERS OF FLUID, ELECTROLYTES AND ACID–BASE BALANCE

Body fluid volume and electrolyte concentration are normally maintained within very narrow limits despite wide variations in dietary intake, metabolic activity and environmental stresses. Homeostasis of body fluids is preserved primarily by the kidneys.

2.4.1 Body fluid compartments

In each organ the internal environment consists of two phases or compartments: an interstitial fluid (ISF) compartment which bathes the cells, and has limited communication with the intracellular fluid (ICF) and the plasma compartment of the blood. These two compartments are separated by the capillaries of the circulatory system. With the exception of proteins, most solutes are readily and rapidly exchanged across the capillaries between the ISF and blood plasma compartments and their compositions are essentially similar. The plasma volume (PV) and the ISF together comprise the extracellular fluid (ECF) compartment of the organ in which the cells exist and function. These three fluid compartments (ISF, PV and ICF) together comprise the total body water (TBW) and account for about 60% of the body weight of the average lean adult male. The remaining 40% is composed of fat and solids.

Functional efficiency depends on the maintenance of homeostasis in the ECF. Because of the mixing of these fluids from the individual organs by the circulation of the blood throughout the body, all organs share an essentially common extracellular environment.

Compartment composition

The body is composed of water, minerals and a wide variety of organic compounds including protein, fat, carbohydrate and other organic substances. All of these substances are distributed in various forms and amounts, some as solids and many in solution, in the ICF and ECF compartments of the body. Some of the dissolved compounds are uniquely restricted to one or another of these compartments, and these compounds, by virtue of their osmotic activity, play a unique role in determining the volume of water in the body and its distribution among the body compartments. Of particular importance in this regard is the restriction of Na^+ to the ECF, of K^+ to the ICF, and of plasma protein, primarily albumin, to the intravascular space or PV.

2.4.2 Disorders of fluid volume

Disorders of fluid volume (or, more appropriately, ECF volume) can be categorised as:

- ECF volume contraction
- ECF volume expansion

ECF volume contraction

ECF volume contraction is a decrease in ECF volume caused by loss of water and total body Na^+ content. A decrease in ECF [ECF volume contraction (hypovolaemia)] is not the same as a decrease in effective plasma volume. Decreased effective plasma volume can occur with decreased ECF, but it can also occur with an increased ECF (eg in heart failure, hypoalbuminaemia, capillary leak syndrome). ECF volume contraction usually involves loss of Na^+. Na^+ loss always causes water loss. Depending on many factors, plasma Na^+ concentration can be high, low, or normal despite the decreased total body Na^+ content.

- Causes include vomiting, sweating, diarrhoea, burns, diuretic use and renal failure (Table 2.9).
- Clinical features include diminished skin turgor, dry mucous membranes, tachycardia and orthostatic hypotension.
- Diagnosis is clinical.
- Treatment involves correction of the cause of volume depletion and administration of fluids to replace existing volume deficits as well as any ongoing fluid losses and to provide daily fluid requirements. Mild-to-moderate volume deficits may be replaced by increased oral intake of Na^+ and water if the patient is conscious and is not vomiting severely. When volume deficits are severe or when oral hydration is impractical, intravenous 0.9% saline is given.

Table 2.9: Common causes of ECF volume depletion	
Extrarenal	Bleeding
	Dialysis: haemodialysis, peritoneal dialysis
	GI: vomiting, diarrhoea, nasogastric suction
	Skin: excessive sweating, burns, exfoliation
	Third-space losses: intestinal lumen, intraperitoneal, retroperitoneal

Table 2.9: continued	
Renal/adrenal	Acute renal failure: diuretic phase of recovery
	Adrenal disease: Addison's disease (glucocorticoid deficiency), hypoaldosteronism
	Bartter's syndrome
	Diabetes mellitus with ketoacidosis or extreme glucosuria
	Diuretics
	Salt-wasting renal disease (medullary cystic disease, interstitial nephritis, some cases of pyelonephritis and myeloma)

ECF volume expansion

An increase in total body Na^+ is the key pathophysiological event leading to ECF volume expansion. It increases osmolality, which triggers compensatory mechanisms that lead to water retention. Movement of fluid between interstitial and intravascular spaces depends on Starling's forces at the capillaries. Increased capillary hydrostatic pressure (as occurs in heart failure), decreased plasma oncotic pressure (as occurs in nephrotic syndrome), or a combination (as occurs in severe cirrhosis) shifts fluid into the interstitial space, producing oedema. In these conditions, subsequent intravascular volume depletion increases renal Na^+ retention, which maintains fluid overload. Common causes of volume overload are listed in Table 2.10.

- Clinical features include weight gain, oedema and orthopnoea. Symptoms and signs, including dependent oedema, are usually diagnostic. Physical findings might suggest a cause. For instance, oedema plus ascites suggests cirrhosis; rales and a third heart sound suggest heart failure.
- Generally, diagnostic testing includes serum electrolytes, urea, creatinine and any other tests directed at the cause (eg chest X-ray for suspected heart failure).
- Causes of isolated lower extremity swelling (eg lymphoedema, venous stasis, venous obstruction, local trauma) should be excluded.
- Treatment aims to correct volume expansion and its cause:
  - In patients with heart failure, maximising left ventricular function (eg by using inotropic agents or afterload reduction) can increase Na^+ delivery to the kidneys and Na^+ excretion.

- Treatment of the causes of nephrotic syndrome depends on the specific renal histopathology:
  - Loop diuretics, such as furosemide, inhibit Na$^+$ reabsorption in the ascending limb of the loop of Henle.
  - Thiazide diuretics inhibit Na$^+$ reabsorption in the distal tubule.
  - Both loop diuretics and thiazide diuretics increase excretion of Na$^+$ and thus water. K$^+$ wasting can be problematic in some patients.
  - K$^+$-sparing diuretics, such as amiloride, triamterene and spironolactone, inhibit Na$^+$ reabsorption in the distal nephron and collecting duct. When used alone, they increase Na$^+$ excretion, but only modestly. Both triamterene and amiloride have been combined with a thiazide to prevent K$^+$ wasting.

Many patients respond insufficiently to diuretics. Common contributing factors include inadequate treatment of the cause of volume overload, non-compliance with dietary Na$^+$ restriction, hypovolaemia and renal disease. Diuresis can frequently be achieved by increasing the dose of a loop diuretic or combining it with a thiazide.

After correction of volume overload, maintenance of euvolaemia might require restriction of dietary Na$^+$ unless the underlying condition can be eliminated. Diets containing 3–4 g/day Na$^+$ are generally adequate, are fairly well tolerated, and work reasonably well in mild-to-moderate volume-overload diets for heart failure. Advanced cirrhosis and nephrotic syndrome often require more severe Na$^+$ restriction (≤1 g/day). K$^+$ salts are often substituted for Na$^+$ salts to make Na$^+$ restriction tolerable; however, care should be taken, especially in patients receiving K$^+$-sparing diuretics or ACE inhibitors and in those with renal disease, because potentially fatal hyperkalaemia can result.

Table 2.10: Common causes of ECF volume expansion

Renal Na$^+$ retention	Cirrhosis
	Drugs: minoxidil, NSAIDs, oestrogens, fludrocortisone
	Heart failure, including cor pulmonale
	Pregnancy and premenstrual oedema
	Renal disease, especially nephrotic syndrome
Decreased plasma oncotic pressure	Nephrotic syndrome
	Protein-losing enteropathy
	Reduced albumin synthesis (liver disease, malnutrition)
Increased capillary permeability	Acute respiratory distress syndrome
	Angioedema
	Burns, trauma
	Idiopathic oedema
	IL-2 therapy
	Sepsis syndrome
Iatrogenic	Administration of excess Na$^+$ (eg 0.9% normal saline IV)

IL = interleukin; NSAIDs non-steroidal anti inflammatory drugs.

2.4.3 Disorders of electrolytes

Sodium

The normal individual consumes 3–5 g NaCl (130–217 mmol Na$^+$) per day. Balance is maintained primarily by the kidneys. Normal Na$^+$ concentration is 135–145 mmol/l (310–333 mg/dl). Potential sources of significant Na$^+$ loss include sweat, urine and GI secretions (Table 2.11). Na$^+$ concentration largely determines the plasma osmolality (P_{osm}), which can be calculated by the following equation:

$$P_{osm}(\text{mosm/l}) = 2[Na^+(\text{mmol/l})$$
$$+ \frac{\text{gluc (mg/dl)}}{18} + \frac{\text{BUN (mg/dl)}}{2.8}$$

Table 2.11: Composition of gastrointestinal secretions

Source	Volume (ml/24 h)[a]	Na$^+$ (mmol/l)[b]	K$^+$ (mmol/l)[b]	Cl$^-$ (mmol/l)[b]	HCO$_3^-$ (mmol/l)[b]
Salivary	1500 (500–2000)	10 (2–10)	26 (20–30)	10 (8–18)	30
Stomach	1500 (100–4000)	60 (9–116)	10 (0–32)	130 (8–154)	0
Duodenum	(100–2000)	140	5	80	0
Ileum	3000	140 (80–150)	5 (2–8)	104 (43–137)	30
Colon	(100–9000)	60	30	40	0
Pancreas	(100–800)	140 (113–185)	5 (3–7)	75 (54–95)	115
Bile	(50–800)	145 (131–164)	5 (312)	100 (89–180)	35

[a]Average volume (range). [b]Average concentration (range).

Normal P_{osm} is 290–310 mosmol/l. In general, hypotonicity and hypertonicity coincide with hyponatraemia and hypernatraemia respectively. However, Na^+ concentration and total body water are controlled by independent mechanisms. As a consequence, hyponatraemia or hypernatraemia can occur in conjunction with hypovolaemia, hypervolaemia, or euvolaemia.

Hypernatraemia

Hypernatraemia is plasma Na^+ concentration >145 mmol/l caused by a deficit of water relative to solute. Hypernatraemia in adults has a mortality of 40%–60%. Hypernatraemia usually implies either an impaired thirst mechanism or limited access to water. The severity of the underlying diseases that usually result in an inability to drink and the effects of brain hyperosmolality are thought to be responsible for the high mortality. The elderly are particularly susceptible, especially in warm weather, due to a reduced thirst response and underlying diseases. Common causes of hypernatraemia are listed in **Table 2.12**.

A major symptom is thirst; other clinical manifestations are primarily neurological (due to an osmotic shift of water out of cells), including confusion, neuromuscular excitability, seizures and coma. Diagnosis is by measuring serum Na^+. Treatment is usually controlled water replacement. If the response is poor, further testing (eg monitored water deprivation or administration of ADH) is directed at detecting the underlying cause.

Hyponatraemia

Hyponatraemia is a decrease in plasma Na^+ concentration to <135 mmol/l caused by an excess of water relative to solute. Common causes include diuretic use, diarrhoea, heart failure and renal disease (Table 2.13). Clinical manifestations are primarily neurological (due to an osmotic shift of water into cells), especially in acute hyponatraemia, and include headache, confusion and stupor; seizures and coma can occur. Diagnosis is by measuring plasma Na^+; plasma and urine electrolytes and osmolality help determine the cause.

Rapid correction of hyponatraemia, even mild hyponatraemia, risks neurological complications. Generally, Na^+ should be corrected no faster than 0.5 mmol/l per hour. The increase should not exceed 10 mmol/l over the first 24 hours. Any identified cause of hyponatraemia is treated concurrently.

Table 2.12: Major causes of hypernatraemia		
Hypernatraemia with hypovolaemia (decreased TBW and Na+; relatively greater decrease in TBW)	Extrarenal losses	GI: vomiting, diarrhoea
		Skin: burns, excessive sweating
	Renal losses	Intrinsic renal disease
		Loop diuretics
	Osmotic diuresis (glucose, urea, mannitol)	
Hypernatraemia with euvolaemia (decreased TBW; near-normal total body Na+)	Extrarenal losses	Respiratory: tachypnoea
		Skin: fever, excessive sweating
	Renal losses	Central diabetes insipidus
		Nephrogenic diabetes insipidus
	Other	Inability to access water
		Primary hypodipsia
		Reset osmostat
Hypernatraemia with hypervolaemia (increased Na+; normal or increased TBW)	Hypertonic fluid administration (hypertonic saline, NaHCO₃, total parenteral nutrition)	
	Mineralocorticoid excess	Adrenal tumours secreting deoxycorticosterone
		Congenital adrenal hyperplasia (caused by 11-hydroxylase defect)
		Iatrogenic

TBW = total body water.

Table 2.13: Major causes of hyponatraemia

Hyponatraemia with hypovolaemia (decreased TBW and Na; relatively greater decrease in Na⁺)	Extrarenal losses	GI: vomiting, diarrhoea	
		Third-space losses	Pancreatitis, peritonitis
			Small-bowel obstruction, rhabdomyolysis
			Burns
	Renal losses	Diuretics	
		Mineralocorticoid deficiency	
		Osmotic diuresis (glucose, urea, mannitol)	
		Salt-losing nephropathies	
Hyponatraemia with euvolaemia (increased TBW; near-normal total body Na⁺)	Diuretics		
	Glucocorticoid deficiency		
	Hypothyroidism		
	Primary polydipsia		
	States that increase release of ADH (post-operative opioids, pain, emotional stress)		
	Syndrome of inappropriate ADH secretion		
Hyponatraemia with hypervolaemia (increased total body Na⁺; relatively greater increase in TBW)	Extrarenal disorders	Cirrhosis	
		Heart failure	
	Renal disorders	Acute renal failure	
		Chronic renal failure	
		Nephrotic syndrome	

Potassium

K^+ is the major intracellular cation, with only 2% of total body K^+ located in the extracellular space. Because most intracellular K^+ is contained within muscle cells, total body K^+ is roughly proportional to lean body mass. An average 70-kg adult has about 3500 mmol of K^+. The normal serum concentration is 3.5–4.5 mmol/l. Approximately 50–100 mmol K^+ is ingested and absorbed daily. Ninety percent of K^+ is renally excreted, with the remainder eliminated in stools.

Hyperkalaemia

- Hyperkalaemia is serum K^+ concentration >5.5 mmol/l resulting from excess total body K^+ stores or abnormal movement of K^+ out of cells. Normal kidneys eventually excrete K^+ loads, so sustained hyperkalaemia usually implies diminished renal K^+ excretion.

- Hyperkalaemia also may be caused by transcellular movement of K^+ out of cells in metabolic acidosis; hyperglycaemia in the presence of insulin deficiency; moderately heavy exercise, particularly in the presence of β-blockade; digoxin intoxication; acute tumour lysis; acute intravascular haemolysis; or rhabdomyolysis. Much more unusual is hyperkalaemic familial periodic paralysis, a rare inherited disorder characterised by episodic hyperkalaemia due to sudden movement of K^+ out of cells, usually precipitated by exercise.

- Hyperkalaemia from total body K^+ excess is particularly common in oliguric states (especially acute renal failure) and with rhabdomyolysis, burns, bleeding into soft tissue or the GI tract, and adrenal insufficiency. In chronic renal failure, hyperkalaemia is uncommon until the glomerular filtration rate (GFR) falls to <10–15 ml/min unless dietary

K^+ intake is excessive or another source of excess K^+ load is present, such as oral or parenteral K^+ therapy, GI bleeding, tissue injury, or haemolysis.

- Other potential causes of hyperkalaemia in chronic renal failure are hyporeninaemic hypoaldosteronism (type 4 renal tubular acidosis), ACE inhibitors, K^+-sparing diuretics, fasting (suppression of insulin secretion), β-blockers, and NSAIDs. If sufficient KCl is ingested or given parenterally, severe hyperkalaemia may result, even with normal renal function. Causes are usually iatrogenic, such as giving K^+ supplements to patients taking ACE inhibitors.
- Other drugs that may limit renal K^+ output, thereby producing hyperkalaemia, include ciclosporin, lithium, heparin and trimethoprim.
- Clinical manifestations are generally neuromuscular, resulting in muscle weakness and cardiac toxicity that, if severe, can degenerate to ventricular fibrillation or asystole.
- Initial ECG changes occur with K^+>5.5 mmol/l, characterised by shortening of the QT interval and tall, symmetric, peaked T waves. K^+>6.5 mmol/l causes nodal and ventricular arrhythmias, widening of the QRS complex, PR interval prolongation and disappearance of the P wave. Finally, the QRS complex degenerates into a sine wave pattern, and ventricular fibrillation or asystole ensues.
- The diagnosis is made by plasma K^+ level >5.5 mmol/l. Because severe hyperkalaemia requires prompt treatment, it should be considered in patients at high risk, such as those with renal failure, advanced heart failure treated with ACE inhibitors and K^+-sparing diuretics, or symptoms of urinary obstruction, particularly if arrhythmias or other electrocardiographic signs of hyperkalaemia are present.
- Diagnosis of the cause of hyperkalaemia includes review of drugs and measurement of electrolytes, urea and creatinine. In cases where renal failure is present, additional tests, including a renal ultrasound to exclude obstruction, are required.
- Treatment involves giving a cation exchange resin and, in emergencies, Ca^{2+} gluconate, insulin and dialysis (Table 2.14).

Table 2.14: Management of hyperkalaemia

Mild hyperkalaemia (plasma $K^+ < 6$ mmol/l)

- Diminish K^+ intake
- Stop K^+-elevating drugs
- Loop diuretic enhances renal K^+ excretion
- Na^+ polystyrene sulfonate (ion exchange resin): acts as a cation exchange resin and removes K^+ through the GI mucosa

Moderate to severe hyperkalaemia (plasma $K^+ > 6$ mmol/l)

- Administration of 10–20 ml 10% Ca^{2+} gluconate (or 5–10 ml 22% Ca^{2+} gluceptate) IV over 5–10 min. Ca^{2+} antagonises the effect of hyperkalaemia on cardiac muscle excitability. *Caution should be used when giving Ca^{2+} to patients taking digoxin because of the risk of precipitating hypokalaemia-related arrhythmias.* If the ECG has deteriorated to a sine wave or asystole, Ca^{2+} gluconate may be given more rapidly (5–10 ml IV over 2 min). CaCl can also be used but can be irritating and should be given through a central venous catheter. The effect occurs within minutes but lasts only 20–30 min. Ca^{2+} infusion is a temporising measure while awaiting the effects of other treatments and may need to be repeated
- Administration of regular insulin 5–10 units IV followed immediately by or administered simultaneously with rapid infusion of 50 ml 50% glucose. Infusion of 10% dextrose in water should follow at 50 ml/h to prevent hypoglycaemia. The effect on plasma K^+ peaks in 1 h and lasts for several hours
- A high-dose β-agonist, such as albuterol 10–20 mg inhaled over 10 min (5 mg/ml concentration), can safely lower plasma K^+ by 0.5–1.5 mmol/l and may be a helpful adjunct. The peak effect occurs in 90 min
- Administration of IV $NaHCO_3$ is controversial. It may lower serum K^+ over several hours. Reduction may result from alkalinisation or the hypertonicity due to the concentrated Na^+ in the preparation. The hypertonic Na^+ that it contains may be harmful for dialysis patients who also may have volume overload. If given, the usual dose is 45 mmol (1 ampoule of 7.5% $NaHCO_3$) infused over 5 min and repeated in 30 min. Bicarbonate therapy has little effect when used by itself in patients with advanced renal insufficiency unless acidaemia is also present
- Na^+ polystyrene sulfonate (ion exchange resin)
- Haemodialysis

Hypokalaemia

Hypokalaemia is a serum K^+ concentration <3.5 mmol/l caused by a deficit in total body K^+ stores or abnormal movement of K^+ into cells. Causes of hypokalaemia are listed in Table 2.15.

- Mild hypokalaemia (plasma K^+ 3.0–3.5 mmol/l) rarely causes symptoms.
- Plasma K^+ < 3 mmol/l generally produces muscle weakness and may lead to paralysis and respiratory failure.

- Other muscular dysfunction includes cramping, fasciculations, paralytic ileus, hypoventilation, hypotension, tetany and rhabdomyolysis.
- Persistent hypokalaemia can impair renal concentrating ability, producing polyuria with secondary polydipsia.
- Cardiac effects of hypokalaemia are usually minimal until plasma K^+ levels are <3 mmol/l. Hypokalaemia causes sagging of the ST segment, depression of the T wave, and elevation of the U wave. With marked hypokalaemia, the T wave becomes progressively smaller and the U wave becomes increasingly larger. Sometimes, a flat or positive T wave merges with a positive U wave, which may be confused with QT prolongation. Hypokalaemia may produce premature ventricular and atrial contractions, ventricular and atrial tachyarrhythmias, and second- or third-degree atrioventricular block. Such arrhythmias become more severe with increasingly severe hypokalaemia; eventually, ventricular fibrillation may occur. Patients with significant pre-existing heart disease

Table 2.15: Causes of hypokalaemia	
GI tract losses	Chronic diarrhoea
	Chronic laxative abuse
	Bowel diversion
	Clay pica
	Vomiting
	Gastric suction (which removes HCl, causing the kidneys to excrete K^+)
	Villous adenoma of the colon
Intracellular shift	Glycogenesis during total parenteral nutrition or enteral hyperalimentation
	Administration of insulin
	Stimulation of the sympathetic nervous system, particularly with β_2-agonists (eg albuterol, terbutaline)
	Thyrotoxicosis
	Familial periodic paralysis
Renal losses	Adrenal steroid excess [Cushing's syndrome, primary hyperaldosteronism, rare renin-secreting tumours, glucocorticoid-remediable aldosteronism (a rare inherited disorder involving abnormal aldosterone metabolism), and congenital adrenal hyperplasia]
	Inhibition of the enzyme 11β-hydroxysteroid dehydrogenase (11β-HSDH)
	Liddle syndrome
	Bartter's and Gitelman's syndromes
	Congenital and acquired renal tubular diseases, such as the renal tubular acidoses and Fanconi syndrome
Drugs	Diuretics
	Amphotericin B
	Antipseudomonal penicillins (eg carbenicillin)
	Acute and chronic theophylline intoxication

and/or those receiving digoxin are at risk of cardiac conduction abnormalities, even with mild hypokalaemia.

- Diagnosis is by serum measurement.
- Treatment is administration of K^+ and addressing the cause. Many oral K^+ supplements are available. Because they cause GI irritation and occasional bleeding, they are usually given in divided doses. Liquid KCl given orally elevates levels within 1–2 hours, but it is poorly tolerated in doses >25–50 mmol due to bitter taste. Wax-impregnated KCl preparations are safe and better tolerated. GI bleeding may be even less common with microencapsulated KCl preparations. Several preparations containing 8 or 10 mmol/capsule are available.

When hypokalaemia is severe, is unresponsive to oral therapy, or occurs in hospitalised patients with active disease, K^+ must be replaced parenterally. Because K^+ solutions can irritate peripheral veins, the **concentration should not exceed 40 mmol/l**. The rate of correction of hypokalaemia is limited because of the lag in K^+ movement into cells. Routine **infusion rates should not exceed 10 mmol/h. A total of 240 mmol of K^+ in a 24-h period should not be exceeded** either. In hypokalaemic-induced arrhythmia, IV KCl must be given more rapidly, usually through a central vein or using multiple peripheral veins simultaneously. Infusion of 40 mmol KCl/h can be undertaken but only with continuous cardiac monitoring and hourly plasma K^+ determinations. Glucose solutions are avoided because elevation in the plasma insulin levels could result in transient worsening of hypokalaemia.

Calcium

Normal total plasma Ca^{2+} levels range from 2.20 to 2.60 mmol/l (8.8–10.4 mg/dl). About 40% of the total blood Ca^{2+} is bound to plasma proteins, primarily albumin. The remaining 60% includes ionised Ca^{2+} plus Ca^{2+} complexed with phosphate (PO_4) and citrate. Total Ca^{2+} (ie protein-bound, complexed and ionised calcium) is usually what is determined by clinical laboratory measurement. Ideally, the ionised or free Ca^{2+} should be determined, because this is the physiologically active form of Ca^{2+} in plasma. However, this determination, because of its technical difficulty, is usually restricted to patients in whom significant alteration of protein binding of plasma Ca^{2+} is suspected. Ionised Ca^{2+} is generally assumed to be roughly 50% of the total plasma calcium.

Ca^{2+} is required for the proper functioning of muscle contraction, nerve conduction, hormone release and blood coagulation. In addition, Ca^{2+} helps regulate many enzymes. Despite its important intracellular roles, roughly 99% of body calcium is in bone, mainly as hydroxyapatite crystals. Roughly 1% of bone Ca^{2+} is freely exchangeable with the ECF and therefore is available for buffering changes in calcium balance.

Maintenance of the body Ca^{2+} stores depends on dietary Ca^{2+} intake, absorption of Ca^{2+} from the GI tract and renal Ca^{2+} excretion. In a balanced diet, roughly 1000 mg of Ca^{2+} is ingested each day. About 200 mg/day is lost in the bile and other GI secretions. Depending on the concentration of circulating vitamin D, particularly $1,25(OH)_2D$ [1,25-dihydroxycholecalciferol, calcitriol, or active vitamin D hormone, which is converted in the kidney from 25(OH)D, the inactive form], roughly 200–400 mg of Ca^{2+} is absorbed from the intestine each day. The remaining 800–1000 mg appears in the stool. Ca^{2+} balance is maintained through renal Ca^{2+} excretion averaging 200 mg/day.

Hypercalcaemia

- Hypercalcaemia is total plasma Ca^{2+} concentration >2.60 mmol/l (>10.4 mg/dl) or ionised plasma Ca^{2+} >1.30 mmol/l (>5.2 mg/dl).
- Principal causes include hyperparathyroidism, vitamin D toxicity and cancer (Table 2.16).
- Clinical features include polyuria, constipation, muscle weakness, confusion and coma.
- Diagnosis is by plasma ionised Ca^{2+} and parathyroid hormone levels.

There are four main strategies for lowering plasma Ca^{2+}: decrease intestinal Ca^{2+} absorption, increase urinary Ca^{2+} excretion, decrease bone resorption and remove excess Ca^{2+} through dialysis. The treatment used depends on both the degree and the cause of hypercalcaemia.

- In mild hypercalcaemia (plasma Ca^{2+} <2.88 mmol/l), in which symptoms are mild, treatment is deferred pending definitive diagnosis. After diagnosis, the underlying cause is treated. If symptoms are significant, treatment aimed at lowering plasma Ca^{2+} is necessary. Oral phosphate can be used. When taken with meals, it binds some Ca^{2+}, preventing its absorption. Urinary Ca^{2+} excretion is increased by giving isotonic saline plus a loop diuretic.
- Moderate hypercalcaemia (plasma Ca^{2+} between 2.88 mmol/l and 4.50 mmol/l) can be treated with isotonic saline and a loop diuretic as previously mentioned or, depending on its cause, agents that decrease bone resorption (usually calcitonin, bisphosphonates, or infrequently plicamycin or gallium nitrate), corticosteroids, or chloroquine.
- In severe hypercalcaemia (plasma Ca^{2+} > 4.50 mmol/l or with severe symptoms), haemodialysis with low-Ca^{2+} dialysate may be needed in addition to other treatments above. Although there is no completely satisfactory way to correct severe hypercalcaemia in patients with renal failure, haemodialysis is probably the safest and most reliable short-term treatment.

Table 2.16: Major causes of hypercalcaemia

Excessive bone resorption	Cancer with bone metastases: particularly carcinoma, leukaemia, lymphoma, multiple myeloma	
	Hyperthyroidism	
	Humoral hypercalcaemia of malignancy, ie hypercalcaemia of cancer in the absence of bone metastases	
	Immobilisation: particularly in young, growing people, in those undergoing orthopaedic casting and/or traction, and in those with Paget's disease of bone; also in elderly with osteoporosis, paraplegics and quadriplegics	
	Parathyroid hormone excess: primary hyperparathyroidism, parathyroid carcinoma, familial hypocalciuric hypercalcaemia, advanced secondary hyperparathyroidism	
	Vitamin D toxicity; vitamin A toxicity	
Excessive GI Ca^{2+} absorption and/or intake	Milk-alkali syndrome	
	Sarcoidosis and other granulomatous diseases	
	Vitamin D toxicity	
Elevated plasma protein concentration	**Uncertain mechanism**	Aluminium-induced osteomalacia
		Infantile hypercalcaemia
		Lithium intoxication, theophylline intoxication
		Myxoedema, Addison's disease, post-operative Cushing's disease
		Neuroleptic malignant syndrome
		Thiazide diuretic treatment
	Artifactual	Exposure of blood to contaminated glassware
		Prolonged venous stasis while obtaining blood samples

Hypocalcaemia

- Hypocalcaemia is total plasma Ca^{2+} concentration < 2.20 mmol/l (<8.8 mg/dl) in the presence of normal plasma protein concentrations, or a plasma ionised Ca^{2+} concentration <1.17 mmol/l (<4.7 mg/dl).
- Important causes include hypoparathyroidism, vitamin D deficiency and renal disease.
- Clinical manifestations of hypocalcaemia are due to disturbances in cellular membrane potential, resulting in neuromuscular irritability. Muscle cramps involving the back and legs are common. Insidious hypocalcaemia can produce mild, diffuse encephalopathy and should be suspected in a patient with unexplained dementia, depression, or psychosis. Papilloedema occasionally occurs, and cataracts may develop after prolonged hypocalcaemia.

- Severe hypocalcaemia with plasma Ca^{2+} <7 mg/dl (<1.75 mmol/l) may cause tetany, laryngospasm, or generalised seizures.
  - Tetany characteristically results from severe hypocalcaemia but can result from reduction in the ionised fraction of plasma Ca^{2+} without marked hypocalcaemia, as occurs in severe alkalosis.
    - Tetany is characterised by sensory symptoms consisting of paraesthesiae of the lips, tongue, fingers and feet; carpopedal spasm, which may be prolonged and painful; generalised muscle aching; and spasm of facial musculature. Tetany may be overt with spontaneous symptoms or latent and requiring provocative tests to elicit. Latent tetany generally occurs at less severely decreased plasma Ca^{2+} concentrations (1.75–2.20 mmol/l).

o Chvostek's and Trousseau's signs are easily elicited at the bedside to identify latent tetany. Chvostek's sign is an involuntary twitching of the facial muscles elicited by a light tapping of the facial nerve just anterior to the exterior auditory meatus. It is present in ≤ 10% of healthy people and in most people with acute hypocalcaemia but is often absent in chronic hypocalcaemia. Trousseau's sign is the precipitation of carpal spasm by reduction of the blood supply to the hand with a tourniquet or BP cuff inflated to 20 mmHg above systolic BP applied to the forearm for 3 minutes. Trousseau's sign also occurs in alkalosis, hypomagnesaemia, hypokalaemia and hyperkalaemia and in about 6% of people with no identifiable electrolyte disturbance.

- Arrhythmia or heart block occasionally develops in patients with severe hypocalcaemia. In hypocalcaemia, the ECG typically shows prolongation of the QT and ST intervals. Changes in repolarisation, such as T-wave peaking or inversion, also occur.

- Many other abnormalities may occur with chronic hypocalcaemia, such as dry and scaly skin, brittle nails and coarse hair. *Candida* infections occasionally occur in hypocalcaemia but most commonly occur in patients with idiopathic hypoparathyroidism. Cataracts occasionally occur with long-standing hypocalcaemia and are not reversible by correction of plasma Ca^{2+}.

- Diagnosis of hypocalcaemia involves measurement of plasma Ca^{2+} level.

- The treatment of hypocalcaemia depends on the cause, the severity, the presence of symptoms, and how rapidly the hypocalcaemia developed.

Acute hypocalcaemia

- Promptly correct symptomatic or severe hypocalcaemia with cardiac arrhythmias or tetany with parenteral administration of calcium salts.

- Administer 1–2 ampoules 10% calcium gluconate (93 mg/10 ml) in 50–100 ml of 5% dextrose in water over 5–10 min.

- Measure serum calcium every 4–6 h to maintain serum calcium levels at 8–9 mg/dl.

- Patients with cardiac arrhythmias or patients on digoxin therapy need continuous ECG monitoring during calcium replacement because calcium potentiates digitalis toxicity.

- Calcium chloride 10% solution (273 mg/10-ml ampoule) delivers higher amounts of calcium and has advantages when rapid correction is needed, but it is very irritating when administered intravenously and probably only should be administered centrally.

- Identify and treat the cause of hypocalcaemia and taper the infusion.

- Start oral calcium and vitamin D treatment early. Patients with postparathyroidectomy hungry bone disease, especially those with osteitis fibrosa cystica, can present with a dramatic picture of hypocalcaemia.

- Treatment with calcium and vitamin D for 1–2 days prior to parathyroid surgery may help prevent the development of severe hypocalcaemia.

Chronic hypocalcaemia

Treatment of chronic hypocalcaemia depends on the cause of the disorder.

- PTH deficiency: Patients with hypoparathyroidism and pseudohypoparathyroidism can be managed initially with the oral administration of calcium supplements. The hypercalcaemic effects of thiazide diuretics may offer some additional benefits. In patients with severe hypoparathyroidism, vitamin D treatment may be required; however, remember that PTH deficiency impairs the conversion of vitamin D to calcitriol. Therefore, the most efficient treatment is the addition of 0.5–2 μg of calcitriol or 1-α-hydroxyvitamin D3.

- Hypocalcaemia in patients on dialysis: Administering calcium carbonate (500 mg elemental calcium) 3 times per day is appropriate therapy. Treat secondary hyperparathyroidism by controlling phosphate levels and by suppressing PTH levels with the oral administration of vitamin D (eg calcitriol, paracalcitriol). For more effective treatment, intravenously administer vitamin D once a week. Increase dose and frequency to reduce the PTH levels to 3 times the levels of a healthy person.

- Nutritional vitamin D deficiency from lack of sunlight exposure or poor oral intake of vitamin D: Ultraviolet light or sunlight exposure can treat these patients. Treat nutritional rickets with vitamin D2. Calcium preparations containing 1–2 g of elemental calcium per day orally can treat patients with a calcium deficiency. For breastfed infants, adjust the dose to 30 mg/kg per day. Calcitriol may be used but has the disadvantages of higher price and the possibility of producing hypervitaminosis D with hypercalcaemia.

2.4.4 Disorders of acid–base balance

Acid–base disorders are changes in arterial $P\mathrm{CO_2}$, serum HCO_3^- and serum pH.

- Acidaemia is serum pH <7.35
- Alkalaemia is serum pH >7.45
- Acidosis refers to physiological processes that cause acid accumulation or alkali loss

- Alkalosis refers to physiological processes that cause alkali accumulation or acid loss
- Actual changes in pH depend on the degree of physiological compensation and whether multiple processes are present

Classification

Acidoses and alkaloses are defined (Table 2.17) as metabolic or respiratory on the basis of clinical context and primary changes in serum HCO_3^- or PCO_2.

- Metabolic acidosis is serum HCO_3^- <24 mmol/l. Causes are increased acid production or acid ingestion, decreased renal acid excretion, and GI or renal HCO_3^- loss
- Metabolic alkalosis is serum HCO_3^- >24 mmol/l. Cause is acid loss or HCO_3^- retention
- Respiratory acidosis is PCO_2 >40 mmHg (hypercapnia) Cause is a decrease in respiratory rate or volume or both (hypoventilation)
- Respiratory alkalosis is PCO_2 < 40 mmHg (hypocapnia) Cause is an increase in respiratory rate or volume or both (hyperventilation)

Metabolic acidosis

Metabolic acidosis is primary reduction in HCO_3^-, typically with compensatory reduction in PCO_2. The pH may be markedly low or slightly subnormal. Metabolic acidoses are categorised as high or normal anion gap, based on the presence or absence of unmeasured anions in serum. Causes include accumulation of ketones and lactic acid, renal failure and drug or toxin ingestion (high anion gap) and GI or renal HCO_3^- loss (normal anion gap). Symptoms and signs in severe cases include nausea and vomiting, lethargy and hyperpnoea. Diagnosis is clinical and with arterial blood gases (ABG) and serum electrolytes. The underlying cause is treated. IV $NaHCO_3$ may be indicated when pH is very low.

Metabolic alkalosis

Metabolic alkalosis is primary increase in HCO_3^- with or without compensatory increase in PCO_2. The pH may be high or nearly normal. Common causes include prolonged vomiting, hypovolaemia, diuretic use and hypokalaemia. Renal impairment of HCO_3^- excretion must be present to sustain alkalosis. Symptoms and signs in severe cases include headache, lethargy and tetany. Diagnosis is clinical and with ABG and serum electrolytes. The underlying cause is treated. Oral or IV acetazolamide is sometimes indicated.

Respiratory acidosis

Respiratory acidosis is primary increase in PCO_2 with or without compensatory increase in HCO_3^-. The pH is usually low but

Table 2.17: Primary acid–base disorders

Disorder	pH	HCO_3^-	PCO_2	Compensation
Metabolic acidosis	<7.35	Primary decrease	Compensatory decrease	1.2-mmHg decrease in PCO_2 for every 1-mmol/l decrease in HCO_3^- or $PCO_2 = (1.5 \times HCO_3^-) + 8\ (\pm 2)$ or $PCO_2 = HCO_3^- + 15$ or PCO_2 = last 2 digits of pH × 100
Metabolic alkalosis	>7.45	Primary increase	Compensatory increase	0.6–0.75 mmHg increase in PCO_2 for every 1 mmol/l increase in HCO_3^-. PCO_2 should not rise above 60 mmHg in compensation
Respiratory acidosis	<7.35	Compensatory increase	Primary increase	*Acute:* 1–2 mmol increase in HCO_3^- for every 10 mmHg increase in PCO_2 *Chronic:* 3–4 mmol increase in HCO_3^- for every 10 mmHg increase in PCO_2
Respiratory alkalosis	>7.45	Compensatory decrease	Primary decrease	*Acute:* 1–2 mmol decrease in HCO_3 for every 10 mmHg decrease in PCO_2 *Chronic:* 4–5 mmol decrease in HCO_3^- for every 10 mmHg decrease in PCO_2

may be near normal. Cause is a decrease in respiratory rate and/or volume (hypoventilation) from CNS, pulmonary, or iatrogenic conditions. Respiratory acidosis can be acute or chronic; the chronic form is asymptomatic, but the acute, or worsening, form causes headache, confusion and drowsiness. Signs include tremor, myoclonic jerks and asterixis. Diagnosis is clinical and with ABG and serum electrolytes. The underlying cause is treated. Oxygen and mechanical ventilation are often required.

Respiratory alkalosis
Respiratory alkalosis is a primary decrease in PCO_2 with or without compensatory decrease in HCO_3^-; pH may be high or near normal. Cause is an increase in respiratory rate and/or volume (hyperventilation). Respiratory alkalosis can be acute or chronic. The chronic form is asymptomatic, but the acute form causes light-headedness, confusion, paraesthesiae, cramps and syncope. Signs include hyperpnoea or tachypnoea and carpopedal spasms. Diagnosis is clinical and with ABG and serum electrolytes. Treatment is directed at the cause.

2.5 BLEEDING AND HAEMOSTASIS

Bleeding, technically known as haemorrhage, is a common problem encountered by surgeons. The average human has around 7%–8% of their body weight made up of blood. The circulating blood volume is approximately 70 ml/kg of ideal body weight, so the average 70-kg male has approximately 5000 ml of circulating blood. Loss of 10%–15% of total blood volume can be endured without clinical sequelae in a healthy person.

2.5.1 Types of bleeding
Haemorrhage is classified in to four types.

- **Class I haemorrhage** involves up to 15% of blood volume. There is typically no change in vital signs and fluid resuscitation is not usually necessary.
- **Class II haemorrhage** involves 15%–30% of total blood volume. This is often associated with tachycardia and a narrow pulse pressure. The body attempts to compensate with peripheral vasoconstriction. Skin may start to look pale and feel cool to touch. Volume resuscitation is typically required.
- **Class III haemorrhage** involves loss of 30%–40% of circulating blood volume. The patient's blood pressure drops, the heart rate increases, peripheral perfusion, such as capillary refill, worsens and the mental status worsens. Fluid resuscitation is mandatory.
- **Class IV haemorrhage** involves loss of >40% of circulating blood volume. The body's compensatory

mechanisms are stretched to the limit and aggressive resuscitation is required to prevent death.

2.5.2 Causes of bleeding
Bleeding may result from abnormalities in platelets, coagulation factors or blood vessels.

Disorders of platelets
Platelets are cell fragments that function in the clotting system. Thrombopoietin, primarily produced in the liver in response to decreased numbers of marrow megakaryocytes and circulating platelets, stimulates the bone marrow to synthesise platelets from megakaryocytes. Platelets circulate for 7–10 days. About one-third are always transiently sequestered in the spleen. The platelet count is normally 150 000 to 450 000/µl. However, the count can vary slightly according to menstrual cycle phase, decrease during near-term pregnancy (gestational thrombocytopenia) and increase in response to inflammatory cytokines (secondary, or reactive, thrombocytosis). Platelets are eventually destroyed, primarily by the spleen.

A decrease in platelet count (thrombocytopenia) and/or platelet dysfunction may cause defective formation of haemostatic plugs and bleeding. The conditions associated with thrombocytopenia are outlined in Table 2.18.

The risk of bleeding is inversely proportional to the platelet count. When the platelet count is <50 000/µl, minor bleeding occurs easily and the risk of major bleeding increases. Counts between 20 000 and 50 000/µl predispose to bleeding with trauma, even minor trauma; with counts under 20 000/µl, spontaneous bleeding may occur; with counts of <5000/µl, severe spontaneous bleeding is more likely. However, patients with counts <10 000/µl may be asymptomatic for years.

Platelet disorders result in a typical pattern of bleeding: multiple petechiae in the skin, typically most evident on the lower legs; scattered small ecchymoses at sites of minor trauma; mucosal bleeding (epistaxis, bleeding in the gastrointestinal and genitourinary tracts, vaginal bleeding); and excessive bleeding after surgery.

Disorders of coagulation
Disorders of coagulation can be acquired or hereditary. The major causes of acquired coagulation disorders are vitamin K deficiency, liver disease, disseminated intravascular coagulation and development of circulating anticoagulants.

Severe liver disease (eg cirrhosis, fulminant hepatitis, acute fatty liver of pregnancy) can disturb haemostasis by impairing clotting factor synthesis.

The most common hereditary coagulation disorders are the haemophilias.

Disorders of blood vessels

Vascular bleeding disorders are caused by defects in blood vessels, typically producing petechiae, purpura and bruising but seldom leading to serious blood loss. Bleeding may result from deficiencies of vascular and perivascular collagen in Ehlers–Danlos syndrome and in other rare hereditary connective tissue disorders (eg pseudoxanthoma elasticum, osteogenesis imperfecta, Marfan's syndrome). Haemorrhage may be a prominent feature of scurvy or of Henoch–Schönlein purpura, a hypersensitivity vasculitis common during childhood. In vascular bleeding disorders, tests of haemostasis are usually normal. Diagnosis is clinical.

2.5.3 Haemostasis

Haemostasis, the arrest of bleeding from an injured blood vessel, requires the combined activity of vascular, platelet and plasma factors. Regulatory mechanisms counterbalance the tendency of clots to form. Haemostatic abnormalities can lead to excessive bleeding or to thrombosis.

Physiology of haemostasis

Haemostasis is initiated almost instantly after an injury to the blood vessel damages the endothelium. Local vasoconstriction is followed immediately by formation of a haemostatic plug at the site of injury, called primary haemostasis. Secondary haemostasis occurs simultaneously due to activation of proteins in the blood plasma, called coagulation factors (Table 2.19). These interact in a complex cascade to form fibrin strands which strengthen the platelet plug. A brief overview of the various factors involved in haemostasis is provided below.

Vascular factors

Vascular factors reduce blood loss from trauma through local vasoconstriction (an immediate reaction to injury) and compression of injured vessels by extravasation of blood into surrounding tissues. Vessel wall injury triggers the attachment and activation of platelets and production of fibrin. The platelets and fibrin combine to form a clot.

Platelet factors

Disruption of the vascular endothelium as a result of injury inhibits the various mechanisms, including production of endothelial cell nitric oxide and prostacyclin, which prevent platelet stasis and dilate intact blood vessels. As a result, platelets adhere to the damaged intima and form aggregates. Initial platelet adhesion is to von Willebrand factor (vWF), previously secreted by endothelial cells into the subendothelium. vWF binds to receptors on the platelet surface membrane (glycoprotein Ib/IX). Platelets anchored to the vessel wall

Table 2.18: Causes of thrombocytopenia		
Cause		*Conditions*
Failed platelet production	Diminished or absent megakaryocytes in marrow	Leukaemia, aplastic anaemia, paroxysmal nocturnal haemoglobinuria (some patients), myelosuppressive drugs
	Diminished platelet production despite the presence of megakaryocytes in marrow	Alcohol-induced thrombocytopenia, thrombocytopenia in megaloblastic anaemias, HIV-associated thrombocytopenia, some myelodysplastic syndromes
Increased platelet destruction or use	Platelet sequestration in enlarged spleen	Cirrhosis with congestive splenomegaly, myelofibrosis with myeloid metaplasia, Gaucher's disease
	Immunological destruction	Idiopathic thrombocytopenia purpura, HIV-associated thrombocytopenia, post-transfusion purpura, drug-induced thrombocytopenia, neonatal alloimmune thrombocytopenia, connective tissue disorders, lymphoproliferative disorders
	Non-immunological destruction	Disseminated intravascular coagulation, thrombotic thrombocytopenia purpura–haemolytic-uraemic syndrome, thrombocytopenia in acute respiratory distress syndrome
	Dilution	Massive blood replacement or exchange transfusion (loss of platelet viability in stored blood)
Drug-induced	Direct myelosuppression	Valproic acid, methotrexate, carboplatin, interferon, other chemotherapy drugs
	Immunological platelet destruction	Quinidine group of drugs, heparin

undergo activation. During activation, platelets release mediators from storage granules, including adenosine diphosphate (ADP). Other biochemical changes resulting from activation include:

- Hydrolysis of membrane phospholipids
- Inhibition of adenylate cyclase
- Mobilisation of intracellular Ca^{2+}
- Phosphorylation of intracellular proteins

Arachidonic acid is converted to thromboxane A_2. This reaction requires cyclooxygenase and is inhibited irreversibly by aspirin and reversibly by many NSAIDs. ADP, thromboxane A_2 and other mediators draw additional platelets to the injured endothelium (platelet aggregation) and activate them. Another receptor is assembled on the platelet surface membrane from glycoproteins IIb and IIIa. Fibrinogen binds to the glycoprotein IIa–IIIb complexes of adjacent platelets, connecting them.

Platelets provide surfaces for the assembly and activation of coagulation complexes and the generation of thrombin. Thrombin converts fibrinogen to fibrin. Fibrin strands bind aggregated platelets to help secure the platelet–fibrin haemostatic plug.

Coagulation factors

Plasma coagulation factors (Table 2.19) interact to produce thrombin, which converts fibrinogen to fibrin. Radiating from and anchoring the haemostatic plug, fibrin strengthens the clot.

In the **intrinsic pathway**, factor XII, high-molecular-weight kininogen, prekallikrein and activated factor XI (factor XIa) produce factor IXa from factor IX. Factor IXa then combines with factor VIIIa and procoagulant phospholipid (present on the surface of activated platelets and tissue cells) to form a complex that activates factor X.

In the **extrinsic pathway**, factor VIIa and tissue factor directly activate factor X (Figure 2.1). Activation of the intrinsic or extrinsic pathway activates the **common pathway**, resulting in formation of the fibrin clot. Three steps are involved:

1 A prothrombin activator is produced on the surface of activated platelets and tissue cells. The activator is a complex of an enzyme, factor Xa, and two co-factors, factor Va and procoagulant phospholipid.
2 The prothrombin activator cleaves prothrombin into thrombin and another fragment.
3 Thrombin induces the generation of fibrin polymers from fibrinogen. Thrombin also activates factor XIII, an enzyme that catalyses formation of stronger bonds between fibrin molecules, as well as factor VIII and factor XI.

Ca^{2+} ions are needed in most thrombin-generating reactions (Ca^{2+}-chelating agents, eg citrate, ethylenediaminetetraacetic acid, are used in vitro as anticoagulants). Vitamin-K-dependent clotting factors (factors II, VII, IX and X) normally cannot bind to phospholipid surfaces through Ca^{2+} bridges or function in blood coagulation when synthesised in the absence of vitamin K.

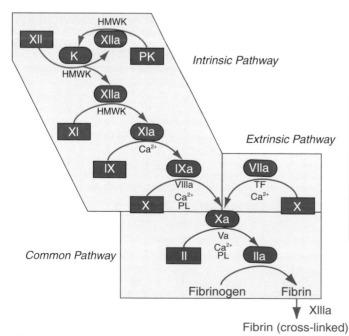

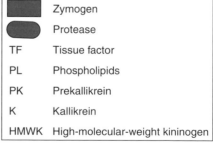

Figure 2.1: Pathways of coagulation

Table 2.19: Coagulation factors and related substances

Number and/or name	Function
I (fibrinogen)	Forms clot (fibrin)
II (prothrombin)	Its active form (IIa) activates I, V, VII, XIII, protein C, platelets
Tissue factor	Co-factor of VIIa (formerly known as factor III)
Calcium	Required for coagulation factors to bind to phospholipid (formerly known as factor IV)
V (proaccelerin, labile factor)	Co-factor of X with which it forms the prothrombinase complex
VI	Unassigned – old name of Factor Va
VII (stable factor)	Activates IX, X
VIII (antihaemophilic factor)	Co-factor of IX with which it forms the tenase complex
IX (Christmas factor)	Activates X; forms tenase complex with factor VIII
X (Stuart-Prower factor)	Activates II; forms prothrombinase complex with factor V
XI (plasma thromboplastin antecedent)	Activates XII, IX and prekallikrein
XII (Hageman factor)	Activates prekallikrein and fibrinolysis
XIII (fibrin-stabilising factor)	Cross-links fibrin
von Willebrand factor	Binds to VIII, mediates platelet adhesion
Prekallikrein	Activates XII and prekallikrein; cleaves HMWK
High-molecular-weight kininogen (HMWK)	Supports reciprocal activation of XII, XI and prekallikrein
Fibronectin	Mediates cell adhesion
Antithrombin III	Inhibits IIa, Xa and other proteases
Protein C	Inactivates Va and VIIIa
Protein S	Co-factor for activated protein C (APC, inactive when bound to C4b-binding protein)
Plasminogen	Converts to plasmin, lyses fibrin and other proteins
Tissue plasminogen activator (tPA)	Activates plasminogen
Urokinase	Activates plasminogen
Plasminogen activator inhibitor-1 (PAI1)	Inactivates tPA and urokinase (endothelial PAI)
Plasminogen activator inhibitor-2 (PAI2)	Inactivates tPA and urokinase (placental PAI)
Cancer procoagulant	Pathological factor X activator linked to thrombosis in cancer

Regulation of coagulation

Several inhibitory mechanisms prevent activated coagulation reactions from amplifying uncontrollably, causing extensive local thrombosis or disseminated intravascular coagulation. These mechanisms include inactivation of procoagulant enzymes, fibrinolysis and clearance of activated clotting factors, especially by the liver.

Inactivation of coagulation factors

Plasma protease inhibitors (antithrombin, tissue factor pathway inhibitor, α_2-macroglobulin, heparin co-factor II) inactivate coagulation enzymes. Antithrombin inhibits thrombin, factor Xa, factor XIa and factor IXa. Heparin enhances antithrombin activity.

Two vitamin-K-dependent proteins, protein C and protein S, form a complex that inactivates factors VIIIa and Va by proteolysis. Thrombin, when bound to a receptor on endothelial cells called thrombomodulin, activates protein C. Activated protein C combines with protein S and phospholipid as co-factors to proteolyse factors VIIIa and Va.

Fibrinolysis

Fibrin deposition and lysis must be balanced to maintain and remould the haemostatic seal during repair of an injured vessel wall. The fibrinolytic system dissolves fibrin by means of plasmin, a proteolytic enzyme. Fibrinolysis is activated by plasminogen activators released from vascular endothelial cells. Plasminogen activators and plasminogen from plasma bind to fibrin. Plasminogen activators catalyse cleavage of plasminogen, creating plasmin (Figure 2.2). Plasmin produces soluble fibrin degradation products that are swept into the circulation. Plasminogen activators are categorised into several types:

- Tissue plasminogen activator (tPA), from endothelial cells, is a poor activator when free in solution but an efficient activator when bound to fibrin in proximity to plasminogen.
- A second type, urokinase, exists in single-chain and double-chain forms with different functional properties. Single-chain urokinase cannot activate free plasminogen but, like tPA, can readily activate plasminogen bound to fibrin. A trace concentration of plasmin cleaves single-chain to double-chain urokinase, which activates plasminogen in solution as well as plasminogen bound to fibrin. Epithelial cells that line excretory passages (eg renal tubules, mammary ducts) secrete urokinase, which is the physiological activator of fibrinolysis in these channels.
- Streptokinase, a bacterial product not normally found in the body, is another potent plasminogen activator. Streptokinase, urokinase and recombinant tPA (alteplase) have all been used therapeutically to induce fibrinolysis in patients with acute thrombotic disorders.

Regulation of fibrinolysis

Fibrinolysis itself is regulated by plasminogen activator inhibitors (PAIs) and plasmin inhibitors that slow fibrinolysis. PAI-1, the most important PAI, inactivates tPA and urokinase and is released from vascular endothelial cells and activated platelets. The primary plasmin inhibitor is α_2-antiplasmin, which quickly inactivates free plasmin escaping from clots. Some α_2-antiplasmin is also cross-linked by factor XIIIa to fibrin during clotting; it may prevent excessive plasmin activity within clots. tPA and urokinase are rapidly cleared by the liver, which is another mechanism of preventing excessive fibrinolysis.

Laboratory testing for disorders of haemostasis

Laboratory testing of coagulation is most likely to be abnormal in patients whose history or examination reveals a bleeding risk. Abnormal results in a patient with no signs or symptoms of excessive bleeding should be repeated to exclude laboratory error. Abnormal results are not always clinically meaningful. For example, patients with deficiencies of factor XII, prekallikrein, or high-molecular-weight kininogen in the intrinsic pathway do not bleed excessively.

Screening tests evaluate the components of haemostasis, including the number of circulating platelets and the plasma coagulation pathways. The most common screening tests for bleeding disorders are the platelet count, prothrombin time (PT) and partial thromboplastin time (PTT). If results are abnormal, a specific test can usually pinpoint the defect. Determination of the level of fibrin degradation products measures in vivo activation of fibrinolysis. Table 2.20 summarises commonly performed laboratory tests for detecting abnormalities of haemostasis.

Disorders of haemostasis

The surgeon is often the first person to be called when a patient experiences ongoing bleeding. To treat such a patient appropriately, the surgeon must identify the cause or source of the bleeding. Causes fall into two main categories: (1) conditions leading to loss of vascular integrity, as in a post-

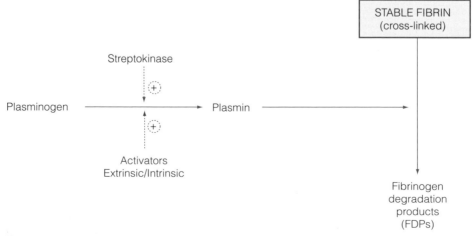

Figure 2.2: Fibrinolytic pathway

Table 2.20: Laboratory tests for detecting abnormalities of haemostasis

Screening test	Normal range	Abnormalities indicated	Most common cause of disorder
PT or INR	12–16 s (PT); 1.0–1.3 (INR)	Extrinsic + common coagulation pathways Deficiency/inhibition of factors VII, X, V, II, and fibrinogen (I)	Liver disease, warfarin therapy, DIC
aPTT/PTTK/kaolin cephalin clotting time	23–31 s	Intrinsic + common coagulation pathways Deficiency/inhibition of one or more of factors XII, IX, VIII, X, V, II and fibrinogen (I)	Liver disease, heparin therapy, haemophilia A + B, DIC
TT	14–16 s	Deficiency or abnormality of fibrinogen; inhibition of thrombin by heparin or FDPs	DIC, heparin therapy, fibrinolytic therapy
FDPs	<10 mg/ml	Accelerated destruction of fibrinogen	DIC
Bleeding time (Ivy method)	3–9 min	Abnormal platelet function	Drugs (eg aspirin), uraemia, von Willebrand's disease

aPTT = activated partial thromboplastin time; DIC = disseminated intravascular coagulation; FDPs = fibrin degradation products; INR = international normalised ratio; PT = prothrombin time; PTTK = PTT with kaolin; TT = thrombin time.

operative patient with an unligated vessel that is bleeding or a trauma patient with a ruptured spleen, and (2) conditions leading to derangement of the haemostatic process.

Surgical bleeding

It is vital for the surgeon to recognise that the most common causes of post-operative bleeding are technical: an unligated vessel or an unrecognised injury is much more likely to be the cause of a falling haematocrit than either a drug effect or an endogenous haemostatic defect. Furthermore, if an unligated vessel is treated as though it were an endogenous haemostatic defect (ie with transfusions), the outcome is likely to be disastrous. For these reasons, in all cases of ongoing bleeding, the first consideration must always be to exclude a surgically correctable cause.

Ongoing bleeding may be surprisingly difficult to diagnose. Healthy young patients can usually maintain a normal blood pressure until their blood loss exceeds 40% of their blood volume (roughly 2 litres). If the bleeding is from a laceration to an extremity, it will be obvious. However, if the bleeding is occurring internally (eg from a ruptured spleen or an intraluminal GI source), there may be few physiological signs.

Even when a technical cause of bleeding has seemingly been excluded, the possibility often must be reconsidered periodically throughout assessment. Patients who are either unresuscitated or under-resuscitated undergo vasospasm that results in decreased bleeding. As resuscitation proceeds, the catecholamine-induced vasospasm subsides and the bleeding may recur. For this reason, repeated reassessment of the possibility of a technical cause of bleeding is appropriate. Only when the surgeon is confident that a missed injury or unligated vessel is not the cause of the bleeding should other potential causes be investigated.

Derangements of haemostasis

Derangements of haemostasis include a broad spectrum of disorders and can be broadly divided into two major categories:

1 Inherited disorders
2 Acquired disorders

Individual disorders of clinical significance in each category are briefly presented below.

Inherited disorders

Numerous congenital abnormalities of haemostasis have been identified. These include, in particular, various abnormalities involving plasma proteins [eg haemophilia and von Willebrand disease (vWD)], platelet receptors (eg Glanzmann thrombasthenia and Bernard–Soulier syndrome) and endothelium (eg telangiectasia).

- Vascular defects (eg haemorrhagic telangiectasias) may carry an increased risk of bleeding as a consequence of dysfunctional fibrinolysis, concomitant platelet dysfunction, or coagulation factor deficiencies.
- Inherited platelet membrane receptor defects are relatively common. Of these, vWD is the one that most frequently causes bleeding. The condition is characterised by von Willebrand factor (vWF) abnormalities, which may take three forms: vWF may be present in a reduced concentration (type I vWD), be dysfunctional (type II vWD), or be absent altogether (type III). Diagnosis of vWD is based on a combination of the patient history (eg previous mucosal bleeding) and laboratory parameters.
- Less common receptor defects include Glanzmann thrombasthenia (a defect in the GPII–IIIa complex), Bernard–Soulier syndrome (a defect in the GPIb–IX

complex) and Scott syndrome (a defect in the platelet's activated surface that promotes thrombin formation); other agonist receptors on the platelet membrane may be affected as well. Intracellular platelet defects are relatively rare but do occur; examples are grey platelet syndromes (eg alpha granule defects), Hermansky–Pudlak syndrome, dense granule defects, Wiskott–Aldrich syndrome and various defects in intracellular production and signalling (involving defects of cyclooxygenase synthase and phospholipase C, respectively).

- Numerous pathological states are also associated with deficiencies or defects of plasma procoagulants. Inherited sex-linked deficiencies of factor VIII (ie haemophilia A) and factor IX (ie haemophilia B and Christmas disease) are relatively common. The clinical presentations of haemophilia A and haemophilia B are similar: haemarthroses are the most common clinical manifestations, ultimately leading to degenerative joint deformities. Spontaneous bleeding may also occur, resulting in intracranial haemorrhage, large haematomas in the muscles of extremities, haematuria and GI bleeding. Factor XI deficiency is relatively common in Jewish people but rarely results in spontaneous bleeding. Such deficiency may result in bleeding after oral operations and trauma, although, there are a number of major procedures (eg cardiac bypass surgery) that do not result in post-operative bleeding in this population.

- Inherited deficiencies of the other coagulation factors are very rare. Factor XIII deficiencies result in delayed post-operative or post-traumatic bleeding. Congenital deficiencies of factor V, factor VII, factor X, prothrombin and fibrinogen may become apparent in the neonatal period (presenting, for example, as umbilical stump bleeding); later in life, they result in clinical presentations such as epistaxis, intracranial bleeding, GI bleeding, deep and superficial bruising, and menorrhagia.

- Defects or deficiencies in the fibrinolytic pathway are also rare and are most commonly associated with thromboembolic events. α_2-antiplasmin deficiencies and primary fibrin(ogen)olysis are rare congenital coagulopathies with clinical presentations similar to those of factor deficiencies. In primary fibrin(ogen)olysis, failure of regulation of tPA and urokinase leads to increases in circulating plasmin levels, which result in rapid degradation of clot and fibrinogen.

Acquired disorders

Acquired coagulopathies are very common, and most do not result in spontaneous bleeding. [Disseminated intravascular coagulation (DIC) is an exception.]

- Acquired platelet abnormalities, both qualitative (ie dysfunction) and quantitative (ie decreases in absolute numbers), are common occurrences. Many acquired thrombocytopathies are attributable to either foods (eg fish oils, chocolate, red wine, garlic and herbs) or drugs (eg aspirin, ibuprofen, other NSAIDs, ticlopidine, various antibiotics, certain antihistamines and phenytoin). Direct anti-platelet receptor drugs (eg abciximab and eptifibatide) block the GPIIb–IIIa complex, thereby preventing platelet aggregation. Thrombocytopenia can be primary or secondary to a number of clinical conditions. Primary bone disorders (eg myelodysplastic or myelophthisic syndromes) and spontaneous bleeding may arise when platelet counts fall below 10 000/mm^3. Thrombocytopenia can be associated with immune causes (eg immune thrombocytopenia purpura or thrombotic thrombocytopenia purpura) or can occur secondary to administration of drugs (eg heparin). Acquired platelet dysfunction (eg acquired vWD) that is not related to dietary or pharmacological causes has been observed in patients with immune disorders or cancer.

- Acquired plasma factor deficiencies are common as well. Patients with severe renal disease typically exhibit platelet dysfunction (from excessive amounts of uraemic metabolites), factor deficiencies associated with impaired synthesis or protein loss (as with increased urinary excretion), or thrombocytopenia (from diminished thrombopoietin production). Patients with severe hepatic disease commonly have impairment of coagulation factor synthesis, increases in circulating levels of paraproteins and splenic sequestration of platelets.

- Haemodilution from massive red blood cell (RBC) transfusions can occur if more than 10 packed RBC units are given within a short period without plasma supplementation.

- Acquired multifactorial deficiencies associated with extracorporeal circuits (eg cardiopulmonary bypass, haemodialysis and continuous venovenous dialysis) can arise as a consequence of haemodilution from circuit priming fluid or activation of procoagulants after exposure to thrombogenic surfaces. Thrombocytopenia can result from platelet destruction and activation caused by circuit membrane exposure, or it can be secondary to the presence of heparin antibody.

- Animal venoms, particularly snake venom, can also cause bleeding. The clinical presentation of coagulopathies associated with snakebites generally mimics that of consumptive coagulopathies.

- Drug-induced factor deficiencies are common, particularly as a result of anticoagulant therapy. The most commonly used anticoagulants are heparin and warfarin. Heparin does not cause a factor deficiency; rather, it accelerates production of antithrombin, which inhibits factor IXa, factor Xa and thrombin, thereby prolonging clot formation. Warfarin reduces procoagulant potential by inhibiting vitamin K synthesis, thereby reducing carboxylation of factor VII, factor IX, factor X, prothrombin and proteins C and S. Newer drugs that can also cause factor deficiencies include direct thrombin inhibitors (eg lepirudin and bivalirudin) and fibrinogen-degrading drugs (eg ancrod).

- Isolated acquired factor deficiencies are relatively rare. Clinically, they present in exactly the same way as inherited factor deficiencies, except that there is no history of earlier bleeding. In most cases, there is a secondary disease (eg lymphoma or an autoimmune disorder) that results in the development of antibody to a procoagulant (eg factor V, factor VIII, factor IX, vWF, prothrombin or fibrinogen).

Disseminated intravascular coagulation

DIC is a complex coagulation process that involves activation of the coagulation system with resultant activation of the fibrinolytic pathway and deposition of fibrin; the eventual consequence is the multiple organ dysfunction syndrome (MODS). The activation occurs at all levels (platelets, endothelium and procoagulants), but it is not known whether this process is initiated by a local stimulus or a systemic one. DIC is an acquired disorder that occurs secondary to an underlying clinical event (eg a complicated birth, severe Gram-negative infection, shock, major head injury, polytrauma, severe burns, or cancer).

DIC is not always clinically evident: low-grade DIC may lack clinical symptoms altogether and manifest itself only through laboratory abnormalities, even when thrombin generation and fibrin deposition are occurring. In an attempt to facilitate recognition of DIC, the disorder has been divided into three phases, distinguished on the basis of clinical and laboratory evidence.

In **phase I DIC**, there are no clinical symptoms, and the routine screening tests (ie INR, aPTT, fibrinogen level and platelet count) are within normal limits. Secondary testing (ie measurement of antithrombin, prothrombin fragment, thrombin–antithrombin complex and soluble fibrin levels) may reveal subtle changes indicative of thrombin generation.

In **phase II DIC**, there are usually clinical signs of bleeding around wounds, suture sites, IV sites, or venous puncture sites, and decreased function is noted in specific organs (eg lung, liver and kidneys). The INR is increased, the aPTT is prolonged, and the fibrinogen level and platelet count are decreased or decreasing. Other markers of thrombin generation and fibrinolysis (eg D-dimer level) show sizeable elevations.

In **phase III DIC**, MODS is observed, the INR and the aPTT are markedly increased, the fibrinogen level is markedly depressed and the D-dimer level is dramatically increased. A peripheral blood smear would show large numbers of schistocytes, indicating RBC shearing resulting from fibrin deposition.

The activation of the coagulation system seen in DIC appears to be primarily caused by tissue factor (TF). The brain, the placenta and solid tumours are all rich sources of TF. Gram-negative endotoxins also induce TF expression. The exposure of TF on cellular surfaces causes activation of factors VII and IX, which ultimately leads to thrombin generation. Circulating thrombin is rapidly cleared by antithrombin. Moreover, the coagulation pathway is downregulated by activated protein C and protein S. However, constant exposure of TF (as a result of underlying disorders) results in constant generation of thrombin, and these regulator proteins are rapidly consumed. Thrombin-activatable fibrinolysis inhibitor (TAFI) and plasminogen activator inhibitor (PAI) also contribute to fibrin deposition by restricting fibrinolysis and subsequent fibrin degradation and clearance. Finally, it is likely that release of cytokines (eg IL-6, IL-10 and TNF) may play some role in causing the sequelae of DIC by modulating or activating the coagulation pathway.

2.5.4 Transfusion

Transfusion practices have changed substantially since the early 1990s. Blood cell transfusions have been shown to have significant immunosuppressive potential, and transmission of fatal diseases through the blood supply has been extensively documented. Traditionally, anaemia by itself was a sufficient indication for transfusion. However, the current consensus is that the threshold for transfusion should be determined by taking into account additional clinical factors besides the haemoglobin concentration.

The decision on whether to transfuse should be based on the patient's current and predicted need for additional oxygen-carrying capacity. A major component of this decision is to determine as promptly as possible whether significant hypovolaemia or active bleeding is present:

- In a hypovolaemic or actively bleeding patient, liberal transfusion is indicated as a means of increasing intravascular volume and preventing the development of profound deficits in oxygen-carrying capacity. Coagulation factors must also be replaced as necessary.
- In a haemodynamically stable patient without evidence of active haemorrhage, it is appropriate to take a more restrictive approach to transfusion, one that is tailored to the symptoms observed and to the specific anticipated risks.

There is therefore no specific haemoglobin concentration or haematocrit (ie transfusion trigger) at which all patients should receive transfusions.

Blood products

Whole blood can provide improved oxygen-carrying capacity, volume expansion and replacement of clotting factors and was previously recommended for rapid massive blood loss. However, because component therapy is equally effective and is a more efficient use of donated blood, whole blood is no longer used for routine transfusion. The following blood products are available in the UK.

Red blood cells (RBCs): Packed RBCs are ordinarily the component of choice with which to increase haemoglobin (Hb). Indications depend on the patient. Oxygen-carrying capacity may be adequate with Hb levels as low as 7 g/l in healthy patients, but transfusion may be indicated with higher Hb levels in patients with decreased cardiopulmonary reserve or ongoing bleeding. One unit of RBCs increases an average adult's Hb by about 1 g/dl and their haematocrit (Hct) by about 3% of the pretransfusion Hct value. When only volume expansion is required, other fluids can be used concurrently or separately. In patients with multiple blood group antibodies or with antibodies to high-frequency RBC antigens, rare frozen RBCs are used.

Washed RBCs are free of almost all traces of plasma, most white blood cells (WBCs) and platelets. They are generally given to patients who have severe reactions to plasma (eg severe allergies, paroxysmal nocturnal haemoglobinuria, or IgA immunisation). In IgA-immunised patients, blood collected from IgA-deficient donors may be preferable for transfusion.

WBC-depleted RBCs are prepared with special filters that remove ≥ 99.99% of WBCs. They are indicated for:

- Patients who have experienced non-haemolytic febrile transfusion reactions
- For exchange transfusions
- For patients who require cytomegalovirus-negative blood that is unavailable
- For the prevention of platelet alloimmunisation

Fresh frozen plasma (FFP): FFP is an unconcentrated source of all clotting factors without platelets. Indications include:

- Correction of bleeding secondary to factor deficiencies for which specific factor replacements are unavailable
- Multifactor deficiency states (eg massive transfusion, DIC, liver failure)
- Urgent warfarin reversal

FFP can supplement RBCs when whole blood is unavailable for exchange transfusion. FFP should not be used simply for volume expansion.

Cryoprecipitate: Cryoprecipitate is a concentrate prepared from FFP. Each concentrate usually contains about 80 units each of factor VIII and WF and about 250 mg of fibrinogen. It also contains fibronectin and factor XIII. Although originally used for haemophilia and von Willebrand's disease, cryoprecipitate is currently used as a source of fibrinogen in acute DIC with bleeding, treatment of uraemic bleeding, cardiothoracic surgery (fibrin glue), obstetric emergencies such as abruptio placentae and HELLP (haemolysis, elevated liver enzymes, and low platelet count) syndrome, and rare factor XIII deficiency. In general, it should not be used for other indications.

WBCs: Granulocytes may be transfused when sepsis occurs in a patient with profound persistent neutropenia (WBCs <500/µl) who is unresponsive to antibiotics. Granulocytes must be given within 24 hours of harvest; however, testing for HIV, hepatitis, human T-cell lymphotropic virus and syphilis may not be completed before infusion. Because of improved antibiotic therapy and drugs that stimulate granulocyte production during chemotherapy, granulocytes are seldom used.

Immune globulins: Rhesus immune globulin (RhIg), given IM or IV, prevents development of maternal Rh antibodies that can result from feto-maternal haemorrhage. The standard dose of intramuscular RhIg (300 µg) must be given to an Rh-negative mother immediately after abortion or delivery (live or stillborn) unless the infant is $Rh_0(D)$ negative or the mother's serum already contains anti-$Rh_0(D)$. If feto-maternal haemorrhage is >30 ml, a larger dose is needed. RhIg is given IV only when IM administration is contraindicated (eg patients with coagulopathy).

Other immune globulins are available for post-exposure prophylaxis for patients exposed to a number of infectious diseases, including cytomegalovirus, hepatitis A and B, measles, rabies, respiratory syncytial virus, rubella, tetanus, smallpox and varicella.

Platelets: Platelet concentrates are used:

- To prevent bleeding in asymptomatic severe thrombocytopenia (platelet count <10 000/µl)
- For bleeding patients with less severe thrombocytopenia (platelet count <50 000/µl)
- For bleeding patients with platelet dysfunction due to antiplatelet drugs but with normal platelet count
- For patients receiving massive transfusion that causes dilutional thrombocytopenia, and sometimes before invasive surgery, particularly with extracorporeal

circulation for >2 hours (which often makes platelets dysfunctional)

One platelet concentrate increases the platelet count by about 10 000/µl, and adequate haemostasis is achieved with a platelet count of about 10 000/µl in a patient without complicating conditions and about 50 000/µL for those undergoing surgery. Therefore, 4–6 random donor platelet concentrates are commonly used in adults.

Platelet concentrates are increasingly being prepared by automated devices that harvest the platelets (or other cells) and return unneeded components (eg RBCs, plasma) to the donor. This procedure, called cytapheresis, provides enough platelets from a single donation (equivalent to 6 random platelet units) for transfusion to an adult, which, because it minimises infectious and immunogenic risks, is preferred to multiple donor transfusions in certain conditions.

Certain patients may not respond to platelet transfusions, possibly because of splenic sequestration or platelet consumption due to HLA or platelet-specific antigen alloimmunisation. These patients may respond to multiple random donor platelets (because of the greater likelihood that some units are HLA compatible), platelets from family members, or ABO- or HLA-matched platelets. Alloimmunisation may be mitigated by transfusing WBC-depleted RBCs and WBC-depleted platelet concentrates.

Other products: Irradiated blood products are used to prevent graft-vs-host disease in patients at risk. Blood substitutes are being developed that use inert chemicals or haemoglobin solutions to carry and deliver O_2 to tissues. Perfluorocarbons are chemically and biologically inactive and are capable of dissolving O_2 and CO_2 under pressure. Because perfluorocarbons are not water-miscible, they are prepared as emulsions. They are undergoing phase II and III clinical trials. Hb-based O_2 carrier solutions are undergoing phase III clinical trials in the US. Hb, human or bovine, is chemically modified, producing a solution capable of O_2 transport. These solutions can be stored at room temperature for up to 2 years, making them attractive for transport to the site of trauma or to the battlefield. However, both perfluorocarbons and Hb-based O_2 carriers are cleared from plasma within 24 hours.

Haematopoietic progenitor cells (stem cells) from autologous or allogenic donors can be transfused as a way of reconstituting haematopoietic function (particularly immune function) in patients undergoing myeloablative or myelotoxic therapy.

Complications of transfusion

The most common complications of transfusion are febrile non-haemolytic and chill-rigor reactions. The most serious complications are acute haemolytic reaction due to ABO-incompatible transfusion and transfusion-related acute lung injury, which have very high mortality rates. The complications of transfusion are discussed below.

Acute haemolytic transfusion reaction (AHTR): AHTR usually results from recipient plasma antibodies to donor RBC antigens. ABO incompatibility is the most common cause of AHTR. Antibodies against blood group antigens other than ABO can also cause AHTR. Mislabelling the recipient's pretransfusion sample at collection or failing to match the intended recipient with the blood product immediately before transfusion is the usual cause, not laboratory error.

Delayed haemolytic transfusion reaction: Occasionally, a patient who has been sensitised to an RBC antigen has very low antibody levels and negative pretransfusion tests. After transfusion with RBCs bearing this antigen, a primary or anamnestic response may result (usually in 1–4 weeks) and cause a delayed haemolytic transfusion reaction. Delayed haemolytic transfusion reaction usually does not manifest as dramatically as AHTR. Patients may be asymptomatic or have a slight fever. Rarely, severe symptoms occur.

Febrile non-haemolytic transfusion reaction: Febrile reaction can occur without haemolysis. Antibodies directed against WBC HLA from otherwise compatible donor blood are one possible cause. This cause is most common in multitransfused or multiparous patients. Cytokines released from WBCs during storage, particularly in platelet concentrates, is another possible cause.

Allergic reactions: Allergic reactions to an unknown component in donor blood are common, usually due to allergens in donor plasma or, less often, to antibodies from an allergic donor. These reactions are usually mild, with urticaria, oedema, occasional dizziness and headache during or immediately after the transfusion. Simultaneous fever is common. Less frequently, dyspnoea, wheezing and incontinence may occur, indicating a generalised spasm of smooth muscle. Rarely, anaphylaxis occurs, particularly in IgA-deficient recipients.

Volume overload: The high osmotic load of blood products draws volume into the intravascular space over the course of hours, which can cause volume overload in susceptible patients (eg those with cardiac or renal insufficiency). RBCs should be infused slowly. The patient should be observed and, if signs of heart failure occur (eg dyspnoea, rales), the transfusion should be stopped and treatment for heart failure begun.

Acute lung injury: Transfusion-related acute lung injury is an infrequent complication caused by anti-HLA and/or anti-granulocyte antibodies in donor plasma that agglutinate and degranulate recipient granulocytes within the lung. Acute respiratory symptoms develop, and the chest X-ray has a characteristic pattern of non-cardiogenic pulmonary oedema. After ABO incompatibility, this is the second most common cause of transfusion-related death. Incidence is 1:5 000–10 000, but many cases are mild. Mild to moderate transfusion-related acute lung injury is probably commonly missed.

Altered oxygen affinity: Blood stored for more than 7 days has decreased RBC 2,3-diphosphoglycerate (DPG), and the 2,3-DPG is absent after >10 days. This absence results in an increased affinity for O_2 and slower O_2 release to the tissues. There is little evidence that 2,3-DPG deficiency is clinically significant except in exchange transfusions in infants, in sickle cell patients with acute chest syndrome and stroke, and in some patients with severe heart failure. After transfusion of RBCs, 2,3-DPG regenerates within 12–24 hours.

Graft–vs–host disease (GVHD): Transfusion-associated GVHD is usually caused by transfusion of products containing immunocompetent lymphocytes to an immunocompromised host. The donor lymphocytes attack host tissues. GVHD can occur occasionally in immunocompetent patients if they receive blood from a donor who is homozygous for an HLA haplotype (usually a close relative) for which the patient is heterozygous. GVHD occurs 4–30 days after transfusion and is diagnosed on the basis of clinical suspicion and skin and bone marrow biopsies. GVHD has >90% mortality because no specific treatment is available. Prevention of GVHD is with irradiation (to damage DNA of the donor lymphocytes) of all transfused blood products.

Complications of massive transfusion: Massive transfusion is transfusion of a volume of blood greater than or equal to one blood volume in 24 hours (eg 10 units in a 70-kg adult). When a patient receives stored blood in such large volume, the patient's own blood may be, in effect, 'washed out'. Complications of massive transfusion include:

- Dilutional thrombocytopenia: the most likely complication. Platelets in stored whole blood are not functional. Clotting factors (except factor VIII) usually remain sufficient. Microvascular bleeding (abnormal oozing and continued bleeding from raw and cut surfaces) may result. Usually 5–8 platelet concentrates (1 unit/10 kg) are enough to correct such bleeding in an adult. FFP and cryoprecipitate may be needed.
- Hypothermia: due to rapid transfusion of large amounts of cold blood, which can cause arrhythmias or cardiac arrest. Hypothermia is avoided by using an IV set with a heat-exchange device that gently warms blood. Other means of warming blood (eg microwave ovens) are contraindicated because of potential RBC damage and haemolysis.

- Citrate toxicity: generally not of concern, even in massive transfusion. However, citrate toxicity may be amplified in the presence of hypothermia. Patients with liver failure may have difficulty metabolising citrate.
- Hypocalcaemia: rarely necessitates treatment (which is 10 ml of a 10% solution of calcium gluconate IV diluted in 100 ml 5% dextrose, given over 10 minutes).
- Hyperkalaemia: patients with renal failure may have elevated potassium if transfused with blood stored for >1 week (potassium accumulation is usually insignificant in blood stored for <1 week). Mechanical haemolysis during transfusion may increase potassium.
- Hypokalaemia: can occur about 24 hours after transfusion of older RBCs (>3 weeks), which take up potassium.

Infectious complications: Bacterial contamination of packed RBCs occurs rarely, possibly due to inadequate aseptic technique during collection or to transient asymptomatic donor bacteraemia. Refrigeration of RBCs usually limits bacterial growth except for cryophilic organisms such as *Yersinia* species, which can produce dangerous levels of endotoxin. All RBC units are inspected before issue for bacterial growth, which is indicated by a colour change. Because platelet concentrates are stored at room temperature, they have greater potential for bacterial growth and endotoxin production if contaminated. To minimise growth, storage is limited to 5 days. The risk of bacterial contamination of platelets is 1:2500 so platelets are routinely tested for bacteria.

Rarely, syphilis is transmitted in fresh blood or platelets. Storing blood for ≥96 hours at 4–10°C kills the spirochaete.

Hepatitis can occur after transfusion of any blood product. The risk has been reduced by viral inactivation through heat treatment of serum albumin and plasma proteins and by the use of recombinant factor concentrates. Tests for hepatitis are required for all donor blood. The estimated risk of hepatitis B is 1:200 000; of hepatitis C, 1:2.6 million. Because its transient viraemic phase and concomitant clinical illness are likely to preclude blood donation, hepatitis A (infectious hepatitis) is not a significant cause of transfusion-associated hepatitis.

HIV infection is another potential infectious complication. The estimated risk of HIV transmission due to transfusion is 1 in 26 million.

Cytomegalovirus (CMV) can be transmitted by WBCs in transfused blood. It is not transmitted through FFP. Because CMV does not cause disease in immunocompetent recipients, routine antibody testing of donor blood is not required. However, CMV can cause serious or fatal disease in immunocompromised patients, who should probably receive CMV-negative blood products that have been provided by CMV antibody-negative donors or by blood depleted of WBCs by filtration.

Human T-cell lymphotropic virus 1 (HTLV-1), which can cause adult T-cell lymphoma/leukaemia, HTLV-1-associated myelopathy and tropical spastic paraparesis, causes post-transfusion seroconversion in some recipients. All donor blood is tested for HTLV-1 and HTLV-2 antibodies. The estimated risk of false-negative results on testing of donor blood is 1:641 000.

Creutzfeldt–Jakob disease has never been reported to be transfusion-transmitted, but current practice precludes donation from a person who has received human-derived growth hormone or a dura mater transplant or who has a family member with Creutzfeldt–Jakob disease. Also new variant Creutzfeldt–Jakob disease (mad cow disease) has not been transmitted by blood transfusion.

Malaria is transmitted easily through infected RBCs. Many donors are unaware that they have malaria, which may be latent and transmissible for 10–15 years. Storage does not render blood safe. Prospective donors must be asked about malaria or whether they have been in a region where it is prevalent. Donors who have had a diagnosis of malaria or who are immigrants, refugees, or citizens from countries in which malaria is considered endemic are deferred for 3 years; travellers to endemic countries are deferred for 1 year. Babesiosis has rarely been transmitted by transfusion.

2.6 SURGICAL ONCOLOGY

Cancer is an unregulated proliferation of cells due to loss of normal controls, resulting in unregulated growth, lack of differentiation, local tissue invasion and, often, metastasis. Cancer can develop in any tissue or organ at any age. There is often an immune response to tumours. Many cancers are curable if detected at an early stage, and long-term remission is often possible in later stages. However, cure is not always possible and is not attempted in some advanced cases in which palliative care provides better quality of life than vigorous but fruitless attempts at tumour eradication.

2.6.1 Nomenclature

The following closely related terms may be used to designate abnormal growths:

Neoplasm: a scientific term which refers to an abnormal proliferation of genetically altered cells.

Tumour: generally means any swelling or mass. However, the vast majority of entities referred to as 'tumours' in common usage are in fact neoplasms. Specifically, a tumour is a **solid**

neoplasm; some neoplasms, such as haematological cancers, are not solid.

Malignant neoplasm: synonymous with cancer. It is a neoplasm characterised by a population of cells that grow and divide without respect to normal limits, invade and destroy adjacent tissues, and which may spread to distant anatomical sites through a process called metastasis.

Malignant tumours are usually named using the Latin or Greek root of the organ of origin as a prefix and the tissue type affected as the suffix. For instance, a malignant tumour of the liver is called **hepatocarcinoma**; a malignant tumour of the fat cells is called **liposarcoma**. For common cancers, the English organ name is used. For instance, the most common type of breast cancer is called **ductal carcinoma of the breast** or **mammary ductal carcinoma**. Here, the adjective **ductal** refers to the appearance of the cancer under the microscope, resembling normal breast ducts.

Benign neoplasm: a neoplasm that has self-limiting growth and does not invade other tissues or metastasise. It is usually not cancerous.

Benign tumours are named using '-oma' as a suffix with the organ name as the root. For instance, a benign tumour of the smooth muscle of the uterus is called **leiomyoma** (the common name of this frequent tumour is **fibroid**). However, some cancers also use this prefix for historical reasons, examples being melanoma and seminoma.

Pre-malignant neoplasm: a non-invasive neoplasm that may not form an obvious mass, but which has the potential to progress to cancer if left untreated. Pre-malignant neoplasms may show distinctive microscopic changes such as dysplasia or atypia.

Metastasis: the transfer of a disease from one organ or part to another organ or part not directly connected with it. Only malignant neoplastic cells have the capacity to metastasise. Cancer cells can break away from a primary tumour, penetrate the lymphatics and blood vessels, circulate through the bloodstream and grow in a distant focus (metastasise) in normal tissues elsewhere in the body.

When cancer cells spread to form a new tumour, it is called a secondary, or **metastatic tumour**, and its cells are like those in the original tumour. This means, for example, that if breast cancer spreads (metastasises) to the lung, the secondary tumour is made up of abnormal breast cells (not abnormal lung cells). The disease in the lung is metastatic breast cancer (not lung cancer).

Cancer cells may spread to lymph nodes (regional lymph nodes) near the primary tumour. This is called nodal involvement, positive nodes, or regional disease. Localised spread to regional lymph nodes near the primary tumour is not normally counted as metastasis, although this is a sign of a worse prognosis.

Dysplasia: refers to an abnormality in maturation of cells within a tissue. This generally consists of an expansion of immature cells, with a corresponding decrease in the number and location of mature cells. Dysplasia is often indicative of an early neoplastic process. The term 'dysplasia' is typically used when the cellular abnormality is restricted to the originating tissue, as in the case of an early, in-situ neoplasm. For example, epithelial dysplasia of the cervix (cervical intraepithelial neoplasia – a disorder commonly detected by an abnormal Pap smear) consists of an increased population of immature (basal-like) cells which are restricted to the mucosal surface, and have not invaded through the basement membrane to the deeper soft tissues.

2.6.2 Classification

Cancers are classified by the type of cell that resembles the tumour and, therefore, the tissue presumed to be the origin of the tumour. Examples of general categories include:

Carcinoma: malignant tumours derived from epithelial cells. This group represents the most common cancers, including the common forms of breast, prostate, lung and colon cancer.

Sarcoma: malignant tumours derived from connective tissue or mesenchymal cells.

Lymphoma and leukaemia: malignancies derived from haematopoietic (blood-forming) cells.

Germ cell tumours: tumours derived from totipotent cells. Totipotent cells have the ability to divide and produce all the differentiated cells in an organism, including extra-embryonic tissues. Germ cell tumours are most often found in adults in the testes and ovary, while in fetuses, babies and young children these are most often found in the body midline, particularly in the sacrococcygeal area.

Blastic tumour: a tumour (usually malignant) which resembles an immature or embryonic tissue. Many of these tumours are most common in children.

Table 2.21 summarises the nomenclature and classification of neoplasms based on the tissue of origin.

2.6.3 Carcinogenesis

Carcinogenesis is the process by which normal cells are transformed into cancer cells. Cell division (Figure 2.3) is a physiological process that occurs in almost all tissues and under many circumstances. Normally, the balance between proliferation and programmed cell death, usually in the form of apoptosis, is maintained by tightly regulating both processes to ensure the integrity of organs and tissues. Genetic mutations are largely responsible for the generation of malignant cells or carcinogenesis. These mutations alter the quantity or function of protein products that regulate cell growth and division and DNA repair.

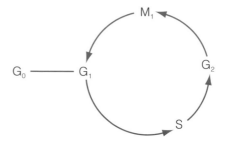

Figure 2.3: The cell cycle. G_0 = resting phase (non-proliferation of cells); G_1 = variable pre-DNA synthetic phase (12 h to a few days); S = DNA synthesis (usually 2–4 h); G_2 = post-DNA synthesis (2–4 h) – a tetraploid quantity of DNA is found within cells; M_1 = mitosis (1–2 h)

Mutated genes

Two major categories of mutated genes are oncogenes and tumour suppressor genes.

Oncogenes are abnormal forms of normal genes (proto-oncogenes) that regulate cell growth. Mutation of these genes may result in direct and continuous stimulation of the molecular biological pathways (eg intracellular signal transduction pathways, transcription factors, secreted growth factors) that control cellular growth and division.

There are >100 known oncogenes that may contribute to human neoplastic transformation. For example, the *ras* gene encodes the Ras protein, which regulates cell division. Mutations may result in the inappropriate activation of the Ras protein, leading to uncontrolled cell growth and division. In fact, the Ras protein is abnormal in about 25% of human cancers. Other oncogenes have been implicated in specific cancers. These include various protein kinases (bladder cancer, breast cancer), *bcr-abl* (chronic myelocytic leukaemia, B-cell acute lymphocytic leukaemia), C-*myc* (small-cell lung cancer), N-*myc* (small-cell lung cancer, neuroblastoma) and C-*erb* B-2 (breast cancer). Specific oncogenes may have important implications for diagnosis, therapy and prognosis.

Oncogenes typically result from acquired somatic cell mutations secondary to point mutations (eg from chemical carcinogens), gene amplification (eg an increase in the number of copies of a normal gene), or from insertion of viral genetic elements into host DNA. Occasionally, mutation of germ cell lines results in vertical transmission and a higher incidence of cancer development in offspring.

Table 2.21: Nomenclature of neoplasms

Tissue of origin			Benign	Malignant
Composed of one parenchymal cell type	Tumours of epithelial origin	Stratified squamous	Squamous cell papilloma	Squamous cell or epidermoid carcinoma
		Basal cells of skin or adnexa		Basal cell carcinoma
		Epithelial lining of glands or ducts	Adenoma	Adenocarcinoma
			Papilloma	Papillary carcinomas
			Cystadenoma	Cystadenocarcinoma
		Respiratory passages	Bronchial adenoma	Bronchogenic carcinoma
		Renal epithelium	Renal tubular adenoma	Renal cell carcinoma
		Liver cells	Liver cell adenoma	Hepatocellular carcinoma
		Urinary tract epithelium (transitional)	Transitional cell papilloma	Transitional cell carcinoma
		Placental epithelium	Hydatidiform mole	Choriocarcinoma
		Testicular epithelium (germ cells)		Seminoma
				Embryonal carcinoma
	Tumours of melanocytes		Naevus	Malignant melanoma
	Tumours of mesenchymal origin	Connective tissue and derivatives	Fibroma	Fibrosarcoma
			Lipoma	Liposarcoma
			Chondroma	Chondrosarcoma
			Osteoma	Osteogenic sarcoma
	Endothelial and related tissues	Blood vessels	Haemangioma	Angiosarcoma
		Lymph vessels	Lymphangioma	Lymphangiosarcoma
		Synovium		Synovial sarcoma
		Mesothelium		Mesothelioma
		Brain coverings	Meningioma	Invasive meningioma
	Blood cells and related cells	Haematopoietic cells		Leukaemias
		Lymphoid tissue		Lymphomas
	Muscle	Smooth	Leiomyoma	Leiomyosarcoma
		Striated	Rhabdomyoma	Rhabdomyosarcoma
More than one neoplastic cell type – mixed tumours, usually derived from one germ cell layer	Salivary glands		Pleomorphic adenoma (mixed tumour of salivary origin)	Malignant mixed tumour of salivary gland origin
	Renal angle			Wilms' tumour
More than one neoplastic cell type derived from more than one germ cell layer – teratogenous	Totipotential cells in gonads or in embryonic rests		Mature teratoma, dermoid cyst	Immature teratoma, teratocarcinoma

Tumour suppressor genes are inherent genes that play a role in cell division and DNA repair and are critical for detecting inappropriate growth signals in cells. If these genes, as a result of inherited or acquired mutations, become unable to function, genetic mutations in other genes can proceed unchecked, leading to neoplastic transformation.

As with most genes, two alleles are present that encode for each tumour suppressor gene. A defective copy of one gene may be inherited, leaving a person with only one functional allele for the individual tumour suppressor gene. If an acquired mutation occurs in the other allele, the normal protective mechanisms of the tumour suppressor gene are lost, and dysfunction of other protein products or DNA damage may escape unregulated, leading to cancer. For example, the retinoblastoma gene (*RB*) encodes for the protein pRB, which regulates the cell cycle by stopping DNA replication. Mutations in *RB* occur in 30%–40% of all human cancers, allowing affected cells to divide continuously.

Another mechanism that results in defective function and transcription of tumour suppressor genes is aberrant methylation of the promoter region of these genes, which inhibits gene transcription. Greater degrees of aberrant methylation and greater numbers of affected genes cause tumours to be more malignant and are associated with shortened survival in lung, bladder and prostate cancer.

Another important regulatory protein, p53, prevents replication of damaged DNA in normal cells and promotes cell death (apoptosis) in cells with abnormal DNA. Inactive or altered p53 allows cells with abnormal DNA to survive and divide. Mutations are passed to daughter cells, conferring a high probability of neoplastic transformation. The *TP53* gene is defective in many human cancers.

2.6.4 Causes of cancer

The causes of cancer can be broadly classified in to three major categories: environmental, immunological and genetic.

Environmental causes

- **Viruses** contribute to the pathogenesis of human malignancies (Table 2.22). This may occur through the integration of viral genetic elements into the host DNA. These new genes are expressed by the host; they may affect cell growth or division, or disrupt normal host genes required for control of cell growth and division. Alternatively, viral infection may result in immune dysfunction, leading to decreased immune surveillance for early tumours.
- **Parasites** of some types can lead to cancer. *Schistosoma haematobium* causes chronic inflammation and fibrosis of the bladder, which may lead to cancer. *Opisthorchis sinensis* has been linked to carcinoma of the pancreas and bile ducts.
- **Chemical carcinogens** can induce gene mutations and result in uncontrolled growth and tumour formation (Table 2.23). Other substances, called co-carcinogens, possess little or no inherent carcinogenic potency but enhance the carcinogenic effect of another agent when exposed simultaneously.
- **Ultraviolet radiation** can induce skin cancer (eg basal and squamous cell carcinoma, melanoma) by damaging DNA. This DNA damage consists of formation of thymidine dimers, which may escape repair due to inherent defects in DNA repair (eg xeroderma pigmentosum) or through rare, random events.
- **Ionising radiation** is also carcinogenic. For example, survivors of the atomic bomb explosions in Hiroshima and Nagasaki have a higher than expected incidence of leukaemia and other cancers. Similarly, the use of X-rays to treat non-malignant disease (acne, thymic or adenoid enlargement, ankylosing spondylitis) results in higher rates of acute and chronic leukaemias, Hodgkin and non-Hodgkin lymphomas, multiple myeloma, aplastic anaemia terminating in acute non-lymphocytic leukaemia, myelofibrosis, melanoma and thyroid cancer. Industrial exposure (eg to uranium by mine workers) is linked to development of lung cancer after a 15- to 20-year latency. Long-term exposure to occupational irradiation or to internally deposited thorium dioxide predisposes people to angiosarcomas and acute non-lymphocytic leukaemia.
- **Chronic skin irritation** leads to chronic dermatitis and, in rare cases, to squamous cell carcinoma. This occurrence is presumably due to random mutations that occur more frequently because of the increased cell turnover.

Immunological causes

Immune system dysfunction as a result of genetic mutation, acquired disease, aging, or immunosuppressants interferes with normal immune surveillance of early tumours and results in higher rates of cancer. Known cancer-associated immune disorders include:

- Ataxia-telangiectasia [acute lymphocytic leukaemia (ALL), brain tumours, gastric cancer]
- Wiskott–Aldrich syndrome (lymphoma, ALL)
- X-linked agammaglobulinaemia (lymphoma and ALL)
- Immune deficiency secondary to immunosuppressants or HIV infection (large-cell lymphoma, Kaposi's sarcoma)
- Rheumatological conditions, such as systemic lupus erythematosus, rheumatoid arthritis and Sjögren's syndrome (B-type lymphoma); and general immune disorders (lymphoreticular neoplasia)

Genetic causes

Most forms of cancer are 'sporadic', and have no basis in heredity. There are, however, a number of recognised syndromes of cancer with a hereditary component, often defective tumour suppressor alleles. Examples include:

- Certain inherited mutations in the genes *BRCA1* and *BRCA2* are associated with an elevated risk of breast cancer and ovarian cancer
- Tumours of various endocrine organs in multiple endocrine neoplasia (MEN types 1, 2A, 2B)
- Li-Fraumeni syndrome (various tumours such as osteosarcoma, breast cancer, soft-tissue sarcoma, brain tumours) due to mutations of *p53*
- Turcot syndrome (brain tumours and colonic polyposis)
- Familial adenomatous polyposis: an inherited mutation of the *APC* gene that leads to early onset of colon carcinoma
- Hereditary non-polyposis colorectal cancer (HNPCC, also known as Lynch syndrome) can include familial cases of colon cancer, uterine cancer, gastric cancer and ovarian cancer, without a preponderance of colon polyps
- Retinoblastoma, when occurring in young children, is due to a hereditary mutation in the retinoblastoma gene

- Down's syndrome patients, who have an extra chromosome 21, are known to develop malignancies such as leukaemia and testicular cancer

Table 2.22: Viruses causing cancer

Virus	Cancer
Cytomegalovirus	Kaposi's sarcoma
Epstein–Barr virus	Burkitt's lymphoma, immunoblastic lymphoma, nasopharyngeal carcinoma
Hepatitis B virus	Hepatocellular carcinoma
Herpesvirus 8	Kaposi's sarcoma
HIV	Kaposi's sarcoma, lymphoma
Human papillomaviruses	Cervical carcinoma
Human T cell lymphotrophic virus	T-cell lymphomas, hairy cell leukaemia

2.6.5 Clinical features of cancer

The clinical features of neoplasms can be divided into three categories of symptoms – local, those due to spread, and sytemic.

Table 2.23: Chemical carcinogens

Chemical carcinogen		Cancer
Occupational carcinogens	Soot and mineral oil	Skin cancer
	Arsenic	Lung cancer, skin cancer
	Asbestos	Lung cancer, mesothelioma
	Hair dyes and aromatic amines	Bladder cancer
	Benzene	Leukaemia
	Nickel	Lung cancer, nasal sinus cancer
	Formaldehyde	Nasal cancer, nasopharyngeal cancer
	Vinyl chloride	Hepatic angiosarcoma
	Painting materials, non-arsenic pesticides, diesel exhaust, chromates, man-made mineral fibres	Lung cancer
Lifestyle carcinogens	Alcohol	Oesophageal cancer, oropharyngeal cancer
	Betel nuts	Oropharyngeal cancer
	Tobacco	Head and neck cancer, lung cancer, oesophageal cancer, bladder cancer
Drug carcinogens	Alkylating agents	Leukaemia
	Diethylstilboestrol	Liver cell adenoma, vaginal cancer in exposed female fetuses
	Oxymetholone	Liver cancer
	Thorotrast	Angiosarcoma

Local symptoms: unusual lumps or swelling, haemorrhage, pain and/or ulceration. Compression of surrounding tissues may cause symptoms such as jaundice.

Symptoms due to spread/metastasis: enlarged lymph nodes, cough and haemoptysis, hepatomegaly, bone pain, fracture of affected bones and neurological symptoms. Although advanced cancer may cause pain, it is often not the first symptom.

Systemic symptoms: weight loss, poor appetite and wasting, excessive sweating (night sweats), anaemia and specific paraneoplastic syndromes, ie specific conditions that are due to an active cancer, such as thrombosis or hormonal changes.

2.6.6 Diagnosis of cancer

A complete history and physical examination may reveal unexpected clues to early cancer.

History: Clinicians must be aware of predisposing factors and must specifically ask about familial cancer, environmental exposure (including smoking history), and prior or present illnesses (autoimmune diseases, previous immunosuppressive therapy, hepatitis B and hepatitis C, HIV infection, abnormal Papanicolaou test, or human papillomavirus infection). Symptoms suggesting occult cancer can include fatigue, weight loss, fevers or night sweats, cough, haemoptysis, haematemesis or haematochezia, change in bowel habits, and persistent pain.

Physical examination: The physical examination should direct particular attention to skin, lymph nodes, lungs, breasts, abdomen and testes. Prostate, rectal and vaginal examinations are also important.

Laboratory investigations: Laboratory tests are performed on patients with symptoms and include serum tumour markers, molecular tests, imaging tests and biopsy.

- **Serum tumour markers** (Table 2.24) may offer corroborating evidence in patients with findings suggestive of a specific malignancy. These markers, however, are not useful for screening. Alpha-fetoprotein may be elevated in hepatocellular carcinoma and testicular carcinomas, carcinoembryonic antigen in colon cancer, β-human chorionic gonadotropin in choriocarcinoma and testicular carcinoma, serum immunoglobulins in multiple myeloma, DNA probes (eg *bcr* probe to identify a chromosome 22 alteration) in chronic myelogenous leukaemia, CA-125 in ovarian cancer, CA 27-29 in breast cancer, and prostate-specific antigen and prostatic acid phosphatase in prostate cancer. Restricting tumour marker testing to specific organ-related evaluations minimises false-positive test results and does not result in missed tumours.
- **Molecular tests** use gene-expression profiling (a genomics microassay method) and proteomics to define tumour

subtypes (eg lymphoma, leukaemias), to delineate the origin of metastatic cancers originating from an unknown primary cancer (eg lung cancer), and to assist in recognising inherent (or acquired) chemotherapy resistance.

- **Imaging tests** often include plain X-rays, sonograms, CT scans and MRIs. These tests assist in identifying abnormalities, determining qualities of a mass (solid or cystic), providing dimensions and establishing relationships to surrounding structures, which may be important if surgery or biopsy is being considered.
- **Biopsy** to confirm the diagnosis and tissue of origin is almost always required when cancer is suspected or detected. The choice of biopsy site is usually determined by ease of access and degree of invasiveness. If lymphadenopathy is present, fine-needle or core biopsy may yield the tumour type; if non-diagnostic, open biopsy is done. Other biopsy routes include bronchoscopy for easily accessible mediastinal or central pulmonary tumours, percutaneous liver biopsy if liver lesions are present and CT- or ultrasound-guided biopsy. If these procedures are not suitable, open biopsy may be necessary.

2.6.7 Screening for cancer

Screening tests (Table 2.25) are performed in asymptomatic patients at risk. The rationale is that early diagnosis may decrease cancer mortality, allow for less radical therapy and reduce costs. Risks, however, include false-positive results, which necessitate confirmatory tests (eg biopsy, endoscopy) that can lead to anxiety, significant morbidity and cost, and false-negative results, which may give a mistaken sense of security, causing the patient to ignore subsequent symptoms. (See also Section 7.1.2)

Screening for cancer should be performed when:

- A distinct high-risk group can be identified (eg those with certain infections, exposures, or behaviour)
- The disease has an asymptomatic period during which treatment would alter outcome
- The morbidity of the disease is significant
- An intervention is available that is acceptable and effective at changing the natural history of the condition

The screening tests themselves should satisfy the following criteria:

- Cost and convenience are reasonable
- Reliability, including accuracy, precision, and person-to-person variability, is high
- Sensitivity and specificity are adequate
- The positive predictive value is high in the population screened
- The test or procedure is acceptable to the patient

Table 2.24: Tumour markers

Tumour marker	Cancer	Additional associations/comments	Significance	Usual sample
AFP (α–fetoprotein)	Liver, germ cell cancer of testes or ovaries	Also elevated during pregnancy	Helps diagnose, monitor treatment, and determine recurrence	Blood
B2M (beta–2 microglobulin)	Multiple myeloma and lymphomas	Present in many other conditions, including Crohn's disease and hepatitis; often used to determine cause of renal failure	Determines prognosis	Blood
BTA (bladder tumour antigen)	Bladder	Gaining acceptance	Helps diagnose and determine recurrence	Urine
CA 15-3 (cancer antigen 15-3)	Breast and others including lung, ovarian	Also elevated in benign breast conditions; can use CA 15-3 or CA 27-29 (two different assays for same marker)	Stage disease, monitor treatment, and determine recurrence	Blood
CA 19-9 (cancer antigen 19-9)	Pancreatic, sometimes colorectal and bile ducts	Also elevated in pancreatitis and inflammatory bowel disease	Stage disease, monitor treatment, and determine recurrence	Blood
CA 72-4 (cancer antigen 72-4)	Ovarian	No evidence that it is better than CA-125 but may be useful when combined with it	Helps diagnose	Blood
CA-125 (cancer antigen 125)	Ovarian	Also elevated with endometriosis, some other diseases and benign conditions; not recommended as a general screen	Helps diagnose, monitor treatment, and determine recurrence	Blood
Calcitonin	Thyroid medullary carcinoma	Also elevated in pernicious anaemia and thyroiditis	Helps diagnose, monitor treatment, and determine recurrence	Blood
CEA (carcino-embryonic antigen)	Colorectal, lung, breast, thyroid, pancreatic, liver, cervix and bladder	Elevated in other conditions such as hepatitis, chronic obstructive pulmonary disease, colitis, pancreatitis, and in cigarette smokers	Helps monitor treatment and determine recurrence	Blood
EGFR (Her-1)	Solid tumours, such as of the lung (non-small-cell), head and neck, colon, pancreas, or breast	Not available in every laboratory	Helps guide treatment and determine prognosis	Tissue

Table 2.24: *continued*

Tumour marker	Cancer	Additional associations/comments	Significance	Usual sample
Oestrogen receptors	Breast	Increased in hormone-dependent cancer	Helps determine prognosis and guide treatment	Tissue
hCG (human chorionic gonadotropin)	Testicular and trophoblastic cancer	Elevated in pregnancy, testicular failure	Helps diagnose, monitor treatment, and determine recurrence	Blood, urine
Her-2/neu	Breast	Oncogene that is present in multiple copies in 20%–30% of invasive breast cancer	Helps determine prognosis and guide treatment	Tissue
Monoclonal immunoglobulins	Multiple myeloma and Waldenström's macroglobulinemia	Overproduction of an immunoglobulin or antibody, usually detected by protein electrophoresis	Helps diagnose, monitor treatment, and determine recurrence	Blood, urine
NSE (neurone-specific enolase)	Neuroblastoma, small-cell lung cancer	May be better than CEA for following this particular kind of lung cancer	Monitor treatment	Blood
NMP22	Bladder	Not widely used	Helps diagnose and determine recurrence	Urine
Progesterone receptors	Breast	Increased in hormone-dependent cancer	Helps determine prognosis and guide treatment	Tissue
PSA (prostate-specific antigen), total and free	Prostate	Elevated in benign prostatic hypertrophy, prostatitis and with age	Helps screen for and diagnose, monitor treatment, and determine recurrence	Blood
Prostate-specific membrane antigen (PSMA)	Prostate	Not widely used, levels increase normally with age	Helps diagnose	Blood
Prostatic acid phosphatase (PAP)	Metastatic prostate cancer, myeloma, lung cancer	Not widely used anymore, elevated in prostatitis and other conditions	Helps diagnose	Blood
S-100	Metastatic melanoma	Not widely used	Helps diagnose	Blood
TA-90	Metastatic melanoma	Not widely used, being studied	Helps diagnose	Blood
Thyroglobulin	Thyroid	Used after thyroid is removed to evaluate treatment	Determine recurrence	Blood

Table 2.25: Cancers in which screening is recommended

Type of cancer	Procedure	Frequency
Breast cancer	Breast self-examination	Monthly after age 20
	Breast physical examination	Every 3 years between ages 20 and 39; then yearly
	Mammography	Yearly, starting at age 40
Cervical cancer	Papanicolaou (Pap) test	Yearly in all women who are sexually active or starting at age 18
Cervical, uterine and ovarian cancers	Pelvic examination	Every 1–3 years between ages 18 and 40; then yearly
Prostate cancer	Rectal examination and blood test for prostate-specific antigen	Yearly after age 50 (or age 45 if in a high-risk group)
Rectal and colon cancer	Faecal occult blood or	Yearly, starting at age 50
	Flexible sigmoidoscopy or	Every 5 years, starting at age 50
	Colonoscopy	Every 10 years, starting at age 50

2.6.8 Staging and grading of cancer

Staging and grading schema have been devised for malignant neoplasms, because the stage and/or grade may determine the treatment and the prognosis. In general, the higher the stage, the larger a neoplasm is and the further it has spread.

Staging

The most common systems for staging employs the TNM classification. A 'T' score is based on the size and/or extent of invasion. The 'N' score indicates the extent of lymph node involvement. The 'M' score indicates whether distant metastases are present.

In Figure 2.4, utilising a lung carcinoma as an example, the principles of staging are illustrated.

Grading

Grading schemes are based on the microscopic appearance of a neoplasm with haematoxylin and eosin (H&E) staining. In general, a higher grade means that there is a lesser degree of differentiation and the worse will be the biological behaviour of a malignant neoplasm. A well-differentiated neoplasm is composed of cells that closely resemble the cell of origin, while poorly differentiated neoplasms have cells that are difficult to recognise as to their cell of origin. Grading schemes have been devised for many types of neoplasms, mainly carcinomas. Most grading systems have three or four grades (designated with numbers or roman numerals).

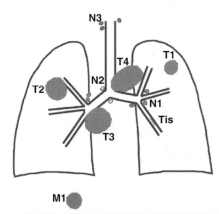

Staging of malignant neoplasms	
Stage	Definition
Tis	In situ, non-invasive (confined to epithelium)
T1	Small, minimally invasive within primary organ site
T2	Larger, more invasive within the primary organ site
T3	Larger and/or invasive beyond margins of primary organ site
T4	Very large and/or very invasive, spread to adjacent organs
N0	No lymph node involvement
N1	Regional lymph node involvement
N2	Extensive regional lymph node involvement
N3	More distant lymph node involvement
M0	No distant metastases
M1	Distant metastases present

Figure 2.4: Staging of malignant neoplasms

Utilising an adenocarcinoma as an example, the principles of grading are illustrated are Figure 2.5

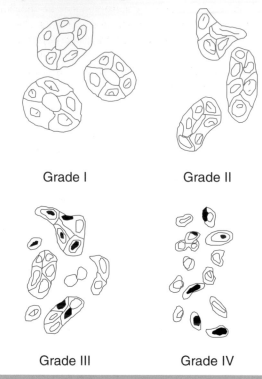

Grade I   Grade II

Grade III   Grade IV

Grading of malignant neoplasms	
Grade	**Definition**
I	Well differentiated
II	Moderately differentiated
III	Poorly differentiated
IV	Nearly anaplastic

Figure 2.5: Grading of malignant neoplasms

2.6.9 Treatment of cancer

Treatment modalities available for cancer include: surgery, chemotherapy, radiotherapy, immunotherapy, monoclonal antibody therapy or other methods. The choice of therapy depends on the location and grade of the tumour and the stage of the disease, as well as the general state of the patient (performance status). A number of experimental cancer treatments are also under development.

Complete removal of the cancer without damage to the rest of the body is the goal of treatment. Sometimes this can be accomplished by surgery, but the propensity of cancers to invade adjacent tissue or to spread to distant sites by microscopic metastasis often limits its effectiveness. The effectiveness of chemotherapy is often limited by toxicity to other tissues in the body. Radiation can also cause damage to normal tissue.

Surgery

In theory, cancers can be cured if entirely removed by surgery, but this is not always possible. When the cancer has metastasised to other sites in the body prior to surgery, complete surgical excision is usually impossible. Examples of surgical procedures for cancer include mastectomy for breast cancer and prostatectomy for prostate cancer. The goal of the surgery can be the removal of either only the tumour, or the entire organ. A single cancer cell is invisible to the naked eye but can regrow into a new tumour, a process called recurrence. For this reason, the pathologist examines the surgical specimen to determine if a margin of healthy tissue is present, thus decreasing the chance that microscopic cancer cells are left in the patient.

In addition to removal of the primary tumour, surgery is often necessary for staging, ie determining the extent of the disease and whether it has metastasised to regional lymph nodes. Staging is a major determinant of prognosis and of the need for adjuvant therapy.

Occasionally, surgery is necessary to control symptoms, such as spinal cord compression or bowel obstruction. This is referred to as palliative treatment.

Radiotherapy

Radiotherapy (also called radiation therapy, X-ray therapy, or irradiation) is the use of ionising radiation to kill cancer cells and shrink tumours. Radiotherapy can be administered externally (external-beam radiotherapy) or internally via brachytherapy. The effects of radiotherapy are confined to the region being treated. Radiotherapy injures or destroys cells in the area being treated (the 'target tissue') by damaging their genetic material, making it impossible for these cells to continue to grow and divide. Although radiation damages both cancer cells and normal cells, most normal cells can recover from the effects of radiation and function properly. The goal of radiotherapy is to damage as many cancer cells as possible, while limiting harm to nearby healthy tissue. Hence, it is given in several fractions, allowing healthy tissue to recover between fractions.

Radiotherapy may be used to treat almost every type of solid tumour, including cancers of the brain, breast, cervix, larynx, lung, pancreas, prostate, skin, stomach, uterus, or soft-tissue sarcomas. Radiation is also used to treat leukaemia and lymphoma. Radiation dosage to each site depends on a number of factors, including the radiosensitivity of each cancer type and whether there are tissues and organs nearby that may be damaged by radiation. Thus, as with every form of treatment, radiotherapy is not without its side-effects.

Chemotherapy

Chemotherapy involves the treatment of cancer with anticancer drugs that can destroy cancer cells. Anticancer drugs interfere with cell division. Most forms of chemotherapy target all rapidly dividing cells and are not specific for cancer cells, although some degree of specificity may come from the inability of many cancer cells to repair DNA damage, while normal cells generally can. Hence, chemotherapy has the potential to harm healthy tissue, especially those tissues that have a high replacement rate (eg intestinal lining). These cells usually repair themselves after chemotherapy.

Because some drugs work better together than alone, two or more drugs are often given at the same time. This is called 'combination chemotherapy'. Most chemotherapy regimens are given in a combination.

The treatment of some leukaemias and lymphomas requires the use of high-dose chemotherapy and total body irradiation. This treatment ablates the bone marrow, and hence the body's ability to recover and repopulate the blood. For this reason, bone marrow, or peripheral blood stem cell harvesting, is carried out before the ablative part of the therapy, to enable 'rescue' after the treatment has been given. This is known as 'autologous stem cell transplantation'. Alternatively, haematopoietic stem cells may be transplanted from a matched, unrelated donor.

Immunotherapy

Cancer immunotherapy refers to a diverse set of therapeutic strategies designed to induce the patient's own immune system to fight the tumour. Contemporary methods for generating an immune response against tumours include intravesical BCG immunotherapy for superficial bladder cancer, and the use of interferons and other cytokines to induce an immune response in patients with renal cell carcinoma and melanoma. Vaccines to generate specific immune responses are the subject of intensive research for a number of tumours, notably malignant melanoma and renal cell carcinoma.

Allogeneic haematopoietic stem cell transplantation ('bone marrow transplantation' from a genetically non-identical donor) can be considered a form of immunotherapy, since the donor's immune cells will often attack the tumour in a phenomenon known as graft-vs-tumour effect. For this reason, allogeneic haematopoietic stem cell transplantation leads to a higher cure rate than autologous transplantation for several cancer types, although the side-effects are also more severe.

Hormonal therapy

The growth of some cancers can be inhibited by providing or blocking certain hormones. Common examples of hormone-sensitive tumours include certain types of breast and prostate cancers. Blocking oestrogen or testosterone is often an important additional treatment. In certain cancers, administration of hormone agonists, such as progestogens, may be therapeutically beneficial.

Targeted therapy

Targeted therapy, which first became available in the late 1990s, has had a significant impact on the treatment of some types of cancer, and is currently a very active research area. This comprises the use of agents specific for the deregulated proteins of cancer cells. Small-molecule-targeted therapy drugs are generally inhibitors of enzymatic domains on mutated, overexpressed, or otherwise critical proteins within the cancer cell. Prominent examples are the tyrosine kinase inhibitors, imatinib, and gefitinib.

Monoclonal antibody therapy is another strategy in which the therapeutic agent is an antibody which specifically binds to a protein on the surface of the cancer cells. Examples include the anti-HER2/neu antibody trastuzumab (Herceptin®) used in breast cancer, and the anti-CD20 antibody rituximab, used in a variety of B-cell malignancies.

Targeted therapy can also involve small peptides as 'homing devices' which can bind to cell surface receptors or affected extracellular matrix surrounding the tumour. Radionuclides which are attached to these peptides eventually kill the cancer cell if the nuclide decays in the vicinity of the cell.

Photodynamic therapy

Photodynamic therapy (PDT) is another treatment modality for cancer involving a photosensitiser, light, tissue oxygen and often use of lasers. A photosensitiser is a chemical compound that can be excited by light of a specific wavelength. This excitation uses visible or near-infrared light. In PDT, either a photosensitiser or the metabolic precursor of one is administered to the patient. The tissue to be treated is exposed to light suitable for exciting the photosensitiser. Usually, the photosensitiser is excited from a ground singlet state to an excited singlet state. It then undergoes intersystem crossing to a longer-lived excited triplet state. One of the few chemical species present in tissue with a ground triplet state is molecular oxygen. When the photosensitiser and an oxygen molecule are in proximity, an energy transfer can take place that allows the photosensitiser to relax to its ground singlet state, and create an excited singlet state oxygen molecule. Singlet oxygen is a very aggressive chemical species and will very rapidly react with any nearby biomolecules. (The specific targets depend heavily on the photosensitiser chosen.) Ultimately, these destructive reactions will result in cell killing through apoptosis or necrosis.

PDT is being used for treatment of basal cell carcinoma and lung cancer.

Peri-operative care and anaesthetics

CONTENTS

Peri-operative care and anaesthetics

Peri-operative care refers to the care provided to patients before, during and after the operation. It is as important as the surgery itself, if not more so. Inadequate peri-operative care and pre-operative preparations can cause considerable morbidity for patients and can ruin potentially successful operations and outcomes. Pre-operative care involves assessing a patient's fitness for surgery as well as identifying any co-morbid conditions that may need optimising. Particular anaesthetics can also be tailored to an individual's clinical requirements. Fluid balance is also a very important consideration that needs to be addressed, especially in patients undergoing major surgery. Post-operative care allows recovery from anaesthesia as well as allowing patients to heal from their surgical procedures. This chapter forms an excellent adjunct to surgery and represents the bare minimum that every student revising for surgery should know. Most sections have been kept extremely short and relevant as this book is intended as a surgical revision guide. Further reading with a textbook on peri-operative medicine and anaesthetics as well as spending time observing anaesthetists in the peri-operative period are essential.

Revision objectives

You should:
- Be familiar with the technique of pre-operative assessment as well as familiar with therapeutic adjuncts administered in the peri-operative period
- Understand fluid management principles and fluid balance in surgical patients
- Be aware of pre-existing medical conditions and how these can affect the surgical patient
- Know how to categorise a patient into ASA grading
- Know the different stages of administering anaesthetics and the medications and methods used in each stage
- Be aware of the common post-operative medical conditions which can affect a patient and be able to investigate and manage these accordingly

3.1 PERI-OPERATIVE CARE IN SURGERY

3.1.1 Pre-operative care
Preparation required prior to going to theatre is determined by:

- How soon surgery is required
    - Emergency: immediate action for a life-threatening condition, eg ruptured abdominal aortic aneurysm (AAA)
    - Urgent: within a few hours, eg appendicitis
    - Elective: planned surgery, eg varicose veins
- The nature of surgery and anaesthesia required. Local anaesthetic (LA) vs regional vs General anaesthesia (GA)
- Where the surgery will be, eg Emergency department or main theatre
- Facilities available (eg surgical equipment, post-op ITU bed availability)

Important aspects of pre-operative care include:

- History
    - This will determine the need for surgery and affects the nature of the anaesthetic used (See Box 3.1).
- Examination
    - A full examination allows the surgical pathology to be confirmed and reveals any further signs of disease elsewhere.
- Investigations
    - These must be appropriate to the surgery and the patient (see Box 3.2).
- Consent
    - Informed consent ensures that patients understand their condition and treatment options.
    - Complications with >1% incidence and life-threatening should be discussed.
    - The clinician performing the treatment process should ideally obtain consent. If this is not possible, an appropriately qualified person with suitable understanding of the procedure and its risks should take this responsibility.
    - If patients lack capacity, a decision can be made by the doctor to proceed if it is thought to be in the best interests of the patient.
- Nutrition
    - Elective patients should avoid solids 6 hours pre-operatively and clear fluids up to 2 hours pre-operatively. Oral medication can and should be taken the morning of the operation unless there are clear reasons not to.
    - In an emergency, the risks of delaying surgery may outweigh the risk of aspiration, so a fasting period is overlooked.
    - A fasting period is required when planning local and/or regional anaesthesia as a GA may be required unexpectedly.

3.1.2 Therapeutic adjuncts

Additional therapeutics to consider at this stage include:

- **Thromboembolic prophylaxis.** This is important as surgical patients may develop a venous thrombosis or pulmonary embolism which is a cause of mortality and/or morbidity. Measures to reduce this include:
  - Compression stockings and pneumatic calf compression, except in cases of patients with peripheral vascular disease
  - Post-operative leg elevation and early ambulation
  - Heparin prophylaxis. Commonly, low-molecular-weight heparin used. Stop 24 hours prior to insertion or removal of an epidural catheter.
- **Premedication.** This reduces patient anxiety and allows for a smoother anaesthetic.
- **Antibiotics.** These may be used for prophylaxis or treatment. Prophylaxis is given peri-operatively depending on the nature of the surgery. The choice is determined by the surgeon.
- **Bowel preparation.** This depends on surgery but usually requires strong laxatives such as Picolax® to ensure the bowel is clean prior to abdominal surgery. Hydration is important as these drugs can cause significant diarrhoea. Minor anal surgery such as haemorrhoidectomy only requires rectal emptying, for which phosphate enemas are sufficient.

Box 3.1: Taking a surgical history: important points

- History of presenting complaint
  - Influences urgency of treatment and anaesthetic management
- Past medical history
  - Determines overall anaesthetic and procedural risk
- Anaesthetic history
  - This can highlight any specific problems with agents used or post-operative nausea and vomiting
- Family history
  - Problems with anaesthetic drugs may be genetic
  - Systemic illness such as porphyria can influence management
- Drug history
  - Interaction with anaesthetic agents can be important
  - Sudden withdrawal of drugs such as steroids can cause problems
  - Previous allergy history is important
- Social history
  - Smoking influences peri-operative course

Box 3.2: Important investigations in the pre-operative period

These are influenced by patient, surgical or medical factors

Patient factors
Screening tests are useful in eliciting occult abnormality in certain groups of patients:
- Urinalysis
- Full blood count, especially if >60 years or an O&G patient
- Urea and electrolytes, especially >60 years
- Electrocardiogram (ECG) for >60 years or major surgery
- Sickle cell test for untested Afro-Caribbeans

Surgical factors
Tests may be needed to plan surgery or anticipate problems:
- Full blood count (FBC) if significant blood loss is expected
- Urea and electrolytes (U&Es) for major surgery or for baseline prior to urological intervention
- Amylase for diagnosis
- ECG for major surgery
- Chest X-ray for assessment, eg in major trauma, suspicion of malignancy
- Coagulation studies for obstructive jaundice or patients on anticoagulants
- Group and save or cross-matching

Medical factors
These may be extensive, depending on co-morbidity and urgency of the surgical intervention
Simple tests may be needed but the pathology will determine others. Some examples include:
- U&Es for diuretic therapy
- ECG in hypertension
- Echocardiography with cardiorespiratory patients
- Lung function tests and arterial blood gases for pre-existing lung disease
- Cervical spine X-ray for rheumatoid arthritis

3.1.3 Fluid balance

It is important to have a good understanding of fluid balance in surgical patients. They must maintain a circulating volume to enable tissue perfusion, healing and function.

Factors affecting fluid and electrolyte balance in surgical patients include:

- Major surgery requires patients to be 'nil by mouth' (NBM), when intravenous hydration is important. Fluid requirements during this period can be supplemented by intravenous fluids.
- Fluid sequesters in the 'third space', a large transcellular space with a layer of epithelium, eg gut, pleura.
- Blood loss may have been underestimated, particularly before surgery.
- Surgery and/or critical illness cause a stress response where the sympathetic drive results in sodium and water retention following aldosterone and ADH release.
- Length of surgery – in a laparotomy approximately 1 litre of fluid is lost per hour through evaporation from viscera.
- Pre- and post-operative fluid loss through nasogastric tube drainage and/or bowel preparation prior to surgery.

Total body water (TBW) measures 60% of an adult's total body weight. It is higher in children. The normal water distribution in a 70-kg male is shown in Box 3.3.

Box 3.3: Normal water distribution in a 70-kg male

Total body water (TBW) = extracellular fluid (ECF) + intracellular fluid (ICF)

Typical values for 70-kg male:

TBW = 42 litres (60% total body weight)

ECF = 14 litres (20% total body weight)

ICF = 28 litres (40% total body weight)

ECF = interstitial fluid + plasma fluid

Interstitial fluid = 11.5 litres

Plasma fluid = 3.5 litres

There is a constant equilibrium maintained between the **intracellular** and **extracellular** fluid. The main cations in **intracellular fluid** are potassium and magnesium. They are in balance with phosphate, proteins and organic ions, the anions. In **extracellular fluid**, sodium is the main cation and chloride is the major anion.

Balance is maintained across the cell membrane (Starling's hypothesis) by:

- The **hydrostatic pressure** of water in the capillary and the tissue
- The **oncotic pressure** exerted by insoluble particles (ie proteins, ions) in the capillary and tissue
- The **permeability** or leakiness of the membrane to substances

An excess of tissue fluid is **oedema** and occurs if there is an imbalance between hydrostatic and oncotic pressure.

To understand the fluid requirements of a surgical patient, consider:

- The normal daily requirements
  - The average 70-year-old takes 2.6 litres a day in food, drink and products of cellular metabolism.
  - A similar volume is lost through the alimentary canal (saliva, gastric juice, bile, intestinal juice), kidneys (filtration) skin (sweating) and lungs (evaporation).
- The clinical state
  - There may be a fluid deficit that needs to be replaced, eg acute bleeding, increased insensible losses during febrile episodes or from bowel preparation.
  - Fluid overload may occur if there is new or old underlying cardiac dysfunction. An overall negative balance should be planned here.
  - Hypoalbuminaemia or capillary leak states such as sepsis make it difficult to maintain an intravascular volume. There may be significant oedema in the face of fluid depletion.
  - Hyperventilation, pyrexia, diarrhoea, vomiting, third-space losses in bowel obstruction, ascites and effusions all cause fluid depletion.
- Renal function and electrolyte measurements
  - Pulmonary oedema may be precipitated.

Fluid management

Fluid restriction
If the overall aim is to achieve a negative balance (eg patient is volume overloaded).

Colloids
These solutions contain molecules that do not pass across the capillary membrane. They are therefore useful for quick intravascular expansion. Commonly used examples include Gelofusin®, Haemaccel®, Hetastarch® and dextrans. Albumin is a naturally occurring colloid.

Crystalloids

These shift across the capillary membrane according to their sodium content.

- Normal saline and Hartmann's solution (Ringer's lactate) have a composition similar to ECF (Na^+ 150 mmol/l) and so this is where the fluid distributes to.
- 5% dextrose acts as pure water and distributes throughout the total body water. The glucose content goes into cells and is burnt or stored as glycogen.
- 'Dextrose/saline' – some of the water stays in the ECF because of its sodium content whilst the rest follows total body water.

Blood products

This is the best fluid to use if it is in deficit. If there is significant active blood loss it should be replaced by whole blood or packed red cells and any coagulopathy or thrombocytopenia should be corrected with the appropriate agent.

Complicating factors with transfusion include:

- Infection
  - Viral (eg HIV)
  - Bacterial (*Staphylococcus*, etc at time of donation)
  - Parasitic (eg malaria)
  - Risk is reduced by donor screening and laboratory testing of blood
- Immunological reactions
  - ABO incompatibility: abdominal pain, vomiting, substernal pain and hypotension, haemorrhage, multiorgan failure and death
  - Strict protocols to ensure the correct patient receives the correct blood are important
  - Rhesus or other red cell antibody incompatibility can also occur
- Pyrexia – milder reactions with a variety of foreign antigenic material. Often white cells and plasma antigens
- Jehovah's witnesses
  - Fundamentalist Christian sect with religious beliefs where autologous blood transfusion is unacceptable
  - Often willing to accept death as a consequence
  - Anaesthetist must be made aware and a clear discussion about what can and cannot be accepted by the patient must be had
  - Autotransfusion in a continuous circuit with the patient may be accepted

3.1.4 Pre-existing medical conditions

There are myriad medical conditions from which a patient may suffer when undergoing surgery. As a basic rule it is important to optimise the condition before surgery.

This is particularly important in **cardiovascular** disease. The anaesthetist in particular must be aware of hypertension, cardiac failure, valvular, ischaemic or dysrhythmic abnormalities. An ECG is imperative and an echocardiogram helpful.

Similarly, **respiratory** patients must be considered by their severity (previous history, current treatments, patient's own opinion). It may be necessary to arrange arterial blood gases and/or lung function tests. Smoking cessation, as little as 12 hours before surgery, has been shown to improve cardiorespiratory function peri-operatively. It should always be encouraged.

Diabetic disease makes patients more prone to infection and can delay healing. Non-insulin-dependent diabetics simply need to stop their hypoglycaemics prior to elective surgery and be operated first on the list; 5% glucose can be used if hypoglycaemia occurs. In major emergency procedures, insulin glucose regimes such as 'sliding scales' will have to be considered. Insulin-dependent patients may omit their insulin for minor routine surgery but again will need an insulin/glucose regime at most other times.

Patients on long-term **steroids** will also need to continue their steroid cover during the peri-operative period and will also need parenteral cover with hydrocortisone injections at times they are 'nil by mouth'. This is essential as patients can go into an Addisonian crisis. Patients who have taken any dose of steroids for less than a 2-week period prior to surgery are not at risk of going into crisis. The steroids can be stopped without a need to taper the dosage as required with long-term administration.

3.2 PRINCIPLES AND PRACTICE OF ANAESTHESIA

3.2.1 Pre-operative anaesthetic assessments

Pre-operative assessments provide the anaesthetist with their first contact with a surgical patient. It enables them to anticipate and reduce any problems that may occur. The important features of this assessment include:

- Determining the state in which the patient will present to theatres, by:
  - Taking a systematic medical history, including any previous problems with the anaesthetic procedure
  - Performing a general examination, including an airway assessment
  - Reviewing investigations, ie blood results, ECG, chest X-ray as appropriate for the surgery

- Discussing the anaesthetic procedure with the patient and minimising anxiety
- Planning the best anaesthetic
- Suggesting any necessary medical interventions to optimise the patient before surgery and prescribing any premedications.

Airway assessments

Airway assessments are important before the anaesthetic is delivered to help predict problems with intubation. There are many indicators based on the anatomy of the head and neck that can be used for this:

- Extent of mouth opening
- State of dentition (overriding upper teeth make intubation more difficult)
- Size of jaw (a smaller jaw makes intubation more difficult)
- Thyromental distance (less than 6 cm makes intubation more difficult)
- Ease of cervical spine movement
- Mallampati classification

The Mallampati classification

This assesses the hypopharynx. The patient is sat upright, told to open the mouth fully and protrude the tongue as far as possible. The examiner then looks into the mouth with a light torch to assess the degree of hypopharynx visible (see Figure 3.1).

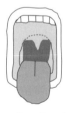 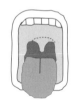

Class I: soft palate uvula, fauces, pillars visible Class II: soft palate uvula, fauces visible

Class III: soft palate base of uvula visible Class IV: hard palate uvula not visible

Figure 3.1: Mallampati classification

ASA score

Anaesthetists use the American Society of Anesthesiologists (ASA) score to indicate the level of peri-operative risk. This is summarised in Box 3.4.

Box 3.4: ASA classification of physical status

Class	Physical state
I	A normal healthy patient
II	A patient with mild systemic disease
III	A patient with severe systemic disease that is not incapacitating
IV	A patient with incapacitating systemic disease that is a constant threat to life
V	A moribund patient who is not expected to survive for 24 hours, with or without the operation
E	Emergency cases are designated by the addition of 'E' to the classification number

---

3.2.2 Types of anaesthesia

Commonly understood to be a state of reversible consciousness.

However, there is more than one type of anaesthesia:

- General anesthesia: achieves complete unconsciousness (narcosis) and analgesia
- Local anaesthesia: topical application, local infiltration or a ring block limits the anaesthetised area
- Regional anaesthestics, major nerve blocks or spinal/ epidural techniques anaesthetise a larger area than a local anaesthetic

The anaesthetist will determine the type of anaesthesia to be used by considering the nature of surgery as well as patient factors. Patient factors include medical status as well as the preferences of the patient.

Local and regional anaesthetics can be combined with general anaesthesia to reduce the overall opiate analgesic and general anaesthesia requirements.

Agents used in local and regional anaesthesia include lidocaine and bupivacaine, which can be combined with adrenaline (epinephrine). Adrenaline causes vasoconstriction, preventing excess spread of the anaesthetising agent and limits its toxicity.

3.2.3 Premedication and induction of anaesthesia

Premedication may be used at the discretion of the anaesthetist. It can:

- Relieve anxiety
- Reduce discomfort
- Cause amnesia

Benzodiazepines such as midazolam are commonly used.

Induction is achieved by administering drugs that cause the patient to become unconscious before surgery. Inducing agents may be:

- Intravenous: requires intravenous access and is the quickest method. Agents include thiopentone, propofol and etomidate
- Inhalational: may be a more suitable method for those who are needle-phobic or for children. Isoflurane or sevoflurane may be used

Induction requires close monitoring of the pulse rate, blood pressure and peripheral oxygen saturations. All agents can cause hypotension, respiratory depression and laryngeal spasm. They may invoke allergies, just like other drugs. The anaesthetist must be aware of these effects prior to, during and after surgery.

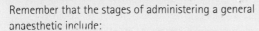

> **Essential note**
>
> Remember that the stages of administering a general anaesthetic include:
> - Premedication
> - Induction
> - Maintenance
> - Reversal

3.2.4 Muscle relaxants

Once anaesthesia has been induced and the anaesthetist is ready to intubate, they will want to paralyse the patient, which:

- Aids endotracheal intubation by relaxing and keeping the vocal cords open
- Prevents involuntary muscle movement during surgery, enabling surgical access and process

Muscle relaxants are classed as competitive or non-competitive:

- **Competitive** (or depolarising): compete with acetylcholine at the neuromuscular junction

- Original example of this group is curare, which was originally used by South Americans as an arrow poison
- Adopted into pancuronium, vecuronium or atracurium
- Choice of drug is determined by its side-effects profile, duration of action and elimination route
- **Non-competitive** (or non-depolarising)
  - Prolong depolarisation of the muscle membrane so that nerve impulses and acetylcholine release cannot initiate contraction
  - Preceded by an initial period of uncoordinated contractions called fasciculations
  - Paralysis that follows is of rapid onset and lasts for about 5 minutes
  - Suxamethonium is the only example in clinical use

3.2.5 Maintaining anaesthesia

This is with the use of an anaesthetic agent that is **inhaled** or **injected intravenously**. Common inhalational agents used include isoflurane and sevoflurane. Propofol is often used as an intravenous agent to maintain anaesthesia.

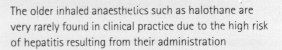

> **Essential note**
>
> The older inhaled anaesthetics such as halothane are very rarely found in clinical practice due to the high risk of hepatitis resulting from their administration

3.2.6 Reversing anaesthesia and extubation

Anaesthetists will try to time administration of their agents to coincide with the end of surgery.

- Inhaled agents are very volatile and will be exhaled with respiration very quickly.
- Intravenous agents are chosen for their short half-lives

As the anaesthetic drug is wearing off, the paralysis must be reversed. This will prevent an inability to self-ventilate in the period of awakening, which would otherwise be extremely distressing. Reversal is achieved by using **anticholinesterases**. These inhibit the breakdown of acetylcholine which can then compete at the neuromuscular junction. **Neostigmine** is often used. To prevent the effect of an excess of acetylcholine at parasympathetic effector organs (eg the vagus nerve causing bradycardia) an antimuscarinic such as **atropine** is used.

Extubation: When complete reversal is achieved and the patient is awake, alert and self-ventilating, the endotracheal tube may be removed safely.

3.2.7 Post-operative monitoring

The patient notes should include a daily review of the following parameters post-operatively, as indicated by the nature of the operation:

- Vital signs
- Antibiotics (course length, suitability)
- Analgesia
- Routine medication
- Mobility status
- Drain output
- Nasogastric tube and urinary catheter output
- Fluid balance status/IV fluid prescription
- Dietary build-up
- Bowel status (not open, flatus only, or stools passed)
- Blood tests
- Breathing progress/CXR as needed
- Wound review/sutures out
- Need for rehabilitation requirements (eg physiotherapy)
- Discharge planning
- Need for additional assistance (eg occupational therapy, home help, district nurse)

3.3 COMMON MEDICAL PROBLEMS IN THE POST-OPERATIVE PERIOD

There are numerous medical problems that can occur in surgical patients. The commonest problems encountered as a junior doctor are discussed here. These represent about 90% of all the conditions you will initially be called to deal with. Use this section to guide your thought process in utilising a logical approach to dealing with post-operative patients.

3.3.1 Pyrexia

The timing of a fever in a post-operative patient may provide useful clues about its cause.

Immediately post-operatively, consider pyrexia to be because of:

- Surgery itself. Mild (<38°C) self-limiting fever in 30% of patients who have had major surgery. Usually present 2 days post-operatively. Due to a systemic response to heat losses in theatre and impaired temperature regulation during anaesthesia.
- Blood transfusion reaction. Occurs in 2% of patients receiving blood transfusion. Often due to an immune reaction to white cells or plasma allergens.
- Malignant hyperthermia. Occurs during anaesthesia or <6 hours after. Due to very rare inherited disorder of striated muscle causing sudden hypercatabolism when anaesthetic is given. Significant pyrexia (>39°C) with

tachycardia, tachypnoea, hypoxia, acidosis and hyperkalaemia.

If more than 2 days have passed since surgery, consider:

- Bacteraemia and sepsis. Common. The spectrum reflects the impact of pathogens on the host's defence system and mortality worsens with severity:
  - Bacteraemia: positive blood cultures
  - Sepsis: evidence of infection with a systemic response such as pyrexia or tachycardia
  - Sepsis syndrome: systemic response to infection with evidence of organ dysfunction, eg confusion, hypoxia, oliguria, metabolic acidosis
  - Septic shock: septic syndrome with hypotension that does not respond to volume replacement.
  - Presentation may depend on the source of bacteraemia, and common sites of infection are shown in Table 3.1.
- Venous thromboembolism. Particular risk factors are orthopaedic and gynaecological surgery. Pyrexia may be the only presentation.

Management of pyrexia will involve an appreciation of the cause:

- Stop blood transfusions associated with persistent pyrexias and treat with simple antipyretics such as paracetamol.
- Malignant hyperpyrexia will need specialist ITU involvement and dantrolene.
- Sepsis requires cultures, including samples of blood for microscopy, culture and sensitivity when febrile. CXR if the chest is suspected. Inflammatory markers such as C-reactive protein (CRP) and white cell count (WCC) may be helpful, though these may be raised in the post-operative period. Dipstick and culture the urine and wound if necessary.
- Take cultures before starting any antibiotics and involve the microbiologists when deciding which to use.
- Thromboembolism must be formally diagnosed and adequately treated as discussed elsewhere.

Essential note

When working as a junior doctor, you will often be asked to perform a septic screen in a patient. This involves a focused clinical assessment with history taking and examination directed at finding the source of the sepsis (chest, urine, wound, cannulae, catheters) as well as ordering specific investigations (eg CXR, urine dip and microculture and sensitivity (MC+S), wound swab, CVP/cannula removal and culture, blood culture, arterial blood gas, stool culture)

Table 3.1: Source of bacteraemia and common sites of infection

Likely source	Likely organism	Culture with most yield
Urinary tract, post-urosurgery	Gram-negatives	Midstream urine (MSU) or sterile catheter sample
Chest	Gram-negatives (incl. *Escherichia coli*, *Haemophilus influenzae*, *Pseudomonas*)	Sputum Tracheostomy site swab if present
Wound	*Staphylococcus*, Gram-negatives, anaerobes	Wound swab Pus
CVP line/venflon site/TPN feeding line	*Staphylococcus*, esp. coagulase-negative; fungi, esp. if on TPN	Wound swab if exit site purulent Consider removal of line and send line tip
Biliary tree sepsis (eg post-ERCP or post-cholecystectomy)	*Pseudomonas*, enterococcus	Bile from drainage bag
Faecal peritonitis	Enterobacteria, anaerobes	Blood cultures Wound swab or pus
Neurosurgical shunt	V-P shunt: Gram-positives V-A shunt: Gram-negatives	CSF from 'button' tap (not LP)
Post insertion of prosthesis	*Staphylococcus aureus* and coagulase-negative *Staphylococcus*	Blood cultures Wound swab
Diarrhoea after antibiotic treatment	*Clostridium difficile*	Stool for *C. difficile* toxin

CSF = cerebrospinal fluid; CVP = central venous pressure; ERCP = endoscopic retrograde cholangiopancreatography; LP = lumbar puncture; TPN = total parenteral nutrition.

3.3.2 Post-operative pain

Inadequate pain relief in the post-operative period can lead to:

- Poor oxygenation due to atelectasis
- Pain on coughing resulting in sputum retention and pneumonia
- Increased sympathetic activity, myocardial work and oxygen consumption
- Altered blood flow to brain, kidney and uterus
- Gastric stasis
- Increased platelet aggregation, decreased venous blood flow and skeletal muscle spasm with splinting and higher risk of deep vein thrombosis and pulmonary embolism
- Psychological effects with anxiety and poor sleep

Assessment of pain includes considering:

- Location
  - Wound pain is worse on movement and in the first 72 hours. If not settling, consider a wound infection.
  - Chest pain may be sharp and worse on respiratory effort, ie **pleuritic**, and this could be the result of pleural infection or infarction following an embolus. Retrosternal pain with or without radiation may be **cardiac** in nature and may represent ischaemia or infarction.
  - Abdominal pain can be the result of:
    - Urinary retention
    - Constipation
    - Leakage of surgical anastomosis
    - Sepsis
    - New abdominal pathology, eg ischaemia
  - Legs: Consider a deep venous thrombosis or sciatica.
- Severity is best assessed by measuring it on a pain score or scale. This enables titration of analgesia to individual needs.
- Existing analgesia. The anaesthetist may have provided:
  - **Patient–controlled analgesia (PCA).** This is a programmable syringe driver with a hand-held trigger switch for intravenous analgesic supply. The patient has usually been loaded with analgesic and is then able trigger the PCA and give themselves more when necessary. The type and concentration of analgesia (usually morphine or fentanyl) are predetermined, as are the bolus doses the patient is able to self administer, the lockout interval and maximum dose. A continuous background infusion may also be set up.

- **Epidural analgesia.** This is most frequently used in thoracotomy or major laparotomy incisions, major limb surgery, in patients with high cardiorespiratory risks and in cancer pain and terminal care. Local anaesthetics and/or opioids are used to block nerve roots and opioid receptors. An epidural syringe can be maintained post-operatively to provide more analgesia if required.

Analgesia can be obtained through various routes, including oral, intramuscular, intravenous or rectal routes. It can be given regularly or as required. Drugs used for analgesia use the 'analgesic ladder', which is a simple guide to administering analgesics. It simply starts at the bottom of the ladder with paracetamol and works up in a stepwise format, with stronger analgesics being used alone or in combination with each other to tackle stronger pains. The top end of the ladder uses opioids in combination with other analgesics. The ladder also makes use of the same drugs with varying frequencies of administration (eg regular morphine is higher up on the ladder than prn morphine). Most hospitals have an acute pain service that can be contacted to assist the patient with regards to analgesia management. In the post-operative period, it is likely that doctors will make use of the analgesic ladder from the top downwards as the pain present from the immediate post-operative period will likely diminish as the days progress. The reason for employing an analgesic ladder is to allow for sufficient analgesia to be given whilst minimising the side-effects profile from more potent analgesics. Why give morphine to a patient who is tolerating the pain with paracetamol and codeine adequately?

Drugs used for analgesia include:

- Opioids such as morphine, diamorphine and fentanyl
  - Most potent and useful in severe pain
  - Common side-effects include nausea and vomiting, delayed gastric emptying and constipation, histamine release with bronchospasm in asthmatics and respiratory depression. Respiratory depression can be reversed by naloxone
  - Can accumulate in renal failure
- Non-steroidal anti-inflammatory drugs (NSAIDs)
  - Good for moderate pain and bony pain
  - Examples are ibuprofen and diclofenac
  - Side-effects include gastric irritation and they are contraindicated when there is a history of gastric or duodenal ulcers. Additionally, there is reduced renal blood flow, retention of sodium and water and chronic renal damage in long-term use. Platelet inhibition can occur and there may be bronchospasm, particularly in the asthmatic
- Paracetamol
  - Useful in mild pain or as adjuncts

- Very high doses can be hepatotoxic
- May be combined with a weak opioid such as codeine or dihydrocodeine, making co-dydramol or co-codamol

3.3.3 Breathlessness

Breathlessness or dyspnoea is commonly caused by hypoxaemia. The cause of hypoxaemia needs to be diagnosed carefully for best treatment and this will involve a history, examination and investigations such as chest radiography and arterial blood gases.

Onset of breathlessness can give clues as to the cause (see Table 3.2).

Table 3.2: Causes of breathlessness	
Time to onset	*Possible causes*
Sudden	Pulmonary oedema
	Pneumothorax
	Pulmonary embolism
	Anaphylaxis
	Aspiration
Hours	Lung collapse and atelectasis
	Fluid overload from left ventricular failure or excess fluids
	Asthma
	Pulmonary contusion
	Acute respiratory distress syndrome (ARDS)
Days	Pleural effusion
	Lung collapse
	Consolidation
	Pneumonia
Non–respiratory	Metabolic acidosis
	Pain
	Anxiety

Basic management should include:

- Ensuring the airway is patent. Remove any obstruction
- Administering high-flow oxygen via a face mask. Remember that hypoxia will kill before hypercapnia
- Ensuring adequate breathing by considering the tidal volume and breath sounds on auscultation. A self-inflating bag can assist respiration
- Checking the pulse and blood pressure for circulation
- Connecting pulse oximetry and possibly arranging blood gases
- Ensuring intravenous access

Remember to arrange an ECG if there is cardiovascular compromise. Chest radiography may be necessary on the basis of your assessment. Determine a plan of action, which may involve calling for help from the anaesthetist, intensivist or on-call physician.

3.3.4 Oliguria/anuria

A urine output of less than 30 ml/hour or 0.5 ml/kg for 3 hours consecutively should alert the clinician to underlying problems.

Ensure there is a patent urethral catheter in situ. This may involve flushing the catheter to make sure it is not blocked. If there is no catheter, a bladder scan should be performed to exclude urinary retention. Patients in urinary retention require urgent catheterisation.

Assess the patient clinically for their fluid status. Hypovolaemia or cardiac failure can lead to a low urine output. Sepsis can cause oliguria. Urgent electrolytes, urea, creatinine and haemoglobin are important for further diagnosis of the underlying cause and subsequent management.

Unless the patient is in frank cardiac failure, a rapid fluid challenge of 500 ml of fluid over 15 minutes should be administered initially. This may improve urine output but may not if the patient is persistently fluid-depleted or has developed a primary renal pathology, eg acute tubular necrosis.

Radiography may be necessary to exclude post-renal problems, for example ureteric damage following pelvic surgery.

Do not use diuretics until there is confidence that hypovolaemia has been corrected. Stop all nephrotoxic drugs such as NSAIDs and angiotensin-converting enzyme (ACE) inhibitors.

It may become necessary to involve the intensive care or renal team, who can then consider inotropic support and high-dose diuretics. Haemofiltration may become necessary, particularly if there is:

- Hyperkalaemia >6.5 mmol/l
- Pulmonary oedema
- Acidosis with pH <7.2
- Rapidly rising urea >30 mmol/l

3.3.5 Cardiac problems

Dysrhythmia requires the ABC response, ie Airway, Breathing, Circulation assessment, as in any urgent assessment. A 12-lead ECG needs to be compared with the pre-operative trace. A rhythm strip will help to determine:

- The presence of a sinus rhythm

- Bradycardia, due to drugs such as β-blockers or right coronary artery infarct. Treat with atropine if haemodynamically compromised
- Tachycardia, that may be:
  - Narrow- or broad-complex (QRS complex >0.12 s or three small squares)
  - Regular or irregular
- Ectopic beats, which may be atrial (usually not necessary to treat unless there is an electrolyte imbalance) or ventricular
  - Ventricular ectopics must be considered seriously if they are frequent (>5/minute), multifocal or occur in runs of two or more
  - Ventricular ectopics are also important if they occur at or just before the T wave (R-on-T phenomenon) and here can precipitate ventricular fibrillation

Atrial fibrillation is common, showing an irregular narrow-complex tachycardia where there are no P waves. Consider if this is long-standing and if there is some medication that may have been missed in the peri-operative period.

A common approach when there is no haemodynamic compromise:

- Treat pain, hypovolaemia and hypoxia
- Check electrolytes including magnesium and treat as necessary
- Slow the rate of atrial fibrillation with digoxin if the above do not help
- Treat a supraventricular tachycardia with vagal manoeuvres and/or adenosine. Seek further help
- Ventricular tachycardia is a medical emergency and requires specialist help
- Ventricular fibrillation occurs in the context of a cardiac arrest and emergency help is required with a crash team alert

Hypotension becomes a cause for concern if the systolic blood pressure is <90 mmHg and compounded by evidence of end-organ dysfunction (such as oliguria or confusion).

There are many causes, which can occur in combination:

- Hypovolaemic shock occurs when there is not enough fluid in the circulation to maintain a satisfactory cardiac output. There may be actual fluid loss, such as in bleeding, GI losses or relative hypovolaemia in a vasodilated state.
- Cardiogenic shock occurs when there is pump failure, often due to pre-existent inefficiency, ischaemia, dysrhythmia or mechanical disorders. Lung pathology, such as a pulmonary embolism or tension pneumothorax, can also cause pump failure.

Peri-operative care and anaesthetics

- Vasodilatation such as in septic shock or due to arteriovenous fistula dilatation. Vasodilatation can also occur in anaphylactic shock, adrenal shock, high spinal or epidural anaesthesia (autonomic blockade) and spinal shock.
- Drug actions. A plethora of drugs can cause hypotension.
- Metabolic disorders such as those with bone profile disorders or acidosis.

Do not forget the vasovagal response and measurement error (for example, using the correct cuff).

Urgent assessment is important with the ABC approach, history and examination. Investigations must include an assessment of fluid status with catheterisation if necessary. FBC, U&Es, cross-match, ECG and/or chest radiograph. Arterial blood gases are important to look for hypoxia and the acid–base balance. Serum cortisol may be necessary to look for adrenal insufficiency.

A clear plan of action is necessary. Unless there is a clear cardiac source, rapid intravenous fluid replacement is required. Look for an improvement with blood pressure or urine output. Frequent reviews are necessary and involve specialist help if the first-line measures do not work.

Hypertension can be a frequent problem. Causes include:

- Pain
- Anxiety
- Drugs such as inotropes, salbutamol, aminophylline
- Hypoxia or hypercapnia (in the early stages due to agitation and vasomotor stimulation)
- Full bladder
- Raised intracranial pressure via the Cushing reflex
- Malignant hyperthermia
- Hormonal, eg phaeochromocytoma, thyroid crisis
- Essential hypertension

An ECG should be performed to look for ischaemia and left ventricular hypertrophy and basic biochemistry to assess renal function.

Repeat the blood pressure with the correctly sized cuff. Then consider and treat the underlying cause. Check that any prescribed antihypertensives have been given. Oral antihypertensives can often be prescribed in most circumstances that are not easily reversible, such as pain. In severe, unresolving hypertension, intensive care support may be required.

Abdominal surgery

CONTENTS

Abdominal surgery represents the bulk of a general surgeon's emergency and elective workload. In the present day, with surgeons specialising within general surgery, it is unusual to find a single general surgeon operating outside their area of expertise within the abdomen. The areas of specialisation and subspecialisation within the abdomen include:

- Upper GI surgery
  - Oesophagogastric surgery
  - Bariatric surgery
  - Benign upper GI/laparoscopic surgery
- Hepatopancreaticobiliary surgery
- Colorectal surgery
  - Inflammatory bowel surgery
  - Pelvic floor disorders/pelvic surgery
  - Cancer surgery
  - Laparoscopic colorectal surgery

Common conditions such as hernias may be covered by any general surgeon as well as acute general surgical conditions such as bowel obstruction, perforation, ischaemia, inflammation and infection.

Abdominal surgery is also very commonly examined in finals and this chapter reflects on those common topics. If it was to be suggested that you skim through any single chapter (out of desperation!) on the night before exams, it would be this one. The revision objectives have been kept short and simple in principle, but should be regarded as extensive in practice and preparation for exams. Good luck!

4.1 INTRODUCTION

Surgery can be an easy topic to learn and requires a logical approach. Whilst a small number of individuals are capable of memorising textbooks, allowing them to achieve high marks in their exams, the vast majority find this very difficult and tend to struggle.

The secret to studying surgery is the ability to pick up key clinical features from the history/examination that will differentiate one condition from another, eg abdominal pain radiating to the back can either be aortic dissection or pancreatitis but from the history, a 35-year-old alcoholic, it should be very easy to know which of the two the question is trying to ascertain.

This is why most doctors and medical textbooks will say '80% of the diagnosis is in the history.' It is the history that will

Revision objectives

- Know the differential diagnosis of common symptoms representing abdominal disease. This includes but is not limited to: dysphagia, reflux symptoms, abdominal pain, vomiting, change in bowel habit, haematemesis, bleeding PR, jaundice, abdominal distension, lump in the groin, anal pain and discharge, and abdominal mass
- Know the common causes, differential diagnosis, clinical features and basic management of acute abdominal conditions. The commonest conditions include, but are not limited to: appendicitis, diverticulitis, cholecystitis, biliary colic, pancreatitis, colitis, gastroenteritis, gastritis and peptic ulcer disease, bowel obstruction, bowel ischaemia, perforated viscus, GI haemorrhage, strangulated hernia, ruptured abdominal aortic aneurysm, ruptured spleen, ectopic pregnancy, renal colic, pyelonephritis, and pelvic inflammatory disease
- Know the epidemiology, common causes, differential diagnosis, clinical features, and management of elective abdominal conditions as defined by region: upper GI, hepatobiliary, colorectal, hernia surgery
- Know how to perform the following examinations for OSCEs or clinical examinations:
  - Inguinoscrotal examination for lumps in the groin
  - Abdominal examination
  - Rectal examination

enable you to extract a patient's symptoms, and in conjunction with examination you will be able to establish an accurate differential diagnosis.

Memorising long lists of investigations is pointless as you will notice that investigations are requested to exclude or confirm a diagnosis. Investigations can be requested from your differential diagnosis which stems from the clinical assessment.

This chapter covers abdominal surgery, which makes up the majority of any general surgeon's workload. The main sections covered in this chapter include acute abdomen, abdominal wall and hernias, oesophagogastric surgery, hepato-pancreaticobiliary surgery and colorectal surgery.

The first section of acute abdomen aims to introduce the topic of peritonitis. The subsequent sections of this initial chapter deal with other non-surgical conditions that may present with an acute abdomen. The remainder of the common acute

Abdominal surgery

abdominal conditions are covered under the specialty sections depending on the organ involved. Abdominal wall surgery and hernias tend to be dealt with by all general surgeons regardless of specialty. When revising any topics in surgery or writing essays, it is helpful to outline the clinical conditions into:

- Anatomy
- Aetiology
- Epidemiology
- Pathophysiology
- Clinical features
- Differential diagnosis
- Investigations
- Management
- Complications
- Follow-up
- Prognosis

4.1.1 Definition

By defining a condition you will be able to appreciate the disease mechanism just from the name, for example anything ending with 'itis' = inflammation.

From the ending -itis you can conclude the following:

- Four cardinal features of inflammation will almost certainly be present (rubor – erythema, calor – temperature, dolor – pain, tumor – swelling).
- Inflammation causes cells to become 'leaky', leaking intracellular products such as in pancreatitis where there is a leak of amylase (an enzyme produced by pancreas) resulting in raised amylase, or in hepatitis where there is a leak of aspartate aminotransferase (AST)/alanine aminotransferase (ALT) (enzymes produced by hepatocytes) resulting in raised AST/ALT. This results in an inflammatory response leading to elevated inflammatory markers (WCC and CRP).

4.1.2 Anatomy

By thinking of the anatomy in simple logical terms of the area involved you should be able to ascertain the cause(s) of the condition you are asked about. For example, when asked give

five causes of large-bowel obstruction, understanding that bowel is a tube it becomes clear that the obstruction can be mechanical (physical block of the tube) or functional (loss of peristalsis, ie ileus).

Mechanical causes of bowel obstruction can then be divided anatomically into extraluminal (eg hernia, compressing masses), luminal (eg tumours), or intraluminal (eg gallstone ileus) causes, whilst functional bowel obstruction results from reduced parasympathetic supply to the bowel such as anticholinergic drugs, general anaesthesia, etc.

4.1.3 Aetiology

This can be approached by utilising the 'surgical sieve' and then applying that to an organ within a medical or surgical setting.

Surgical sieve

- Organic
  - Hereditary
    - Congenital
    - Familial
    - Genetic
- Acquired
  - Infection
    - Acute or chronic
    - Type (bacterial, viral, fungal, or parasitic)
  - Inflammation
  - Iatrogenic: medically, radiologically or surgically
  - Autoimmune
  - Metabolic
  - Endocrine
  - Degenerative
  - Vascular
  - Neoplastic: benign or malignant
- Idiopathic
- Psychogenic (functional)

Organ source: the acute abdomen (pain that is often serious or life-threatening) can be classified as a medical or surgical abdomen depending on the pathology arising from the organ involved (Table 4.1).

Table 4.1	
Causes of acute abdominal pain	*Non-surgical causes of acute abdominal pain*
Inflammation and infection	**Intra–abdominal**
Appendicitis	Diseases of the liver
Cholecystitis	Tumours
Diverticulitis	Abscesses
Pancreatitis	Primary peritonitis
Salpingitis	Bacteria/TB
Mesenteric adenitis	*Candida*

Table 4.1 *continued*

Causes of acute abdominal pain	Non-surgical causes of acute abdominal pain
Primary peritonitis	Glove lubricants
Crohn's disease	Infections
Ulcerative colitis	Viral gastroenteritis
Pyelonephritis	Food poisoning
Terminal ileitis	Typhoid
Yersinia infection	Mesenteric adenitis
Meckel's diverticulitis	*Yersinia*
Obstruction	Curtis–Fitz-Hugh syndrome (*Chlamydia* causing right upper quadrant pain)
Renal colic	**Neurological**
Biliary colic	Spinal disorders
Small-bowel obstruction	Tabes dorsalis
Congenital (bands, atresia)	**Abdominal wall pain**
Meconium ileus	Rectus sheath haematoma
Malrotation of gut	Neurovascular entrapment
Adhesions	**Retroperitoneal**
Hernia	Pyelonephritis
Intussusception	Acute hydronephrosis
Gallstone	**Infections**
Tumours	Infectious mononucleosis (EBV)
Crohn's disease	Epstein–Barr virus
Large-bowel obstruction	Herpes zoster
Tumour	**Metabolic disorders**
Volvulus	Diabetes
Inflammatory stricture	Addison's disease
Perforation	Uraemia
Gastric ulcer	Porphyria
Duodenal ulcer	Haemochromatosis
Diverticular disease	Hypercalcaemia
Colon cancer	Heavy metal poisoning
Ulcerative colitis	**Immunological**
Lymphoma	Polyarteritis nodosa
Foreign body perforation	Systemic lupus
Perforated cholecystitis	**Haematological**
Perforated appendicitis	Sickle cell
Perforated oesophagus	Haemolytic anaemia
Perforated strangulated bowel	Henoch–Schönlein purpura
Abdominal trauma	Leukaemia
Haemorrhage	Lymphomas
Rupture of aortic aneurysm	Polycythaemia
Mesenteric artery aneurysm	Anticoagulant therapy
Aortic dissection	**Intrathoracic**
Ruptured ovarian cyst	Myocardial infarction
Ruptured ectopic pregnancy	Pericarditis
Ovarian bleed	Pneumothorax, pleurisy
Endometriosis	Coxsackievirus B
Rupture of liver tumour	Strangulation of diaphragmatic hernia
Rectus sheath haematoma	
Abdominal trauma	

Causes of acute abdominal pain	Non-surgical causes of acute abdominal pain
Infarction Torsion of a viscus Ischaemic bowel (arterial thrombosis/embolus) Venous thrombosis Aortic dissection	Aortic dissection Boerhaave syndrome Right heart failure

4.1.4 Epidemiology

Certain conditions are more commonly found in particular types of people. This can be related to gender, age, ethnicity, or population. It becomes easier to arrive at a diagnosis by knowing whether a condition is commoner in females or males, the young or old, or how common it is in the population (common things are common!). For example, if a question begins by stating that a 9-year-old boy presents to A&E with severe lower abdominal pain worse on the right, we can conclude from the age (child) and sex (M) and site of pain (RLQ) that this is very likely to be one of two conditions – acute appendicitis or mesenteric adenitis.

- Incidence/prevalence
- Age
- Sex
- Geography (ethnicity)

4.1.5 Pathophysiology

This is the disease mechanism, which will aid understanding of how conditions present and why we manage them the way we do, eg mechanical bowel obstruction results in venous congestion and third space losses leading to dehydration, hence why IV fluids ('drip') are given.

4.1.6 Clinical features

Symptoms

Most common symptom is abdominal pain to which **SOCRATES** is applied:

- **Site:** knowing anatomically what structures are within that area (Figure 4.1), you will be able to produce a list of differentials. Using key features from the history you will be able to narrow down your differentials and formulate a diagnosis:
  - **Localised** (can patient point to site with one finger?)
  - **Generalised**
- **Onset:** sudden or gradual
  - Classifying the onset of pain can allow conditions to be easily diagnosed

> **Essential note**
>
> Conditions with gradual onset usually are inflammatory in nature. A sudden onset of pain usually implies an obstruction or perforation of a viscus or blood vessel. Examples include aneurysm rupture, ulcer perforation, bowel obstruction, biliary and ureteric colic, acute limb ischaemia, testicular torsion (vessel obstruction due to torsion)

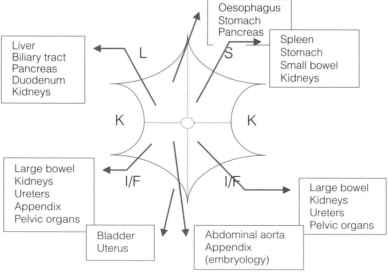

Figure 4.1: Structures in the abdomen

- **Character:** dull/aching/crampy/sharp/stabbing
  - Dull pains are usually visceral, whereas sharp pains are usually peritoneal
- **Radiation**
  - Back, eg pancreatitis, aortic dissection
  - Scapular tip pain, eg cholecystitis
  - Shoulder tip pain, eg acute cholecystitis/biliary pain, splenic rupture, peritonitis, ectopic pregnancy
- **Associations**
  - Nausea and vomiting (colour, blood, volume, frequency, duration)
  - Fevers/chills (hot/cold, shakes, measure temperature)
  - Anorexia and weight loss (intentional, quantity, duration)
  - PR bleeding or discharge (start/during/end of motion, colour, quantity, frequency, duration)
  - Diarrhoea (colour, blood, quantity, frequency, duration, recent travel, recent eat out, dietary habits, normal bowel habits)

- Constipation (normal bowel habits)
- Tenesmus (sensation of incomplete emptying)
- Change in bowel habit (loose stool)
- Difficulty swallowing (dysphagia; food and water; to what level)
- Painful swallowing (odynophagia; food and water; to what level)
- Bloating (frequency, associated with food)
- Acid brash/waterbrash (change in taste/increased saliva respectively)
- Eating and drinking (before or after meals)
- Urinary symptoms (dysuria, frequency, haematuria)
- Gynaecological symptoms including LMP (periods' quality, timing, nature)
- **Timing**
  - Constant or intermittent (waxes and wanes or colicky)
  - Frequency (how often)
  - Duration (how long it lasts each time it comes about)
  - Period (how long this problem has been going on for)

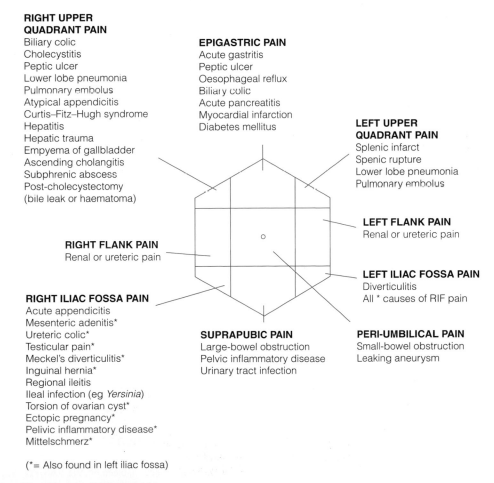

RIGHT UPPER QUADRANT PAIN
Biliary colic
Cholecystitis
Peptic ulcer
Lower lobe pneumonia
Pulmonary embolus
Atypical appendicitis
Curtis–Fitz–Hugh syndrome
Hepatitis
Hepatic trauma
Empyema of gallbladder
Ascending cholangitis
Subphrenic abscess
Post-cholecystectomy
(bile leak or haematoma)

EPIGASTRIC PAIN
Acute gastritis
Peptic ulcer
Oesophageal reflux
Biliary colic
Acute pancreatitis
Myocardial infarction
Diabetes mellitus

LEFT UPPER QUADRANT PAIN
Splenic infarct
Spenic rupture
Lower lobe pneumonia
Pulmonary embolus

LEFT FLANK PAIN
Renal or ureteric pain

RIGHT FLANK PAIN
Renal or ureteric pain

LEFT ILIAC FOSSA PAIN
Diverticulitis
All * causes of RIF pain

RIGHT ILIAC FOSSA PAIN
Acute appendicitis
Mesenteric adenitis*
Ureteric colic*
Testicular pain*
Meckel's diverticulitis*
Inguinal hernia*
Regional ileitis
Ileal infection (eg *Yersinia*)
Torsion of ovarian cyst*
Ectopic pregnancy*
Pelivic inflammatory disease*
Mittelschmerz*

(*= Also found in left iliac fossa)

SUPRAPUBIC PAIN
Large-bowel obstruction
Pelvic inflammatory disease
Urinary tract infection

PERI-UMBILICAL PAIN
Small-bowel obstruction
Leaking aneurysm

Figure 4.2: Sites of acute abdominal pain

- Exacerbating/relieving
  - Exacerbating factors
    - Eating and drinking (E+D), eg alcohol (exacerbates pancreatitis)
    - Movement, eg peritonitis
  - Relieving factors
    - Lying still, eg peritonitis
    - Movement, eg renal colic
    - Leaning forwards, eg acute pancreatitis
    - Bowels opening, eg constipation
    - Medication, eg analgesia, antiemetics
- Severity
  - How severe on a scale of 0–10 (0 = no pain, 10 = worst pain imaginable)

Signs

- **Observations:** temperature, blood pressure (BP), heart rate (HR), respiratory rate (RR), saturation, urine output, fluid chart (input vs output) weight chart
- **General inspection:** well/unwell, dry, jaundice, sweating, alert or drowsy, distress
- Abdomen examination
  - **Inspect:** distension, scars, bruising, symmetry, visible masses or pulsations
  - **Palpate:** tenderness, guarding, rebound (percussion) tenderness, masses, collections, organomegaly
  - **Percuss:** resonant, tympanic, dull, ascites, bladder, liver edge
  - **Auscultate:** hyperactive ('tinkling'), reduced, absent
  - **Digital rectal examination (DRE):** stool, blood, mucus, masses, tenderness
  - **Vaginal examination (VE):** cervical excitation, masses, tenderness
- Peritonism
  - Guarding
  - Rebound tenderness
  - Percussion tenderness
  - Positive cough sign (ask patient to cough: ↑pain ± drawing up of knees)
  - Paralytic ileus (hypoactive/absent bowel sounds and distension)
- Shock
  - ↓Systolic BP <90 mmHg
  - Postural drop (↓SBP or DBP >15 mmHg)
  - ↑HR
  - ↓Capillary refill
  - ↓JVP/CVP
  - ↓Urine output (oliguria/anuria)
  - Cold and clammy, sweating, dry mucous membranes, pre-syncope/syncope

4.1.7 Differential diagnosis

Think of the sites involved (Figure 4.2) and use the key clinical features to aid you in narrowing down your differential and formulating your impressions.

4.1.8 Investigations

- Bloods: FBC, U&E, liver function tests (LFT), amylase, CRP, blood cultures
- Urinalysis:
  - Dipstick
  - MC+S
  - Pregnancy test (βhCG)
- Radiology:
  - Radiography:
    - AXR (erect and supine)
    - CXR (erect) – to assess for free air under the diaphragm
    - Left lateral decubitus (for assessing presence of free intraperitoneal air if erect CXR is equivocal)
  - Ultrasonography (organ-specific, eg appendix scan)
  - CT abdomen
  - MRI
- Other (as appropriate to system involved) eg mesenteric angiogram for GI bleeding

4.1.9 Management

- Conservative
  - Wait and watch
  - NBM + IV fluids + catheterise + fluid measurement + analgesia
- Medical
  - Analgesia, eg paracetamol, tramadol
  - Antiemetic, eg cyclizine
  - Antibiotics, eg cefuroxime + metronidazole
  - Antispasmodic, eg buscopan, mebeverine
  - DVT prophylaxis, eg LMWH (Clexane®) + TEDS
- Surgical
  - Laparoscopy + proceed
  - Endoscopy + proceed
  - Laparotomy + proceed
- Radiological
  - USS-guided drainage
- Endoscopic
  - 'Top and/or tail' oesophagogastroduodenoscopy ([OGD] and colonoscopy)

4.1.10 Complications

- Operative
  - General: infection, bleeding, VTE (DVT/PE), wound dehiscence, incisional hernia

- Specific: depends on condition named, eg mesh infection from a hernia repair
- **Non-operative:** depends on condition named, eg acute appendicitis can lead to perforation if untreated

4.1.11 Follow-up
- Arrangements for discharge
  - Dressing changes by district nurse
  - Antibiotic therapy duration
- Suture removal/wound care
- Referral to other specialists
- Clinic follow-up date

4.1.12 Prognosis
- Mortality
- Morbidity

4.2 THE ACUTE ABDOMEN

4.2.1 Peritonitis

Definition
Periton- – serosal membrane that lines the abdominal cavity and which is reflected over the contained viscera, the greater and lesser omentum, and the transverse mesocolon; **-itis** = inflammation.

Anatomy
The peritoneum contains vascular and lymphatic capillaries, nerve endings and immune-competent cells, particularly lymphocytes and macrophages.

The parietal peritoneum: forms a closed sac.

- **Anterior and lateral:** lines the interior surfaces of the abdominal wall
- **Posterior:** forms the boundary to the retroperitoneum
- **Inferior:** covers the extraperitoneal structures in the pelvis
- **Superior:** covers the undersurface of the diaphragm

The visceral peritoneum: formed by the reflection of the parietal layer of the peritoneum onto the abdominal viscera.

The peritoneal cavity: potential space between the two layers (parietal and visceral peritoneum), containing peritoneal fluid <50 ml (plasma ultrafiltrate).

Aetiology
Peritonitis can be classified as primary (spontaneous), secondary (related to a pathological process in a visceral organ) or tertiary (persistent or recurrent infection despite adequate therapy).

- **Primary**
  - **Spontaneous bacterial peritonitis (SBP):** occurs extensively in patients with ascites from chronic liver disease but can also occur in nephrotic syndrome (both are hypoalbuminaemic states) and is thought to result from translocation of bacteria (commonly Gram-negative organisms) across the gut wall
- **Secondary**
  - **Localised (transmural)**
    - Bowel inflammation
      - Inflammatory bowel desease (IBD; ulcerative colitis and Crohn's disease)
    - Visceral inflammation
      - Appendicitis
      - Diverticulitis
      - Pancreatitis
      - Cholecystitis
      - Gynaecological conditions (salpingitis, tubo-ovarian cyst, PID)
    - Bowel ischaemia
      - Incarcerated hernia
      - Mesenteric ischaemia
      - Volvulus
    - Trauma
      - Intraperitoneal bleeding
      - Rupture of a viscus
  - **Generalised (diffuse)**
    - Perforation
    - Pancreatitis
    - Any localised peritonitis
    - Any abdominal surgery

Pathophysiology
Compartmentalisation of the peritoneal cavity, in conjunction with the greater omentum, affects the localisation and spread of peritoneal infections. This occurs by confining the area involved and may lead to abscess formation. This process can, however, lead to persistent infection and life-threatening sepsis.

Clinical features
- **Symptoms (SOCRATES)**
  - S – depends on organ unless generalised
  - O – acute or gradual (depends on cause)
  - C – depends on cause but usually sharp
  - R – depends on underlying cause
  - A – nausea, vomiting, anorexia
  - T – progressive
  - E – exacerbated by movement, relieved by lying still
  - S – severe pain

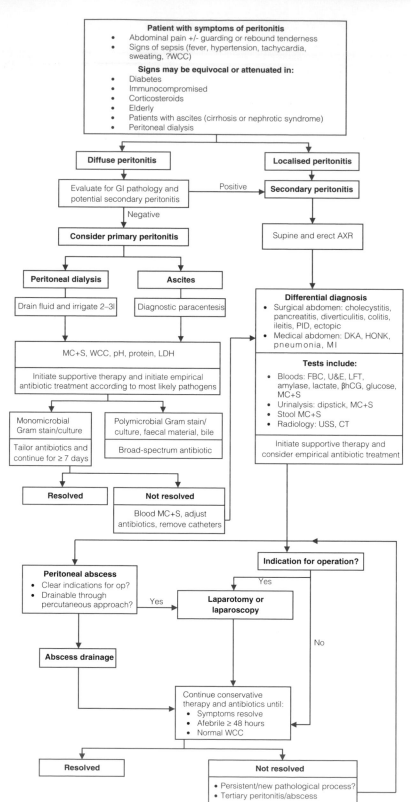

Figure 4.3: Management of peritonitis

- **Signs**
  - **Observations:** ↑T (swinging pyrexia = abscess), ↓BP, ↑ HR, ↑RR
  - **Inspect:** appears toxic, distended, lying still, positive cough test
  - **Palpate:** guarding, generalised tenderness, rebound tenderness
  - **Percuss:** percussion tenderness
  - **Auscultate:** hypoactive-to-absent bowel sounds
  - **DRE:** anterior tenderness and increased abdominal pain

Differential diagnosis

Any acute abdomen unless localised, at which point look at area involved and review.

Investigations

- **Bloods:** FBC, U&E, LFT, CRP, LDH, amylase, cross-match G+S
- **Urinalysis:** dipstick, MC+S, pregnancy test (βhCG)
- **Radiology**
  - **Erect CXR:** perforation
  - **AXR (plain erect and supine):** bowel obstruction, oedema
  - **Transabdominal ultrasound scan (USS):** intra-abdominal collections
  - **CT abdomen:** collection, leak
- **Paracentesis (primary peritonitis; therapeutic and diagnostic):** MC+S, WCC, protein, pH, etc

Management

See Figure. 4.3.

- **Conservative**
  - IV fluids + NBM + observe
- **Medical**
  - **Antibiotics,** eg cefuroxime (aerobic cover) and metronidazole (anaerobic cover)
  - **Analgesic,** eg paracetamol, tramadol, oral morphine (Oramorph®) (prn)
  - **Antiemetic,** eg cyclizine, ondansetron, metoclopramide (unless obstruction)
- **Surgical**
  - **Laparoscopy/laparotomy**
- **Radiological**
  - **USS/CT–guided drainage:** abscess or fluid collection

Complications

- Septicaemia
- Shock and collapse

Prognosis

- Poor if untreated; prognosis worsens with time

4.2.2 Acute pyelonephritis

Definition

Pyelo– = kidney; **nephr–** = nephron; **–itis** = inflammation.

Anatomy

Retroperitoneal organ.

The hilum of the kidney contains:

- Renal artery
- Renal vein
- Lymph nodes
- Ureter (dilates to form the pelvis, which divides into calyces)

Aetiology

- **Classification**
  - **Acute pyelonephritis:** ascending infection into the kidneys
  - **Chronic pyelonephritis:** incompetent ureteric valves leading to reflux of urine back up the ureters (vesico-ureteric reflux)
- **Causes**
  - Gram negative
    - *Escherichia coli* (commonest)
    - *Klebsiella*
    - *Pseudomonas aeruginosa*
    - *Enterobacter*
  - Gram positive
    - *Staphylococcus aureus*
    - Coagulase-negative staphylococci (*S. saprophyticus*)
    - Group B streptococci
    - *Enterococcus faecalis*
- **Risk factors**
  - **Female:** short urethra
  - **Pregnancy:** elevated progesterone causes decreased ureteral peristalsis and increases bladder capacity
  - **Urinary tract obstruction:** urinary stasis impeding urinary flow, leading to ascending infection into the kidney
    - **Mechanical**
      - Extraluminal, eg abdominal/pelvic masses, retroperitoneal fibrosis, constipation
      - Luminal, eg tumours (renal/ureteric/bladder/urethral), stricture
      - Intraluminal, eg renal tract stone, sloughed renal papilla, blood clot
    - **Functional**
      - Iatrogenic, eg anticholinergics, antidepressants
      - Neurogenic, eg diabetes mellitus (autonomic bladder neuropathy), multiple sclerosis, spinal cord disease

- **Diabetes mellitus:** glucosuria leads to increased bacterial growth
- **Immunosuppression**
- **Intercourse:** local mechanical trauma
- **Spermicidal:** inhibits growth of lactobacilli, which produce hydrogen peroxide (antiseptic)

Epidemiology

Sex: acute pyelonephritis is more often seen in females due to their shorter urethra.

Pathophysiology

The cleansing mechanism of urine flow and bladder emptying prevents urinary stasis and hence bacterial colonisation of the urinary tract.

E. coli [commonest cause of urinary tract infection (UTI)] expresses adhesins that enable it to adhere to urinary tract epithelial cells, thereby resisting the action of urinary flow. As a result, individuals with reduced flow rates are at an increased risk of developing UTI.

Therefore, obstruction is the most important factor in developing UTI as it negates the flushing effect of urine flow. As acute pyelonephritis results from bacterial invasion of the renal parenchyma, individuals with risk factors for UTI are at an increased risk of developing it.

After the acute infection the kidney can respond in one of four ways:

- Suppuration
- Scarring
- Granulomata formation
- Resolution

Clinical features

- Symptoms
  - General
    - ○ Dysuria
    - ○ Urgency
    - ○ Frequency
    - ○ Strangury
    - ○ Lower abdominal pain
    - ○ Macroscopic haematuria
  - Specific
    - ○ **Acute pyelonephritis**
      - □ Site – unilateral loin pain
      - □ Onset – abrupt onset
      - □ Character – dull ache
      - □ Radiation – suprapubic area and iliac fossa
      - □ Associated with fever, rigors, vomiting, sweating, cloudy offensive urine
      - □ Timing – constant
      - □ Relieved by movement
    - ○ Cystitis
      - □ Suprapubic pain and tenderness
    - ○ Prostatitis
      - □ Perineal and low-back pain
      - □ Flu-like symptoms
      - □ Bladder outflow tract obstruction
        - – Hesitancy
        - – Poor stream
        - – Strangury
        - – Sense of incomplete emptying
        - – Terminal dribbling
- Signs
  - **Observations:** ↑T, ↑HR
  - **Inspect:** cloudy, offensive urine
  - **Palpate:** loin tenderness (unilateral over affected kidney – costovertebral angle tenderness), suprapubic tenderness, rebound tenderness, guarding, distended bladder, renal mass
  - **Percuss:** distended bladder
  - **Auscultate:** bowel sounds normal
  - **DRE:** swollen, tender prostate is suggestive of prostatitis

Differential diagnosis

See Figure 4.4.

Investigations

- **Bloods:** FBC, U&E, Cr, CRP, MC+S (septic)
- **Urinalysis**
  - Dipstick (leucocytes, nitrites, proteinuria, haematuria)
  - MSU MC+S (three procedures for collecting MSU sample: clean catch, urethral catheterisation or suprapubic aspiration)
  - Pregnancy test (βhCG)
- **Radiology**
  - USS (transabdominal)
  - AXR (plain)
  - CT abdomen

Management

- **Conservative**
  - ↑Oral fluid intake ± IV fluids
- **Medical**
  - **Antibiotics**, eg cefuroxime + gentamicin, 10–14 days
  - **Analgesic**, eg tramadol, Oramorph® (prn)
  - **Antipyretic**, eg paracetamol, NSAIDs
  - **Antiemetic**, eg cyclizine
- **Surgical**
  - **Elective:** aim is to reverse conditions that predispose the kidney to recurrent infections and renal damage, eg

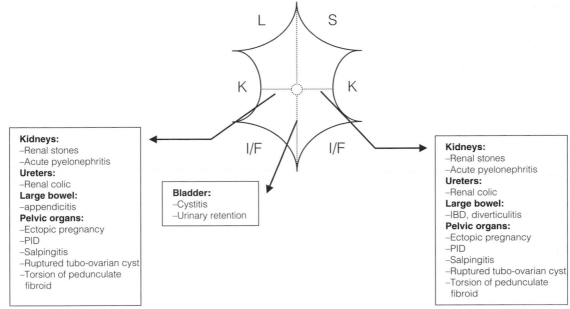

Figure 4.4: Differential diagnoses for acute pyelonephritis

congenital anomalies, fistulas involving the urogenital tract, benign prostatic hyperplasia (BPH), renal calculi, and vesico-ureteric reflux

- Emergency
  - o Incision and drainage: abscess
  - o Nephrectomy: emphysematous pyelonephritis
  - o Nephrostomy or ureteric stent = obstructed ureter with infection

Complications
- Septicaemia
- Hydronephrosis
- Pyonephrosis
- Abscess (cortical/corticomedullary/perinephric): swinging pyrexia
- Acute renal failure
- Chronic renal injury: leading to hypertension and chronic renal failure
- Renal papillary necrosis: mostly occurs in diabetics. CT-guided drainage if not responding to antibiotic therapy
- Emphysematous pyelonephritis: necrotising acute bacterial nephritis leading to air within the kidney parenchyma and perinephric space

Follow-up
Discharge on 14 days of oral antibiotics with follow-up in Outpatients.

- Prophylactic advice
  - Frequent voiding
  - Wipe front to back (females)
  - Post-coital voiding
  - Void before going to bed
  - Cranberry juice (inhibits adherence of *E. coli* to bladder cells)

Prognosis
Prognosis is excellent.

4.2.3 Ectopic pregnancy

Definition
Any pregnancy outside the uterine cavity.

Aetiology
- **Tubal damage:** salpingitis, PID, tubal surgery
- **Previous ectopic pregnancies**
- **Hormonal factors**
  - Endometriosis
  - Progesterone only pill
  - In vitro fertilisation (IVF)
  - Gamete intrafallopian transfer (GIFT)
  - Induction of ovulation
  - Delayed ovulation

Classification
- **Subacute:** typically severe, generalised, constant abdominal pain, vaginal bleeding, amenorrhoea
- **Acute (rupture):** typically shock, collapse, peritonism

Clinical features

Always suspect ectopic pregnancy, miscarriage or viable intra-uterine pregnancy in females of reproductive age presenting with an acute abdomen (abdominal pain), amenorrhoea and vaginal bleeding.

- **Symptoms**
  - Site – lower abdomen
  - Onset – sudden
  - Character – sharp
  - Radiation to shoulder tip (diaphragmatic irritation)
  - Associated with vaginal bleeding (dark red – 'prune juice', or fresh), dysuria
  - Timing – constant
  - Exacerbated by movement and relieved by lying still
- **Signs**
  - **Shock:** ↓BP, postural drop, ↑HR, ↓capillary refill, ↓JVP, cold and clammy, sweating
  - **Peritonism:** guarding, rebound tenderness, positive cough sign
  - **VE:** cervical excitation, adnexal tenderness/mass

Differential diagnosis

Any unilateral acute abdomen.

Investigations

- **Bloods:** FBC, cross-match, serum βhCG
- **Urinalysis:** dipstick, MC+S, pregnancy test (βhCG)
- **Radiology:** transvaginal USS

Management

- **Medical**
  - **Resuscitate and treat shock**
    - IV fluids
      - Colloids, eg Gelofusine® if SBP <90 mmHg
      - Crystalloids, eg normal saline for hydration
    - RBC transfusion
  - **Treat peritonitis**
    - **Antibiotics,** eg cefuroxime (aerobic cover) and metronidazole (anaerobic cover)
    - **Analgesia,** eg paracetamol, tramadol, Oramorph® (prn)
    - **Antiemetics,** eg cyclizine, ondansetron
  - **Rh isoimmunisation prophylaxis**
    - **Anti-D prophylaxis** (Rh D negative)
- **Surgical**
  - **Laparoscopy/laparotomy:** salpingectomy or salpingotomy

Complications

- Haemorrhagic shock
- Further ectopic pregnancy
- Infertility

- Rh sensitisation
- Maternal death
- Fetal death

Prognosis

Prognosis is excellent if ectopic pregnancy is removed without peritonitis and shock progressing. Death can occur if left untreated.

4.2.4 Pelvic inflammatory disease (PID)

Definition

Acute/chronic inflammatory condition affecting the uterus, fallopian tubes and ovaries, secondary to infection.

Aetiology

- **Risk factors**
  - Promiscuity
  - Unprotected intercourse
  - Young age at first intercourse
  - Intrauterine device (IUD)
- **Causes**
  - **Ascending**
    - Sexually transmitted infection
      - *Chlamydia trachomatis*
      - *Neisseria gonorrhoeae*
    - Childbirth
    - Uterine instrumentation, eg termination of pregnancy, IUD
  - **Descending**
    - Appendicitis, eg Gram-negative anaerobes
    - Blood-borne, eg tuberculosis

Clinical features

- **Symptoms**
  - Site – lower abdominal pain
  - Onset – gradual
  - Character – spasmodic
  - Radiation to groin
  - Associated with fever, vaginal discharge, recent menses
  - Timing – 1- to 3-day history
  - Exacerbated by intercourse, movement
- **Signs**
  - **Inspect:** looks unwell
  - **Palpate:** diffuse lower abdominal tenderness, guarding, rebound tenderness
  - **Percuss:** percussion tenderness
  - **Auscultate:** normal bowel sounds
  - **VE:** cervical excitation, adnexal tenderness, purulent cervical discharge

Differential diagnosis

- Any acute unilateral lower abdominal pain

- Appendicitis (especially if pain in RIF)
- Diverticulitis
- UTI
- Gynaecological pathology (endometriosis, ovarian cyst, tumours)

Investigation

- **Bloods:** FBC, U&E, LFT, CRP, serum HCG
- **Urinalysis:** dipstick, MC+S, pregnancy test (βhCG)
- **Swabs:** endocervical, cervical, urethral and high vaginal swabs (HVS) for MC+S
- **Radiology:** USS

Management

- **Conservative**
  - Barrier contraception
  - Education
  - Contact tracing
- **Medical**
  - Antibiotics, eg cefuroxime, metronidazole, ciprofloxacin, doxycycline
  - Analgesia, eg paracetamol, tramadol, oxycodone, Oramorph®
- **Surgical**
  - Laparoscopy
    - Diagnostic laparoscopy
  - Drainage of abscess

Complications

- Subfertility
- Ectopic pregnancy
- Tubo-ovarian abscess (severe pain, high/swinging fever, nausea/vomiting, peritonism, sepsis)
- Chronic PID
- Chronic pelvic pain syndrome
- Fitz-Hugh-Curtis syndrome (perihepatitis with RUQ pain)

Follow-up

- Prevention of ectopic: barrier contraception
- Prevention of PID: combined oral contraceptive pill, barrier contraception

4.3 HERNIA SURGERY

4.3.1 Introduction to hernia surgery

This section deals with conditions affecting the abdominal wall, including hernias. Hernias alone make up a considerable volume of any general surgeon's workload and are very commonly found in the community. They are also one of the only conditions guaranteed to come up on both written and clinical exams at any level from undergraduate to exit exams. The importance of learning this cannot be stressed enough and

the following objectives make up the bare minimum of knowledge required before stepping into any new surgical firm or examination.

- Hernia definition
- Know how to describe a hernia
- Know the general causes of hernias
- Be able to define the differences between the common hernias
- Know the anatomical location of each of the hernias
- Be aware of rarer and eponymous hernias
- Know the anatomy of the inguinal and femoral canals
- Know the clinical presentations of hernias
- Be able to clinically examine a lump or hernia and diagnose it
- Know the management of hernias briefly
- Be able to know and differentiate between the causes of lumps in the groin

Hernia definition and facts

A hernia is a protrusion of any viscus or part of a viscus through its coverings into an abnormal situation.

Examples of hernias include:

- Abdominal wall (external) hernias, such as inguinal, femoral, umbilical, paraumbilical, incisional, ventral and epigastric
- Internal hernias, such as an internal bowel-loop hernia or brainstem herniation through the foramen magnum

Hernias are very common and can occur in men, women and children of all ages. The commonest hernias are inguinal groin hernias.

In the UK alone there are an estimated 70 000 hernia repair operations performed each year and groin hernias are mostly found in males.

Describing hernias

Hernias are best described by using the following characteristics:

- Location (eg inguinal/femoral or other)
- Variety if possible (eg direct or indirect for inguinal hernias)
- Pain (tender or non-tender)
- Reducibility (reducible, or irreducible = incarcerated)
- Strangulated (strangulated or not)
- Obstruction (obstructed or not)

An example of describing a hernia in an exam setting would be: "There appears to be a non-tender incarcerated indirect inguinal hernia which is not strangulated or obstructed."

Structurally, a hernia consists of a neck and a sac containing its contents. The neck is usually passing through the anatomical defect that has led to the hernia in the first place and this often defines the anatomical type of hernia (eg a neck passing through the femoral canal is a femoral hernia). Hernias can also be described by their contents and nearly all eponymous hernias are defined by these (eg, Littre's hernia containing a Meckel's diverticulum).

Causes of hernias

Hernias can occur at sites of weaknesses or defects in their surrounding regions. Weaknesses can be congenital, or can occur at sites where other structures penetrate the surrounding walls, or even areas of weakness caused by surgical incisions. The weakness itself may not be apparent until combined with a precipitating factor that reveals it. The majority of hernias are abdominal wall defects and the remainder of the chapter will concentrate on these rather than on the rarer internal hernias.

Causes of weakness
- Congenital
- Abdominal wall structure penetration
- Incisions
  - Poor closure
  - Poor healing
    - Haematoma
    - Infection
- Weak abdominal wall muscles
  - Damage to nerves following surgery causing weak muscles
  - Cachexia
  - Obesity

Precipitating factors
- Raised intra-abdominal pressure
  - Pregnancy
  - Ascites
  - Chronic cough
  - Constipation
  - Urinary obstruction
  - Heavy lifting

4.3.2 Common hernias and their locations

This section introduces the key features of each of the hernias to help you understand the differences before clinically assessing hernias in general (Box 4.1). Clinical presentations are dealt with later on in this chapter.

The commonest abdominal wall hernias encountered in clinical practice and exams include:

- Inguinal hernia
- Femoral hernia
- Umbilical hernia
- Paraumbilical hernia
- Incisional hernia
- Epigastric hernia
- Sliding hernia
- Parastomal hernia

Inguinal hernia

- This type of hernia is caused by abdominal contents pushing through into the inguinal canal.
- The inguinal canal is defined as an oblique intermuscular slit situated along the medial half of the inguinal ligament through which the spermatic cord passes in males and the round ligament in females.
- There are two types of inguinal hernia, namely direct and indirect:
  - Direct hernias directly pass through an acquired weakness in the posterior wall of the inguinal canal
  - Indirect hernias pass through the deep inguinal ring into the inguinal canal alongside the cord structures and can even pass into the scrotum in men.
- **Direct hernias**
  - Are acquired defects and tend to occur in adulthood
  - Neck lies MEDIAL to the inferior epigastric artery
  - Incidence increases with age
  - 35% of adult male inguinal hernias are direct
  - 5% are both direct and indirect = pantaloon inguinal hernia
  - Commoner in:
    - Males
    - Old age
    - Increased straining and raised intra-abdominal pressure
    - Patients with aortic aneurysms (associated collagen defect)
    - Smokers.
- **Indirect hernias**
  - Thought to be caused by a congenital failure of the closure of the processus vaginalis
  - Neck lies LATERAL to the inferior epigastric artery as it passes through the deep inguinal ring
  - Commonest cause of groin hernia in children
  - Commoner in:
    - The right side
    - Young men
    - African origin
    - Premature or low-birthweight babies
    - Increased intra-abdominal fluid, eg ascites
    - Testicular feminisation syndrome
  - Account for 60% of adult male inguinal hernias
  - 4% of all male infants have an indirect hernia.

Femoral hernia

A femoral hernia occurs when a hernia passes through the femoral ring to enter the femoral canal.

Hernia contents may include extraperitoneal fat, peritoneal sac, or even abdominal contents.

- 35%–50% of all strangulated groin hernias in adults are femoral
- Commoner in:
  - Women (10:1) although the commonest groin hernia in a woman is still the inguinal hernia
  - Parous women
  - Incidence increases with age, especially if the person was fat in middle age
  - The right side

Umbilical and paraumbilical hernia

A true umbilical hernia is a hernia that occurs through the umbilical defect directly. This should be distinguished from a paraumbilical hernia, which occurs through the linea alba directly adjacent to the umbilical defect. The distinction between the two is purely academic as most clinicians call them 'umbilical hernias'.

True umbilical hernias

- Occur as a congenital defect much more commonly in children
- Most close spontaneously by the age of 1 year
- Are commoner in black children
- Adult umbilical hernias are usually secondary to raised intra-abdominal pressure

Paraumbilical hernias

- Occur as an acquired defect
- Occur beside the umbilicus rather than coming through it directly
- Defects in the linea alba often lead to multiple small hernias occurring adjacent to the main presenting paraumbilical hernia

Incisional hernia

Abdominal incision hernias are hernias that occur through acquired scars in the abdominal wall from previous surgery or injury. Any hernia found in the vicinity of a scar, even if not directly under it, should be regarded as incisional until proved otherwise. Conversely, any patient presenting with a hernia should be examined closely for a scar lying near to the lump.

Epigastric hernia

An epigastric hernia is a hernia caused by a defect in the linea alba somewhere between the xiphisternum and umbilicus.

They are more common in men. They may be extremely painful in presentation or present with 'indigestion'.

Sliding hernia

Any hernia in which bowel wall (usually colon) forms the posterior wall of the sac.

- Usually occurs in the elderly
- Occurs as part of an anatomically defined hernia (eg inguinal)
- When on the right side of the abdomen usually contains caecum
- When on the left side of the abdomen usually contains sigmoid colon

Parastomal hernia

Hernia occurring around a stoma site through the weakness in the abdominal wall created by the co-existing stoma. Not uncommon in elderly patients with stomas.

Uncommon hernias

Spigelian – occurs through the linea semilunaris at the lateral border of the rectus sheath.

Richter's hernia – any hernia in which part of the circumference of the bowel becomes trapped in the defect. This is usually the antimesenteric border of bowel.

Littre's hernia – hernia that contains a Meckel's diverticulum in the sac.

Lumbar hernia – hernia occurring through Petit's lumbar triangle or Grynfeltt's space below the 12th rib in the lumbar region.

Maydl's hernia – a hernia with two adjacent loops of bowel in the sac forming a type of 'W' shape.

Obturator hernia – hernia occurring through the obturator foramen

- More common in elderly women
- May be difficult to feel clinically and can present at laparotomy for bowel obstruction
- Clinically it may put pressure on the obturator nerve, causing referred pain down the medial thigh (Howship-Romberg sign).

Amyand's hernia – an inguinal hernia with an acute appendicitis occurring in the sac.

Internal hernias – occur through defects left in the mesentery or adhesions following operations. They can also occur into intra-abdominal fossas (eg paracolic) or through the epiploic foramen of Winslow. They may be asymptomatic or present with bowel obstruction if trapped.

Box 4.1: Anatomical locations of hernias – summary

Inguinal – neck of sac above and medial to the pubic tubercle

Femoral – neck of sac below and lateral to the pubic tubercle

Umbilical – neck through the umbilical defect

Paraumbilical – neck through the linea alba adjacent to the umbilicus

Incisional – neck passing through an abdominal incision or site of injury

Epigastric – neck passing through the linea alba between xiphisternum and umbilicus

Spigelian – neck passing through linea semilunaris at level of posterior rectus sheath edge

Parastomal – neck passing through a weakness formed by the creation of a stoma

Lumbar – neck and sac in the lumbar triangle posteriorly

Obturator – neck passing through obturator foramen

4.3.3 Anatomy of the inguinal and femoral canals

The inguinal canal

The inguinal canal is defined as an oblique intermuscular slit situated along the medial half of the inguinal ligament through which the spermatic cord passes in males and the round ligament in females.

Structures passing into the inguinal canal start from the deep ring and emerge at the superficial ring. The canal structures in the spermatic cord consist of:

Three coverings
- External spermatic fascia
- Cremasteric fascia
- Internal spermatic fascia

Three arteries
- Testicular artery
- Cremasteric artery
- Artery to the vas deferens

Three nerves
- Ilioinguinal nerve (lies superficial to the cremasteric fascia in the canal)

- Genital branch of the genitofemoral nerve
- Sympathetic and visceral nerve afferents

Three others
- Pampiniform plexus (testicular veins)
- Lymphatics
- Vas deferens

Important anatomical landmarks – try to demonstrate them in clinical exams:

- Inguinal ligament – an inward rolled aponeurosis of the external oblique which attaches to the anterior superior iliac spine (ASIS) and the pubic tubercle (PT)
- Superficial ring location – above and medial to the pubic tubercle
- Deep ring location – 2 cm above the **midpoint** of the **inguinal ligament** (halfway between the ASIS and PT). [Note that this differs from the location of the femoral artery which is found at the **midinguinal point** (halfway between ASIS and pubic symphysis) and can easily be confused.]

Further anatomy, such as the boundaries of the inguinal canal and muscle attachments are often forgotten by students and are best learnt through anatomy textbooks, dissections and assisting inguinal hernia operations. Although such anatomical knowledge is important for surgeons treating the hernia, it is not essential to understanding and clinically assessing inguinal hernias.

The femoral canal

The femoral canal is a 1- to 2-cm gap that lies medial to the femoral sheath containing the femoral vein and artery. The entrance to the femoral canal is the **femoral ring** and its boundaries are as follows:

Anteriorly – the inguinal ligament

Posteriorly – the pectineal ligament over the superior pubic ramus

Medially – the lacunar part of the inguinal ligament

Laterally – the femoral vein within the femoral sheath

4.3.4 Clinical presentation and assessment of hernias

Clinical symptoms and signs of hernias

Hernias most commonly present with a **lump** in the patient regardless of their location. Groin lumps are common and can represent inguinal, femoral, or other hernias. They may often have a **cough impulse** if they are not strangulated and may even be **reducible**. Occasionally, hernias present with **pain** after which a clinical examination reveals a lump in the associated area. If this is not picked up on assessment in certain individuals (obesity, etc) then a scan may pick it up as a radiological diagnosis.

Hernias may also present acutely with a **tender mass** which may or may not be reducible. Other presentations include **obstruction** and **strangulation** which usually require urgent surgery if the patient is a suitable candidate for anaesthesia. Occasionally, hernias may cause **local pressure symptoms** such as dysuria in a femoral hernia containing bladder wall.

Assessment of hernias

Hernia assessments are best learnt at the bedside or in the clinical setting with an experienced surgeon. Hernia patients are also found in batches in the day case unit as they are awaiting surgery. Hernia examinations are beyond the scope of this revision book, but a few key points must be mentioned:

- Establish rapport and consent from patient.
- Adequately position and expose.
- Observe from a distance and then closer.
- Ask the patient to show you any lumps that they are aware of (it's allowed!).
- Look for any scars and then ask if you can touch them provided they aren't too tender.
- Feel the hernia, with the patient preferably standing if it is difficult to find, and determine the following:
  - Position
  - Tenderness
  - Reducibility
  - Size
  - Tension
  - Composition.
- Percuss and auscultate the hernia if indicated.
- Define the close-by anatomical landmarks (eg deep ring, inguinal ligament, etc in a patient with an inguinal hernia).
- Examine the opposite side if relevant (mostly for groin hernias).
- Offer to examine the scrotum in men to see the extent of hernias.
- Offer to examine the cardiovascular and respiratory symptoms to assess the patient's fitness for surgery and to reveal any underlying disorder which may have predisposed to the hernia (eg chronic cough from chronic obstructive pulmonary disease).

4.3.5 Management of hernias

Management strategy

Hernia repair should be offered to patients if the hernia is troublesome and causing symptoms. For asymptomatic patients, repair should also be offered if the patient would like one and they are anaesthetically fit to undergo surgery. This is to prevent any future complications such as strangulation or obstruction which may arise from the hernia. Also, hernias may tend to enlarge with time and may become incarcerated, making repair more difficult when necessary. Management of elective abdominal wall hernias uses a general approach regardless of the hernia being treated.

Conservative management

- Wait and watch
- Truss (if unfit for surgery or waiting for surgery and hernia is uncomfortable)

Surgical repair

- Open repair (under local anaesthetic if suitable or general anaesthetic)
  - Mesh repair (for most hernias, especially inguinal and incisional hernias)
  - Simple suturing (eg for small umbilical or femoral hernia where a mesh is not needed)
- Laparoscopic mesh repair
  - Extraperitoneal approach (total extraperitoneal patch or TEPP)
  - Intraperitoneal approach (transabdominal pre-peritoneal or TAPP)

Principles of surgical repair

The principles of surgical repair of abdominal wall hernias are to:

- Isolate the hernia and dissect the sac
- Clear the abdominal wall and free the neck
- Reduce the hernia
  - With or without sac excision
  - Resect strangulated bowel if necessary (in emergency)
- Suture or plicate the abdominal wall defect (in open repair)
- Insert a synthetic, semisynthetic, or biological mesh if indicated and suture/staple this in – tension-free method

Specific complications of hernia repair

- Scar
- Bleeding and haematoma
- Infection – wound or mesh
- Pain
- Recurrence of hernia
- Nerve damage – paraesthesia or anaesthesia
- Damage to cord or other organs (bowel, bladder), especially with laparoscopic approach
- Testicular infarction/atrophy (especially in recurrent inguinal hernia repairs)
- Urinary retention

4.3.6 Lumps in the groin

Groin lumps are common in clinical practice and can be caused by a variety of clinical conditions. They are also very commonly found in clinical examinations. An understanding of the anatomical structures in the groin as well as the pathological processes which can affect the them is essential in clinical assessment.

Although there are many causes of lumps in the groin, the following list represents the commonest causes found, both clinically and in written final exams. The list has been kept simple and has six main categories in which lumps may form.

Hernias (abdominal wall)
- Inguinal
- Femoral

Cord structures
- Hydrocoele of the cord (men)
- Hydrocoele of the canal of Nuck (women)
- Lipoma of the cord
- Ectopic testis
- Rhabdomyosarcoma of the cremasteric muscle

Vessels
- Femoral artery aneurysm
- Saphena varix
- Groin haematoma

Lymph nodes
- Neoplastic (secondary) lymph nodes
- Lymphoma
- Inflammatory lymph nodes

Skin lesions
- Sebaceous cyst
- Lipoma

Retroperitoneal
- Psoas abscess
- Psoas bursa

4.4 OESOPHAGEAL DISEASE

4.4.1 Clinical features

Dysphagia is defined as difficulty in swallowing. This must be distinguished from odynophagia, which is pain on swallowing.

One needs to identify:

- If the patient's symptoms are intermittent or progressive
- Whether dysphagia is for solids, liquids or both
- The timing of regurgitation or coughing following ingestion of solids or liquids, which can also aid diagnosis,

eg with pharyngeal pouch, when the patient may regurgitate minutes to hours following ingestion

Dysphagia can be associated with other systemic disorders, so associated symptoms such as dysarthria, neurological symptoms or vocal symptoms can all be of relevance. Muscle weakness or rheumatological symptoms are also of relevance in the case of myasthenia gravis and systemic sclerosis, which are important causes of dysphagia.

Regurgitation and reflux are terms which are often used interchangeably. **Regurgitation** refers to the expulsion of oesophageal contents above a level of functional or mechanical obstruction. **Reflux** is the inappropriate return of gastric contents.

When trying to list the **causes of dysphagia**, they are most easily classified into (Box 4.2):

- Intraluminal – within the lumen of the oesophagus
- Intramural – within the wall of the oesophagus
- Extramural – outside the wall of the oesophagus

Clinical assessment of a patient with dysphagia:

- History
- Examination
- Blood tests
- Upper GI endoscopy and biopsy/barium swallow
- Oesophageal manometry studies/24-hour pH
- CT scan

Box 4.2: Causes of oesophageal obstruction/dysphagia

Intraluminal
- Foreign body: acute onset, marked retrosternal discomfort, dysphagia even to saliva is characteristic

Intramural
- Carcinoma of the oesophagus: progressive course, associated weight loss and anorexia, low-grade anaemia, possible small haematemesis
- Reflux oesophagitis and stricture: heartburn, progressive course, nocturnal regurgitation
- Achalasia: onset in young adulthood or old age, liquids disproportionately difficult to swallow, frequent regurgitation, recurrent chest infections, long history
- Congenital atresia/tracheo-oesophageal fistula: recurrent chest infections, coughing after drinking. Present in childhood (congenital) or late adulthood

[post trauma, deep X-ray therapy (DXT) or malignant]. Can lead to polyhydramnios in utero
- Chagas' disease (*Trypanosoma cruzi*): South American prevalence, associated with dysrhythmias and colonic dysmotility
- Caustic stricture: examination shows corrosive ingestion, chronic dysphagia, onset may be months after ingestion
- Plummer–Vinson syndrome: oesophageal web associated with iron deficiency anaemia
- Scleroderma: slow onset, associated with skin and hair changes

Extramural
- Pulsion diverticulum: intermittent symptoms, unexpected regurgitation
- External compression: mediastinal lymph nodes, left atrial hypertrophy, bronchial malignancy, thoracic aortic aneurysm, retrosternal goitre, rolling hiatus hernia

4.4.2 Swallowed foreign bodies
- Foreign bodies may end up in the oesophagus due to accidental ingestion or deliberate ingestion, as in psychiatric patients.
- Swallowed objects tend to lodge at one of the three narrowest points within the oesophagus: the cricopharyngeus, the crossing of the left bronchus (extrinsic narrowing), or the diaphragmatic hiatus.
- Although it is advisable to remove foreign bodies (especially sharp objects) through endoscopic means, the general rule is that if the foreign body has passed through the pylorus, it will usually be passed out through the rectum.
- Removal is generally advised to prevent perforation into the mediastinum for sharp objects lodged in the thorax or stomach.
- Smooth items can be left to pass out with stools, provided they are not caustic.
- Monitoring is by serial X-rays.
- A gastrografin swallow may be requested if perforation is suspected.

4.4.3 Plummer–Vinson syndrome
- This condition (also known as Patterson–Brown–Kelly syndrome) is the triad of a pharyngeal web, dysphagia and iron deficiency anaemia.
- Patients are often middle-aged females.
- Other signs which may be present include smooth tongue and koilonychia.

- The syndrome is important as patients are at risk of developing a post-cricoid oesophageal carcinoma.
- Oesophageal dilation may be required to relieve symptoms.
- Endoscopic monitoring is advised for carcinoma surveillance.

4.4.4 Achalasia
This condition is characterised by an inability of the lower oesophageal sphincter to relax appropriately. This is a neuromuscular condition secondary to a loss of ganglionated cells (Auerbach's plexus) in the lower oesophagus. The lower oesophageal sphincter fails to relax and is uncoordinated following a normal peristaltic wave. The oesophagus becomes progressively dilated proximally and hypertrophied. The cause is unknown in most cases but the condition Chagas' disease is extremely similar, and is a result of *Trypanosoma cruzi* infection and commonly occurs in South America.

Clinical features
- The patient describes initial difficulty in finishing a meal and later progresses to dysphagia.
- The dysphagia is progressive and the patient later regurgitates food following a meal.
- Dysphagia may be worse for liquids than solids.
- There may be resultant weight loss. Some features mean that this disease is clinically difficult to distinguish from oesophageal carcinoma.
- If long-standing there may be stasis of food, which may result in mucosal oedema. It is thought that this may be the process by which long-standing achalasia can predispose to malignant change.

Investigation
- Barium swallow is usually helpful in establishing the diagnosis and shows a dilated and tortuous oesophagus with a narrowed segment at the lower oesophageal sphincter. This is also termed a 'bird's beak' appearance.
- Upper gastrointestinal endoscopy is essential for excluding malignancy and may reveal a dilated oesophagus with stasis of oesophageal contents.
- Oesophageal manometry may demonstrate failure of lower oesophageal relaxation during swallowing.

Management
There are no effective medical treatments for achalasia. There are two interventional methods that achieve some resolution of symptoms:

- Endoscopic balloon dilatation is a less invasive procedure and involves forcibly dilating the gastro-oesophageal junction. There is a small risk of oesophageal rupture.

- Longitudinal myotomy of the cardia (or lower oesophageal junction) can be performed via an open or laparoscopic approach. This operation is traditionally known as Heller's cardiomyotomy.

4.4.5 Pharyngeal pouch

A pharyngeal pouch is a diverticulum that protrudes through the inferior pharyngeal constrictor muscles via an area posteriorly known as Killian's dehiscence. It is an example of a false diverticulum as it is a mucosal protrusion and does not have a muscle layer. It usually protrudes to the left side and posteriorly.

Clinical features
- Most patients are middle-aged or elderly.
- Dysphagia and regurgitation of food shortly after eating are the predominant symptoms.
- There may be halitosis due to collection of food within the pouch.
- The patient is at risk of aspiration.
- On examination there may be a swelling on the left side of the neck behind the sternomastoid at the level of the thyroid cartilage.

Investigations
- Barium swallow will identify the pouch.
- Upper GI endoscopy should be avoided as there is a risk of perforation.

Management
- Surgical excision of the pouch is usually undertaken via an open myotomy of cricopharyngeus muscle or endoscopic division of the muscle may be possible (Dohlman's procedure).

4.4.6 Reflux disease

Gastro-oesophageal reflux disease (GORD) is extremely common in the community. GORD results in acid reflux from the stomach back into the oesophagus and patients may present with a variety of symptoms. There is no definite cause found for GORD although a few patients may have a hiatus hernia which can result in reflux. The two conditions discussed within the topic of GORD include reflux oesophagitis and hiatus hernia.

Reflux oesophagitis

This is produced by the reflux of gastric juice causing inflammation of the lower oesophagus and may be secondary to inappropriate relaxation of the lower oesophageal sphincter. Inflammation may progress to ulceration or stricture formation. Barrett's oesophagus (gastric metaplasia of the oesophageal mucosa) may develop as a result, which predisposes to dysplasia and occasionally carcinoma.

GORD is associated with: obesity, smoking, and hiatus hernia (sliding).

Investigations
- Upper GI endoscopy will identify oesophagitis and exclude carcinoma.
- 24-hour ambulatory pH studies – demonstrates acid reflux and can be correlated with patient's symptoms.
- Barium swallow is used occasionally and will identify hiatus hernia.

Medical management
- Weight loss
- Postural modification (avoidance of stooping or lying flat)
- Elevation of the head end of the bed (bricks under the legs of the bed rather than more pillows!)
- Dietary modification (small, frequent meals and avoidance of late meals)
- Alginate antacids
- H_2-receptor antagonists or proton-pump inhibitors
- *Helicobacter pylori* eradication

Surgical management

Anti-reflux surgery/fundoplication involves repair of the lax/stretched diaphragmatic hiatus and wrapping of the fundus of the stomach around the lower oesophagus to act as a valve (Nissen fundoplication).

4.4.7 Hiatus hernia

This is herniation of part of the stomach via the oesophageal hiatus of the diaphragm.

- These can be considered as sliding (approximately 90%) or rolling/paraoesophageal (10%). They are secondary to degeneration and weakening of the musculature of the diaphragmatic hiatus. They are more common in the elderly, females and patients who are overweight.

Sliding hernia

- In this situation the gastro-oesophageal junction passes above the diaphragm, resulting in the reflux of gastric contents.
- This generally presents with symptoms secondary to the intrathoracic mass, such as dyspnoea, hiccoughs, cough.
- There are also symptoms of reflux and regurgitation due to disruption of the lower oesophageal sphincter.
- Severe reflux symptoms may lead to reflux oesophagitis with ulceration or stricture formation and ultimately Barrett's oesophagus (columnar cell metaplasia in the

distal oesophagus which can lead to dysplasia and adenocarcinoma).

Paraoesophageal (rolling) hernia

This hernia tends to produce symptoms relating to a mass in the chest and leads to dysphagia, distension and compressive symptoms. Patients may present with cardiac arrhythmias, respiratory difficulties, or hiccoughs.

- There is usually an absence of reflux symptoms as there is no disruption to the lower oesophageal sphincter.
- Paraoesophageal hernias are prone to complications such as incarceration and gastric volvulus and therefore require surgical treatment.

Investigations

- CXR may reveal a mass or fluid level within the chest
- Barium swallow and meal
- Oesophagogastric duodenoscopy (OGD)
- Oesophageal pH manometry

Management

- For sliding hiatus hernias the mainstay of treatment is medical management of reflux symptoms with proton-pump inhibitors or H_2 antagonists and lifestyle changes.
- Surgical treatment is considered following failure of medical therapy, severe oesophagitis with Barrett's metaplasia, or if a younger patient is reluctant to remain on lifelong proton-pump inhibitors. Surgery is generally indicated in paraoesophageal hernias due to the risk of strangulation.
- Surgery involves reduction of the hernia to the abdominal cavity and repair of the diaphragmatic hiatus followed by fundoplication (Nissen's) and may be performed open or laparoscopically.

4.4.8 Oesophageal perforation

Perforation of the oesophagus may be caused by:

- Swallowed foreign bodies
- Iatrogenic – at endoscopy, especially therapeutic procedures (dilation) or surgery
- Trauma – penetrating wound
- Boerhaave syndrome – spontaneous perforation following a forceful vomit after a large meal

Clinical presentation

- Sharp pain in the chest or epigastrium
- Pyrexia, sepsis
- Shock
- Surgical emphysema (air 'rice krispies' under the skin) in the thorax/neck

- CXR may reveal air in the mediastinum/neck and/or effusion
- Gastrografin swallow will confirm the site and presence of a perforation

Treatment

- Resuscitate patient with IV fluids and ITU/HDU close monitoring
- Treat with broad-spectrum antibiotics
- Nil-by-mouth
- Consider surgical repair for large perforations or for Boerhaave syndrome

4.4.9 Oesophageal tumours

Oesophageal carcinoma is a relatively common tumour, with an incidence of 14 per 100 000 population. It carries a generally poor prognosis. The majority of tumours are squamous carcinoma but there is an increasing number of adenocarcinomas located in the distal oesophagus which may be associated with Barrett's metaplasia. Squamous cell carcinomas are the commonest, occurring in the upper two-thirds of the oesophagus. Adenocarcinomas tend to occur in the lower one-third of the oesophagus, usually arising from Barrett's oesophagus.

Predisposing factors

- Barrett's oesophagus
- Smoking
- Excess alcohol intake
- Achalasia of the cardia
- Male to female ratio 1.8:1

Clinical features

Dysphagia (difficulty in swallowing) is the predominant symptom. The patient may describe a 'sticking' sensation which may occur at a particular level. It tends to be progressive from solids to liquids.

There may be associated regurgitation of solids or liquids, which may result in aspiration. Weight loss may be dramatic and appetite is usually diminished (anorexia).

Examination may reveal cachexia or anaemia. There may be features of metastatic disease such as a palpable liver, pleural effusions, or supraclavicular lymphadenopathy.

Modes of spread

- Local invasion of structures – trachea, lung and pleura, recurrent laryngeal nerve
- Lymphatic – to local lymph nodes (paraoesophageal, supraclavicular, or coeliac)
- Blood-borne – to liver and lung

Investigations

- OGD/upper GI endoscopy is the primary investigation and allows identification and biopsy of the lesion
- Endoscopic ultrasound and laparoscopy to assess for staging of the carcinoma
- Barium swallow may demonstrate an irregular filling defect or stricture
- CXR and USS abdomen – being done less frequently if CT is planned
- CT thorax and abdomen for staging of disease and assessment of metastatic disease

Management

- Curative treatment involves surgical resection, which may be performed via a thoracic, abdominal or thoraco-abdominal approach. The diseased segment is excised and the remaining stomach is usually mobilised into the thoracic cavity, with interposition of the removed oesophagus with small bowel, colon or stomach.
- Chemotherapy (using platinum-based agents) may be given prior to or following surgery and has improved survival rates.
- Palliation may be achieved by radiotherapy, laser debulking of tumours or endoscopic stenting.

Mean survival is very poor and few patients survive 1 year following diagnosis. Even with resection the 5-year survival rate is <25%.

4.5 GASTRIC DISEASE

4.5.1 Peptic ulcer disease

An ulcer is a break in an epithelial surface. Ulcers can occur anywhere within the GI tract, vascular endothelium, or the skin. Peptic ulceration is seen most commonly in the stomach and duodenum but also in the oesophagus, jejunum or at sites of ectopic gastric mucosa (eg Meckel's diverticulum).

Peptic ulceration occurs because of an imbalance between the mucosal defence mechanisms and acid secretion. If defences are broken down or there is an excess of acid, an ulcer can form. Peptic ulcers most commonly occur in the stomach and duodenum. It is easy to appreciate that the stomach is a highly acidic environment naturally and therefore any breakdown in mucosal defences will lead to gastric ulceration. The duodenum on the other hand is neutralised by pancreatic bicarbonate and ulcers will form in situations leading to excess acid production (Zollinger–Ellison, H. pylori).

Aetiological factors

- Cigarette smoking and alcohol
- Non-steroidal anti-inflammatory drugs and steroids
- Zollinger–Ellison syndrome
- Hyperparathyroidism
- Stress
- H. pylori

Helicobacter pylori deserves special mention here as discovery of this organism has been revolutionary in the management of peptic ulceration and gastric carcinoma. It is a Gram-negative, spiral, shaped rod bacterium, which is highly specialised to survive in the gastric environment. It has urease activity and splits urea to produce ammonia and acts to neutralise the acidity of the stomach. This affects the release of gastrin from the G cells in the gastric antrum and results in oversecretion of gastric acid.

H. pylori is associated with chronic gastritis, gastric and duodenal ulceration. There is an association with gastric carcinoma.

H. pylori detection is via three modalities:

- Serology – detection of serum antibodies
- Endoscopic urease test – performed on biopsy samples taken at endoscopy (CLO test = Campylobacter-like organism)
- ^{13}C-urea breath test – urease activity on ingested ^{13}C-urea produces bicarbonate which is exhaled and detected as $^{13}CO_2$

Treatment or eradication of H. pylori involves administration of a proton-pump inhibitor and two antibiotics (often amoxicillin and metronidazole) for a 2-week course. Heli-clear® packs are available to prescribe as part of most hospital formularies.

Clinical features

It is often difficult to differentiate between gastric and duodenal ulceration based on clinical features (Table 4.2).

Epigastric pain is often intermittent and periodic and may be related to food intake or fasting.

- Vomiting and nausea may occur in gastric ulcers (vomiting relieves pain in gastric ulcers).
- Weight loss may occur in gastric ulcers as patients are afraid to eat due to pain.
- There are usually no signs on examination but there may be epigastric tenderness occasionally.

Table 4.2: Clinical features of gastric ulcer vs duodenal ulcer

Gastric ulcer	Duodenal ulcer
• Epigastric pain worsened by eating • Pain relieved by vomiting • Weight loss • Possible epigastric tenderness • Iron deficiency anaemia	• Epigastric pain relieved by food • Worse at night (hunger pains) • Periodic and seasonal (spring/autumn) • Vomiting is uncommon unless pyloric stenosis occurs

Peptic ulceration will generally present to the general surgeon as a result of complications of chronic ulceration or acutely when the ulcer bleeds or perforates.

Complications
- Bleeding
- Perforation – sudden onset, severe generalised abdominal pain with development of peritonitis and board-like rigidity
- Gastric outflow obstruction
- Gastric malignancy/malignant change

Investigations
Mainstay of investigation is upper GI endoscopy or OGD. It can be diagnostic as well as therapeutic. Barium swallow and meal are used infrequently. Ulcers are usually found along the lesser curve in the stomach and on the anterior or posterior surface of the first part of the duodenum (D1). Gastritis is usually found in the antrum and biopsy samples are taken from here for *H. pylori* testing (CLO test).

Management
The approach to the management of peptic ulceration depends on the extent of disease. Preventative measures such as lifestyle changes and *H. pylori* eradication are the mainstay of mild chronic disease.

Antacids, H_2 blockers, or proton-pump inhibitor along with other ulcer-treating medications (sucralfate) remain the initial treatment for peptic ulcers. A repeat endoscopy may be warranted to ensure healing of the ulcer.

Once surgical treatment was a big part of the general surgeon's workload before the era of proton-pump inhibitors. Now gastric surgery is rare for the treatment of peptic ulcers. Operations used to treat ulcers included:

- Truncal vagotomy with pyloroplasty or gastrojejunostomy
- Highly selective vagotomy (more popular)
- Partial gastrectomy (Billroth I and II)

Surgical treatment is now reserved for the management of the complications of peptic ulceration, such as perforation or bleeding and gastric outlet obstruction. These conditions will be considered below.

4.5.2 Gastrointestinal haemorrhage
Bleeding from the gastrointestinal tract may be due to general causes or local sources within the GI tract. General causes are anticoagulants, thrombocytopenia and bleeding diatheses.

Local causes may be considered anatomically:

- Upper GI (Figure 4.5)
- Lower GI
  - Diverticular disease
  - Colonic tumours
  - Angiodysplasia
  - Colitis (ischaemic, infective, inflammatory)
  - Meckel's diverticulum

General presentation of gastrointestinal haemorrhage
The patient may present with haematemesis, which may be fresh red or altered by the gastric environment ('coffee grounds'). Melaena is the passage of altered blood per rectum, which is described as tarry, offensive, black stools and represents blood that has been digested by the GI tract. Bright fresh red blood per rectum may signify a brisk upper GI bleed but may also signify a lower GI source.

As this section deals with disorders of the stomach and duodenum, a special topic concentrating on upper GI bleeding will be dealt with here.

Upper gastrointestinal bleeding

Aetiology
Peptic ulcer disease (commonest): duodenal more common than gastric ulcers.

- Drugs (NSAIDs, aspirin, bisphosphonates, steroids)
- Stress ulcer
  - Head injury leading to ↑ICP (Cushing ulcer)
  - Burns (Curling ulcer)
- Mallory–Weiss tear
- Oesophageal varices (portal hypertension)
  - Extrahepatic
    - Malignant occlusion
    - Hypercoagulable state
    - Budd–Chiari syndrome (hepatic vein obstruction)
    - Portal vein thrombosis
  - Intrahepatic
    - Cirrhosis
    - Schistosomiasis

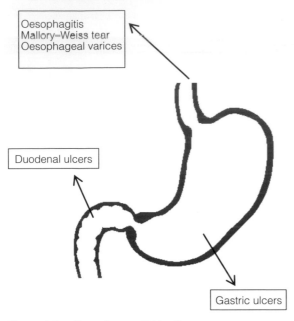

Oesophagitis
Mallory–Weiss tear
Oesophageal varices

Duodenal ulcers

Gastric ulcers

Figure 4.5: Sites of upper GI bleeding

Clinical features

- **Symptoms**
  - Depend on cause. Haematemesis, fresh PR bleeding, or melaena. Epigastric pain which may be exacerbated (gastric) or relieved (duodenal) by eating and antacids. Nausea and vomiting as well as symptoms of iron deficiency anaemia may occur (gastric)

- **Signs**
  - **Observations:** ↓BP (postural hypotension), ↑HR, RR, Sats
  - **Inspect:** pallor, sweating
  - **Palpate:** cold peripheries, epigastric tenderness usually absent
  - **Percuss:** normal
  - **Auscultate:** normal bowel sounds
  - **DRE:** melaena

Differential diagnosis
See Figure 4.6.

Investigations

- **Bloods:** FBC, U&E, Cr, LFT, Coagulation screen (INR, aPTT, PT), cross-match 4 units
- **Urinalysis:** dipstick
- **Endoscopy:**
  - OGD and colonoscopy ('top and tail')
- **Radiology:** if endoscopy equivocal
  - CT venous/arterial flow
  - CT angiography
  - Red cell scan

Management
See Figure 4.7.

Complications

- Haemorrhagic shock
- Rebleeding
- Disseminated intravascular coagulation

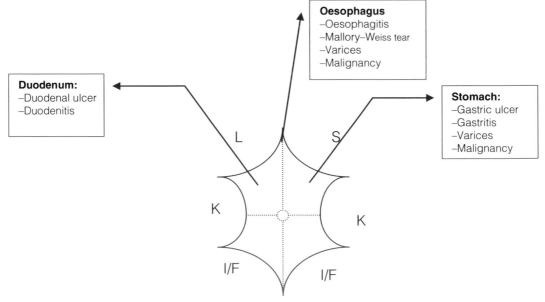

Oesophagus
–Oesophagitis
–Mallory–Weiss tear
–Varices
–Malignancy

Duodenum:
–Duodenal ulcer
–Duodenitis

Stomach:
–Gastric ulcer
–Gastritis
–Varices
–Malignancy

Figure 4.6: Differential diagnosis of upper GI bleeding

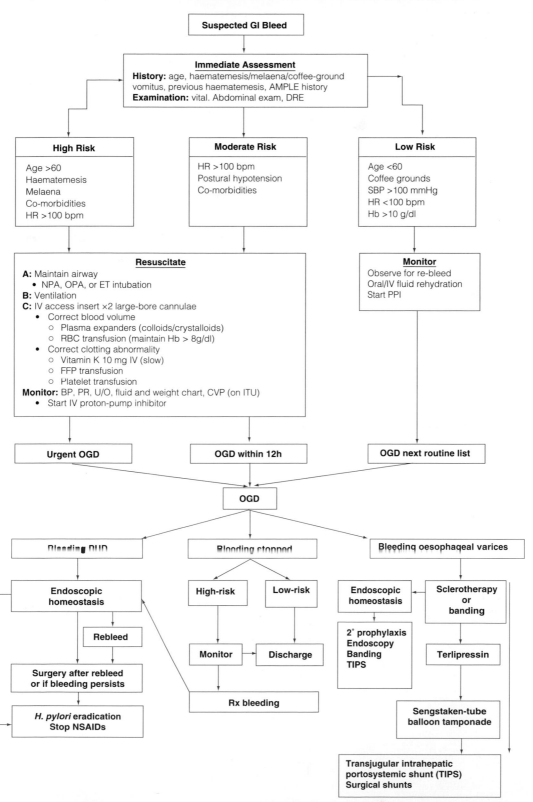

Figure 4.7: Management of upper GI bleeding

Prognosis
- Mortality 10%
- Poor prognostic factors include:
  - ↑Age
  - Shock
  - Varices
  - Rebleeding

4.5.3 Perforated ulcer

This is a common surgical emergency and is usually secondary to an anterior duodenal ulcer but gastric perforation is also commonly seen. Leakage of acid and gastric contents leads initially to localised and then generalised peritonitis.

Clinical features
- Presents with sudden onset of epigastric pain which becomes progressively generalised
- Patient may have signs of dehydration, tachycardia and tachypnoea
- Abdominal examination will usually reveal rigidity and generalised abdominal tenderness with guarding or rebound
- Bowel sounds will be typically absent
- There may be a history of NSAID use or prior dyspepsia

Investigations
- Inflammatory markers (white cell count and C-reactive protein) are usually elevated.
- Erect chest X-ray may reveal free subdiaphragmatic gas, but the absence of this finding does not exclude a perforation.

Management
- Resuscitation of the patient with intravenous fluids, intravenous antibiotics and close monitoring essential
- IV proton pump inhibitor
- Nil by mouth (NG tube to drain stomach contents)
- Surgery or conservative management

There is a place for conservative management with intravenous antibiotics in the case of localised perforation where the patient shows some sign of improvement. If this line of management is adopted then there must be close observation for any sign of deterioration.

In almost all cases treatment is surgical:

- Laparotomy with oversew and omental patching of smaller perforations.
- If the perforation is large then partial gastrectomy and gastrojejunostomy may be performed.
- Laparoscopic repair may be possible for some cases.
- Post-operatively patients should be placed on intravenous proton-pump inhibitors and have subsequent *H. pylori* eradication therapy.

4.5.4 Gastric tumours

Benign tumours of the stomach are rare and are usually adenomas or leiomyomas. The majority of gastric tumours are malignant and mainly adenocarcinomas. Some tumours may be lymphomas in origin. Gastric tumours represent 3% of all cancers in the UK, with an incidence of approximately 10 per 100 000 population. The incidence appears to be decreasing.

Causative factors are summarised in Table 4.3.

Pathology
Currently increasing incidence of proximal gastric tumours situated near the oesophagogastric junction. May vary in macroscopic appearance:

- Ulcerated lesion
- Polypoid lesion protruding into gastric lumen
- Colloid tumour

Table 4.3: Causative factors of gastric tumours	
Proved association	• Familial • Chronic atrophic gastritis • Pernicious anaemia • Blood group A • Gastric surgery • Gastric ulcer and polyps (long-standing) • Ménétrier's disease • Geographical factors – marked increased incidence in Japan (dietary nitrates)
Unproved association but links possible	• Diet high in nitrates • Alcohol • Smoking • *Helicobacter pylori*

- Linitis plastica (leather bottle stomach). Generally anaplastic carcinoma with a submucosal proliferation of tumour; leads to fibrosis

Clinical features

- Generally associated with epigastric pain, which may radiate to the back.
- Vomiting may be predominant with a pyloric tumour causing gastric outlet obstruction.
- Dysphagia may be seen with more proximal tumours near the oesophagogastric junction.
- Weight loss and anorexia is a predominant clinical feature.
- Less commonly gastric carcinomas may present with haemorrhage or perforation.
- Abdominal mass may be present in advanced disease.
- The patient may present with signs of metastatic disease:
  - Jaundice
  - Ascites
  - Hepatomegaly
  - Lymph nodes (Troisier's sign = Virchow's lymph node in left supraclavicular fossa)
  - Chest infection = possible lung metastases
  - Bone pain = bony metastases.

Investigations

- OGD allows detection and biopsy of suspicious tumours or lesions
- Staging investigations such as CT scan of chest and abdomen
- Staging laparoscopy
- Endoscopic ultrasound (EUS)

Management

- Partial or total gastrectomy with lymphadenectomy and resection of local structures depending on extent of invasion (duodenum, pancreas, spleen)
- Chemotherapy may be used pre- or post-operatively
- Radiotherapy is poorly tolerated

4.5.5 Post-gastrectomy complications

Specific immediate and early complications:
- Haemorrhage
- Anastomotic leak
- Chest infection
- Pulmonary embolus
- Wound infection

Late complications:
- Dumping syndrome (early) – occurs shortly after eating a meal. It is due to hyperosmolar contents of a meal rapidly passing into duodenum which exerts an osmotic pressure within the lumen of the duodenum. This leads to

hypersecretion of fluid into the duodenum and a hypovolaemia results. Features include sweating, palpitations, dizziness, flushing, tachycardia, abdominal pain, nausea, and diarrhoea
- Dumping syndrome (late) – rapid absorption of glucose followed by excess insulin secretion. After a few hours this results in hypoglycaemia which causes the symptoms of faintness, sweating and dizziness a few hours after a meal
- Diarrhoea
- Anaemia
  - Vitamin B_{12} deficiency due to lack of intrinsic factor secretion by stomach
    - Treat with B_{12} injections/3 monthly
  - Iron deficiency due to lack of gastric acid
- Calcium deficiency
- Early satiety
- Malnutrition
  - Protein and fat malabsorption
- Carcinoma of gastric remnant
- Pancreatitis

4.6 THE LIVER

4.6.1 Hepatomegaly

- The liver is normally impalpable in adults although the tip may be palpable in thin people.
- It enlarges below the costal margin, moves with respiration and is dull to percussion.
- Hepatic enlargement can have a range of causes (Box 4.3).
- Characteristics of the palpable liver edge, such as consistency, surface texture, pulsatility, tenderness and presence of bruit can give indications of the underlying cause. For example:
  - A smooth tender liver is found in hepatitis and right heart failure
  - A knobbly, hard, irregular liver with audible bruit suggests malignancy
  - A pulsatile liver indicates tricuspid incompetence.

Essential note

An enlarged liver has the following features on clinical examination:

- Enlarges towards the right iliac fossa
- Moves with respiration
- Is dull to percussion

Remember to percuss the upper border of the liver if it appears to be enlarged on clinical examination

Box 4.3: Causes of hepatic enlargement

Haematological
Sickle cell disease
Haemolytic anaemias
Leukaemia
Lymphoma
Myelofibrosis

Inflammatory
Alcoholic liver/cirrhosis
Autoimmune hepatitis
Primary biliary cirrhosis

Infective
Acute viral hepatitis
Malaria
Glandular fever
Abscess
Hydatid cyst
Ebstein–Barr virus

Infiltration
Amyloid
Haemochromatosis

Cardiovascular
Right ventricular failure
Tricuspid incompetence
Hepatic vein thrombosis
Portal vein thrombosis

Malignant
Hepatocellular cancer
Secondary metastatic cancer

4.6.2 Ascites

- Defined as accumulation of free fluid within the peritoneal cavity.
- Characterised by shifting dullness and fluid thrill on examination.
- Should be distinguished from the other common causes of abdominal distension including the other 'F's: fat, flatus, faeces and fetus (in women).
- Investigation involves abdominal ultrasound and sending peritoneal fluid (obtained by ascitic tap) for:
  - White cell count: >250 cells/mm^3 indicates (usually spontaneous) bacterial peritonitis
  - Gram stain and culture for bacteria and acid-fast bacilli (AFBs)
  - Cytology for malignant cells
  - Amylase to exclude pancreatic aetiology
  - Protein: used to subdivide the underlying causes (Box 4.4) into:
    - Transudates (protein <30 g/l)
    - Exudates (protein >30 g/l).

Essential note

Causes of transudates are easily remembered by failure of the three main organs: heart, liver and kidneys

Both pleural effusions and ascites have many similar causes. Learn them well once, apply them twice easily

4.6.3 Jaundice

Aetiology

- Jaundice (icterus) is one of the commonest symptoms of liver disease.
- It presents as yellowing of the skin and sclera as visualised in natural light.

Box 4.4: Causes of ascites

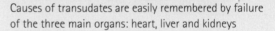

	Transudate			Exudate
Hypoalbuminaemia	Increased venous pressure	Other		Increased leakiness of blood capillaries
Cirrhosis	Heart failure	Hypothyroidism		Infection, eg TB
Nephrotic syndrome	Fluid overload	Meigs' syndrome (triad of ascites, ovarian fibroma and pleural effusion)		Inflammation, eg pancreatitis, appendicitis, or other organ inflammation
Malabsorption	Constrictive pericarditis			Malignancy, eg pancreatic cancer or any advanced abdominal cancer
Protein-losing enteropathy				

- It is caused by accumulation of the pigment bilirubin in the tissues and blood.
- Is clinically recognisable when bilirubin levels exceed 35 µmol/l.
- Classification is classically based on the stage of metabolism of bilirubin (pre-hepatic, hepatic and post-hepatic):
  - Most common causes are alcoholic liver disease and gallstone obstruction
  - Hepatic and post-hepatic forms often co-exist as hepatocellular damage can lead to intrahepatic impairment of conjugated bile flow.

Enterohepatic circulation of bile

Knowledge of bile pigment metabolism is important in understanding the pathogenesis, presentation, investigation and management of jaundice (Figure 4.8).

- Haem component of haemoglobin is broken down (in the spleen and bone marrow) to biliverdin and then bilirubin
- Bilirubin is transported to the liver bound to albumin (bilirubin–albumin). This complex is insoluble in water and thus not excreted in urine
- Bilirubin is conjugated with glucuronic acid by glucuronyl transferase in the liver to form bilirubin–glucuronide

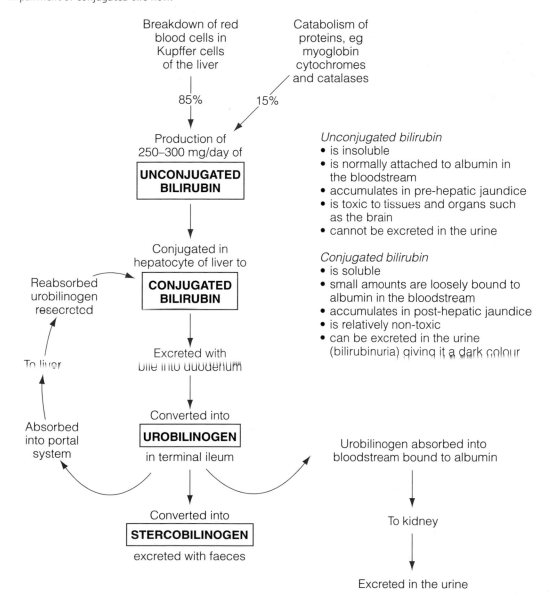

Unconjugated bilirubin
- is insoluble
- is normally attached to albumin in the bloodstream
- accumulates in pre-hepatic jaundice
- is toxic to tissues and organs such as the brain
- cannot be excreted in the urine

Conjugated bilirubin
- is soluble
- small amounts are loosely bound to albumin in the bloodstream
- accumulates in post-hepatic jaundice
- is relatively non-toxic
- can be excreted in the urine (bilirubinuria) giving it a dark colour

Figure 4.8: Bilirubin metabolism

- Bilirubin–glucuronide is water-soluble and secreted in the bile into the gut
- Gut bacteria convert bilirubin–glucuronide to urobilinogen, which follows one of the following paths:
  - Converted to pigmented stercobilinogen, which gives stools the normal brown colour
  - Reabsorbed via the terminal ileum into the portal vein and taken up by the liver, where it is re-excreted into the bile
  - Taken up by the systemic circulation and excreted by kidneys in the urine
- This process is called the enterohepatic circulation (Figure 4.9).

Classification of jaundice

- **Pre-hepatic**
  - Due to excess bilirubin production secondary to increased bilirubin production:
    - Haemolytic anaemia (eg sickle cell disease and thalassaemia)
    - Dyserythropoiesis
    - Incompatible blood transfusion
    - Rhabdomyolysis and haematoma resorption
  - Results in unconjugated hyperbilirubinaemia and high urobilinogen
    - Water-insoluble, not excreted by kidneys and does not enter urine

- **Hepatic**
  - Reduced bilirubin conjugation and hepatocyte dysfunction
    - Gilbert's and Crigler–Najjar syndromes
    - Hepatitis:
      - Viral (hepatitis A & B, EBV, CMV)
      - Alcoholic
      - Autoimmune
      - Drug-induced: paracetamol overdosage, statins, TB medications
    - Cirrhosis
    - Other
      - Hepatocellular cancer
      - Haemochromatosis
      - Wilson's disease
      - α_1-antitrypsin deficiency
      - Budd–Chiari syndrome
      - Congestive cardiac failure (due to hepatic congestion)
  - There is usually a varying degree of cholestasis and so both conjugated and unconjugated bilirubin appear in the blood
- **Post-hepatic**
  - Results from impaired excretion of bile from the liver into the gut
    - Conjugated bilirubin is therefore reabsorbed into the blood, increasing serum and urine levels, making the urine dark

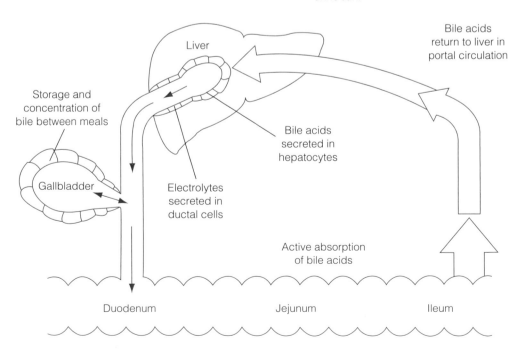

Figure 4.9: Enterohepatic circulation of bile

○ Less conjugated bilirubin in the bowel leads to reduced stercobilinogen and the stools become pale
- Obstruction of the common bile duct may be due to
  ○ Intraluminal factors:
    □ Gallstones
    □ Infestation (*Clonorchis, Schistosomia*)
  ○ Mural obstruction:
    □ Congenital atresia of the bile duct
    □ Cholangiocarcinoma
    □ Sclerosing cholangitis
    □ Mirizzi's syndrome (gallbladder mass associated with chronic cholecystitis)
    □ Benign stricture
      – Post-inflammatory
      – Post-operatively
  ○ Extramural obstruction
    □ Pancreatitis
    □ Carcinoma of head of pancreas
    □ Carcinoma of ampulla of Vater
    □ Lymphadenopathy at the porta hepatis
      – Metastatic
      – Lymphoma

Diagnosis

Diagnosing the cause of jaundice requires a thorough history, well-conducted examinations and detailed investigations.

History

History should include enquiries on:

- Presenting symptoms, in particular
  - Nature of pain (SOCRATES)
  - Colour of stool and urine
  - Previous episodes of jaundice or anaemia
  - Non-specific symptoms, including pruritus, dyspepsia, anorexia, weight loss
- Risk factors:
  - Drug use and medications
  - Anaemia
  - Splenectomy
  - Gallstones
  - Alcohol consumption
  - Jaundiced contacts
  - Family history
  - Blood transfusions
  - Intravenous drug use
  - Sexual activity
  - Tattoos
  - Occupation (farm workers – leptospirosis)

Box 4.5: Signs of chronic liver disease

Signs of chronic liver disease:

Hands:
- Leuconychia
- Terry's nails
- Telangiectasia
- Palmar erythema
- Clubbing
- Dupuytren's contracture

Abdomen:
- Spider naevi
- Hepatomegaly (tender or not)
- Splenomegaly
- Ascites

Elsewhere:
- Xanthelasmas
- Scleral jaundice
- Parotid enlargement
- Testicular atrophy
- Gynaecomastia
- Purpura

Examination

Important examination findings may include:

- Colour of jaundice: the lemon-yellow tinge is more marked in pre-hepatic jaundice compared with hepatic and post-hepatic jaundice, where it is deeper
- Signs of chronic liver disease (Box 4.5)
- Evidence of malignancy, eg lymphadenopathy
- Palpable gallbladder

Investigations

Initial investigations are aimed at determining the type of jaundice (Table 4.4) with subsequent tests used to determine the underlying cause.

If **pre-hepatic jaundice** suspected:

- LFTs with conjugated/unconjugated bilirubin differential
- Urine testing for urobilinogen
- Blood film
- Reticulocyte count
- Coombs' test

If **hepatic jaundice** suspected:

- Viral hepatitis: hepatitis A, B, EBV and CMV serology
- Autoimmune hepatitis: antinuclear and smooth muscle antibody

Abdominal surgery

- Haemochromatosis: raised ferritin and iron, reduced total iron-binding capacity
- Wilson's disease: reduced copper and caeruloplasmin
- α_1-antitrypsin deficiency: reduced serum α_1-antitrypsin
- Hepatocellular cancer: AFP

If **post-hepatic jaundice** suspected:

- Blood tests
  - LFTs
  - Clotting studies
  - Amylase
  - Urinary bilirubin (academic)
- Ultrasound:
  - Shows presence of gallstones within the gallbladder, thickening of gallbladder wall in inflammation and dilation of the common bile duct (diameter of >7 mm is suggestive of ductal obstruction)
  - If common bile duct dilation found, endoscopic retrograde cholangiopancreatography (ERCP) or preferably magnetic resonance cholangiopancreatography (MRCP) is the next investigation of choice
  - If common bile duct not dilated, obstructive cause is unlikely and needle biopsy of the liver is often the next investigation in the absence of other explanations for jaundice
- ERCP:
  - Shows location and nature of obstruction
  - Used to remove obstructing gallstones and stent-obstructing lesions by passing a tube through or placing a nasobiliary drain
  - Also used to obtain brushings for cytology in ampullary or head of pancreas tumours
  - Complications: perforation, bleeding, pancreatitis and cholangitis
- MRCP:
  - Gives more detailed imaging of the biliary system and main pancreatic duct compared with ERCP
  - Non-invasive
  - Cannot obtain brushings, perform stone retrieval, or stenting
  - Is replacing diagnostic (but not therapeutic) ERCP

Table 4.4: Investigations of jaundice

Type of jaundice		Pre-hepatic	Hepatic	Post-hepatic
Haemoglobin		Low	Normal	Normal
Reticulocytes		Raised in haemolysis	Normal	Normal
Liver function tests:	ALP	Normal	Normal/high	Very high
	γGT	Normal	Normal/high	Very high
	ALT	Normal	Very high	Normal/high
	AST	Normal	Very high	Normal/high
	LDH	Normal	Very high	Normal
Serum bilirubin	Conjugated	Normal	Normal/high	High
	Unconjugated	High	Normal/high	Normal
Urinary bilirubin		Absent	Normal/high	High
Urobilinogen		High	Variable	Absent
Prothrombin time		Normal	May be increased	May be increased
			Due to poor hepatic function	Due to vitamin K malabsorption
			Uncorrected with vitamin K	Corrected with vitamin K
Ultrasound		Normal	May show structural or parenchymal abnormality of liver	Shows gallstones ± dilated bile ducts or other obstruction

ALP = alkaline phosphatase; ALT = alanine aminotransferase; AST = aspartate aminotransferase; γGT = gamma-glutamyl transferase; LDH = lactate dehydrogenase

4.6.4 Portal hypertension

- Normal pressure in the portal system is 8–10 mmHg or 80–150 mmH$_2$O
- Portal hypertension results from obstruction of portal vein flow:
  - Leads to formation of portosystemic collateral vessels between the portal and systemic venous circulation
  - The result is diversion of blood into the collaterals
  - Most important site of collateral formation is the gastro-oesophageal junction, as varices here are superficial and are prone to bleeding

Causes can be subdivided according to the site of pathology (Box 4.6):

- Pre-hepatic (obstruction of flow of portal vein into liver), eg portal vein thrombosis
- Intrahepatic (obstruction of flow of portal vein in the liver), eg cirrhosis
- Post-hepatic (obstruction of outflow of portal vein), eg hepatic vein obstruction (Budd–Chiari syndrome)

Box 4.6: Causes of portal hypertension

Pre-hepatic:
- Portal vein thrombosis
- Portal vein compression
  - Lymph node
  - Pancreatitis
- Splenic vein thrombosis

Intrahepatic:
- Cirrhosis
- Schistosomiasis
- Haemochromatosis
- Wilson's disease
- Primary biliary cirrhosis
- Hepatic metastases
- Veno-occlusive disease

Extrahepatic:
- Hepatic vein thrombosis (Budd–Chiari)
- Right heart failure
- Constrictive pericarditis
- Tricuspid incompetence
- Pulmonary hypertension
- IVC obstruction

Increased portal blood flow (rare)
- Hepatic arteriovenous fistulas
- Splenic arteriovenous fistulas

- Cirrhosis is the commonest cause in the West; worldwide, schistosomiasis may be more important
- **Clinical features:**
  - GI bleeding (haematemesis and melaena)
  - Ascites
  - Splenomegaly
  - Hepatic failure and its sequelae
- **Management** involves:
  - Treating the underlying cause
  - Management of variceal bleeding, see Figure 4.7

4.6.5 Management of variceal bleeds

Treatment of a bleeding of oesophageal varices is based on:

- Immediate resuscitation (see Box 4.7)
- Endoscopy for diagnosis and to stop the bleeding
- Banding involves placing small bands around the varices
- Sclerotherapy involves injection of a sclerosant solution (eg ethanolamine) into the varices
- Pharmacological treatment with IV terlipressin infusion reduces the portal pressure and can be used as a holding measure if banding and sclerotherapy are unsuccessful or unavailable
- Balloon tamponade is used if bleeding continues, but has serious complications, including oesophageal perforation, aspiration pneumonia and mucosal ulceration. Airway must be protected and it should not be left in place for more than 12 hours. A Sengstaken–Blakemore tube is used for tamponade

Box 4.7: Immediate resuscitation

1. ABC including high-flow oxygen
2. Raise foot of bed/head-down position
3. Insert two large-bore IV cannulae (14–16 G)
4. Send blood for FBC, U&E, LFT, clotting, cross-match 6 units
5. Start IV infusion of crystalloids while waiting for blood cross-match
6. Place a CVP line and catheterise the patient
7. Adjust fluid replacement according to BP, CVP pressure and hourly urinary output
8. Correct clotting abnormalities (vitamin K, platelets, fresh frozen plasma)
9. Start on IV proton-pump inhibitor
10. Make patient NBM in preparation for endoscopy
11. Endoscopy (urgent if continuing bleeding) for diagnosis and stopping of bleeding

- Transjugular intrahepatic portosystemic shunt (TIPS) placement involves placing a stent into the liver parenchyma through the internal jugular vein, thereby forming a shunt between the portal and hepatic veins and reducing the portal pressure
- Additional treatment:
  - Prophylactic antibiotics (eg ciprofloxacin)
  - Lactulose to prevent portosystemic encephalopathy
  - Sucralfate to reduce oesophageal ulceration
- Prophylactic measures: given the high recurrence rate of variceal bleeds (70% in 2 years) treatment to prevent further bleeds is essential
  - Propranolol: reduces portal pressure and is also given to patients with varices which have never bled (primary prophylaxis)
  - Repeat endoscopic banding
  - TIPS if medical and endoscopic therapy failed

4.6.6 Hepatic abscesses

Aetiology

Abscesses of the liver are of two types:

- **Pyogenic abscess** can be caused by the following sources of infection:
  - Biliary system
    - From an ascending cholangitis
    - *E. coli* and anaerobic Gram-negative organisms
  - Haematogenous (arterial and portal systems)
    - From septic bacteraemia or infected portal drainage
    - Staphylococcal and streptococcal organisms in arterial bacteraemia
    - Gram-negative enterococci in portal infections
  - Local infections
    - Spreading to the liver
    - For example, subphrenic collections, acute cholecystitis
  - Spontaneous
    - No obvious cause
    - *Peptostreptococcus* and *Streptococcus milleri*
  - Penetrating injury
- **Amoebic abscesses** are caused by *Entamoeba histolytica*, which spreads from the colon, where it often causes an acute diarrhoeal illness, to the liver via the portal veins. Treat with metronidazole and possibly percutaneous radiologically guided drainage if not responding to antibiotic therapy

Hydatid disease of the liver is caused by *Echinococcus granulosus*. This is a cyst and not an abscess. Clinical presentation and investigations are the same as for abscess. Treat with albendazole and/or surgery

Clinical features

- Fevers, rigors and sweating
- Right upper quadrant pain
- Tender hepatomegaly
- Jaundice

Investigations

- Blood cultures: before commencement of treatment therapy identify causative organism and sensitivity to antibiotic
- US/CT: used to identify the site and size of the abscess

Management

- Medical: involves antibiotic therapy – initially blind (eg ciprofloxacin and metronidazole) and tailored once organ is identified or pathogen cultured
- Interventional: radiologically guided percutaneous drainage of liver abscess
- Surgical: used in cases where there is no improvement with medical management

4.6.7 Liver tumours

Liver tumours can be subdivided into four main categories: benign tumours, primary hepatocellular carcinoma, cholangiocarcinoma and metastatic cancer of the liver.

Benign liver tumours

- Adenoma
  - Seen in young women and associated with use of the oral contraceptive pill
  - May present with bleeding following rupture
  - Remove if diagnosis in doubt or if expands/ruptures
- Cavernous haemangioma
  - Can lead to bleeding or be mistaken for tumours
  - These are best left alone if they are asymptomatic

Hepatocellular carcinoma

Aetiology

- Malignant tumour of hepatocytes
- Accounts for 90% of primary liver cancers
- Rare in the UK (incidence of 1/100 000) but there is significant variation worldwide
- It is around 25 times more prevalent in Africa and south-east Asia, reflecting the higher incidence of hepatitis B and C in these regions
- In the west, alcohol is the most important aetiological factor. Others include chronic active hepatitis, haemochromatosis, parasites and anabolic and contraceptive steroids
- Nearly 80% occur on a background of hepatitis, although normal non-cirrhotic livers can be affected

Clinical features
- Initially asymptomatic
- General: anorexia, weight loss, malaise and fatigue
- Abdominal mass and fullness
- Right upper quadrant pain due to liver capsule stretch
- Knobbly, hard, irregular liver on palpation
- Dyspnoea, from direct involvement of diaphragm
- Metastatic effects, eg lymphadenopathy, pleural effusion

Investigations
- Serum AFP levels are significantly raised (>500 ng/ml). Smaller rises occur in cirrhosis
- CT, MRI and hepatic angiography may be used for tumour localisation, staging purposes and determining operability

Management
- Surgical resection:
  - If confined to one lobe can be treated with hepatic lobectomy
  - Best results in small, well-differentiated tumours in the absence of cirrhosis
  - 5-year survival of around 35%
  - 50% have recurrence by 3 years
- Liver transplantation in those with a cirrhotic liver and a small adenoma (<3 cm) and for multifocal cancers
- Chemotherapy in those with inoperable tumours
- Prognosis is poor with 5% 5-year survival

Metastatic cancer of the liver
- 90% of liver tumours are secondary tumours (Box 4.8)
- Liver is the commonest site of metastatic disease
- These are blood-borne deposits and are typically multiple
- Clinical features are generally similar to those of primary hepatocellular carcinoma
- Treatment is usually palliative, except in rare cases of colorectal cancers with small solitary nodular metastases confined to one lobe, where surgical resection may be indicated

---

Box 4.8: Primaries of liver metastases

- Lung
- Breast
- Stomach
- Colon
- Uterus
- Pancreas
- Leukaemia
- Lymphoma

Cholangiocarcinoma

Aetiology
- Adenocarcinomas of the biliary tree
- Rare, representing around 1% of all cancers
- May develop anywhere in the intra- or extrahepatic ductal system
- Associated conditions:
  - Sclerosing cholangitis
  - Ulcerative colitis
  - Choledochal cyst
  - Chronic infection of the biliary tree, particularly with *Clonorchis sinensis*
- Causes obstruction of the extrahepatic bile duct, leading dilation of the intrahepatic ducts and hepatomegaly, which can in turn progress to liver atrophy or cirrhosis

Clinical features
- General: malaise, anorexia and weight loss
- Painless jaundice with pale stools, dark urine and pruritus
- Right upper quadrant pain is a feature of advanced disease
- Hepatomegaly
- Spread occurs through liver substance and regional nodes

Management
- 70% are not operable; of those that are, 70% recur
- Extrahepatic tumours may be treated by pancreaticoduodenectomy
- Intrahepatic tumours may be resected by partial hepatectomy
- Chemotherapy and radiotherapy post-surgery may improve prognosis
- Palliative therapy includes stenting of obstructed extra-hepatic tree
- Survival rate is 30%–40% after complete resection

4.7 THE GALLBLADDER

4.7.1 Gallstones
Gallstones are calculi formed in the gallbladder. They are very common, occurring in up to 20% of the western population, although 80% remain asymptomatic and require no treatment. They can however cause a range of disorders depending on their position in the gallbladder, bile ducts or the gut (Box 4.9).

Abdominal surgery

Box 4.9: Clinical conditions resulting from gallstones

In the gallbladder	**In the bile ducts**	**In the gut**
Biliary colic	Obstructive jaundice	Gallstone ileus
Acute cholecystitis	Cholangitis	
Chronic cholecystitis	Pancreatitis	
Mucocoele		
Empyema		
Carcinoma of gallbladder		

Types of gallstones

There are three main types of stones:

- **Pigment (5%):** small and irregular, consisting of bilirubin polymers and calcium bilirubinate. Pure pigment stones are rare and are found in haemolytic conditions such as sickle cell anaemia and hereditary spherocytosis due to excess bilirubin production. They are radiolucent.

- **Cholesterol (20%):** large, smooth and often solitary, and result from an excess of cholesterol in relation to bile salts and phospholipids in bile. This may be due to a deficiency of bile salts after interruption of the intra-hepatic circulation, for example as a result of terminal ileal disease or resection, or high blood cholesterol. Other risk factors include increasing age, obesity, pregnancy and the contraceptive pill. They are radiolucent.

- **Mixed (75%):** hard and faceted and often multiple. These have a mixture of mainly cholesterol, but also bile pigments and calcium salts. Their metabolic origin is largely similar to that of cholesterol stones; 10% of them are radio-opaque.

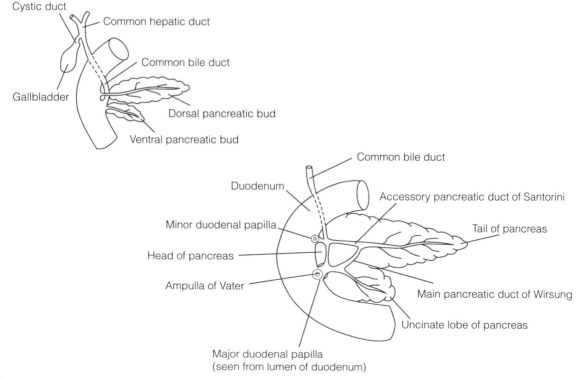

Figure 4.10: Structure of the biliary tree

Risk factors

Gallstones are rare in children and usually occur during middle life, with the incidence increasing with age. They are twice as common in women and often follow pregnancy. Other predisposing factors include drugs (fibrates, oral contraceptive pill), obesity, haemolysis and terminal ileal disease. The typical patient said to be the 'fair, fat, fertile, female of forty'. Most patients, however, do not fit this profile!

Structure of the biliary tree

- The right and left hepatic ducts join in the porta hepatis to form the common hepatic duct.
- The union of the cystic duct from the gallbladder and the common hepatic duct forms the common bile duct.
- The pancreatic duct joins the common bile duct, which runs to the duodenum (Figure 4.10).

4.7.2 Biliary colic

Biliary colic is a symptom caused by obstruction of a stone in the gallbladder outlet (Hartmann's pouch) or cystic duct. The complaint is that of a colicky right upper quadrant or epigastric pain which occurs in association with nausea or vomiting. The symptom settles as the stone falls back into the gallbladder or advances along the duct without further impaction.

Clinical features

- Right upper quadrant pain:
  - Caused by contraction of the gallbladder muscle and cystic duct
  - Severe, typically raising to a peak intermittently, but continuing unrelentingly
  - Radiating to the back and at times referred to the region of the right scapular tip
  - Patient typically curls up in bed, continuously changing position to get comfortable
- Jaundice (if common bile duct obstructed)
- Nausea and vomiting and tachycardia
- Other symptoms associated with gallstones, including dyspepsia, flatulence and intolerance of fatty foods may also be present

Differential diagnosis

- Other causes of sever upper abdominal pain:
  - Acute cholecystitis
  - Acute pancreatitis
  - Perforated peptic ulcer
  - Ruptured aneurysm
- The absence of inflammatory features (increased WCC, fever and local peritonism) differentiate this from acute cholecystitis

- An attack that does not settle within 24 hours suggests acute cholecystitis as the more likely diagnosis

Investigations

- Ultrasound to confirm gallstones

Management

- Many cases are safely managed at home or with a short inpatient stay for analgesia
- Analgesia (often a single injection of an opiate is adequate). Morphine should be avoided as it can stimulate contraction of the sphincter of Oddi.
- Antiemetics
- Cholecystectomy: may be performed immediately or electively at a later date (in which case patients are advised on a low-fat diet in the intervening time)

4.7.3 Acute cholecystitis

Aetiology

Acute cholecystitis is acute inflammation of a gallbladder caused by several factors including physical and chemical irritation, and occasionally later in the episode secondarily bacterial infection.

The majority (99%) of cases are caused by gallstones (calculus cholecystitis). Obstruction of the cystic duct leads to filling of the gallbladder with mucus or pus (commonly sterile on culture) and irritation of the gallbladder wall by the concentrated bile. Occasionally acalculous cholecystitis can occur in association biliary stasis, including major surgery, sepsis, typhoid fever, prolonged total arenteral nutrition and gas gangrene infection.

Clinical features

In contrast to biliary colic the patient is systemically unwell:

- Epigastric or right upper quadrant pain
  - Radiating to the back or right scapula
  - Continuous and exacerbated by breathing
- Nausea and vomiting
- Fever
- On examination, there is local peritonism, with the patient lying still and taking shallow breaths
- Tenderness and guarding in the right upper quadrant, more marked on inspiration
  - Murphy's sign: pain and arrest of inspiration as an inflamed gallbladder strikes the fingers placed at the tip of the 9th rib. This is only positive if the same test does not result in pain in the left upper quadrant
- Inflammatory gallbladder mass may be palpable in cases of empyema or mucocoele

- Tachycardia
- Pyrexia and rigors
- Jaundice may be present in a minority of cases due to an enlarged gallbladder pressing against the adjacent common bile duct or stones passing into the common bile duct

Investigations
- Bloods
  - FBC may show leucocytosis
  - U&E, LFTs and amylase or lipase to exclude acute pancreatitis and assess renal and liver function
  - CRP may be raised
- Abdominal X-ray
  - Only shows radio-opaque stones (10% of cases)
  - May reveal air in the biliary tree – indicates a cholecystoduodenal fistula or recent instrumentation of the biliary tree (ERCP). Also, gas-forming bacteria (eg *E. coli* and clostridial) can cause air in the biliary tree and is associated with increased mortality
- Ultrasound shows:
  - Gallstones as strongly echogenic foci
  - Increased gallbladder wall thickness caused by inflammation
  - Dilatation of the common bile duct (diameter more than 7 mm suggests distal obstruction)
- Hepatobiliary scintigraphy:
  - A radio-isotope scan that is only used if diagnosis remains uncertain after US
  - Typically, contrast is taken up by the liver and excreted in the bile
  - If the cystic duct is patent, gallbladder fills and is visualised, excluding cholecystitis

Management
Most cases resolve with conservative management:

- Patient is kept NBM and resuscitated with IV fluids
- Antiemetic and analgesia
- Antibiotics (eg metronidazole and cefuroxime)
- Elective cholecystectomy after 6–12 weeks when the inflammation has completely settled
  - Cholecystectomy is the only definite treatment
  - Early operations, within 72 hours of the onset are becoming more common due to the reduced risk of recurrent attacks or other gallstone complications such as acute pancreatitis
  - Routinely performed laparoscopically

In the minority of cases where the patient fails to improve early surgical intervention is indicated.

Complications
An empyema is an abscess of the gallbladder, where the gallbladder becomes distended with pus and may be palpable; and is often accompanied by a swinging fever.

Other worrying signs include increasing tachycardia and temperature with worsening or generalised peritonitis. These are suggestive of gallbladder perforation or infarction (gangrenous cholecystitis).

4.7.4 Chronic cholecystitis
Aetiology
Chronic cholecystitis is chronic recurrent inflammation of the gallbladder almost always caused by gallstones, resulting in fibrosis and thickening of the gallbladder.

Clinical features
- Patients complain of vague abdominal discomfort and pain
- Nausea
- Flatulence
- Symptoms particularly present after fatty meals

Differential diagnosis
Distinguish from other causes of chronic dyspepsia, including:

- Gastro-oesophageal reflux
- Peptic ulcer disease
- Irritable bowel syndrome
- Hiatus hernia
- Relapsing pancreatitis

Investigations
- US may show gallstones and increased gallbladder wall thickness
- If the diagnosis is unclear, other investigations for dyspepsia including an OGD may be necessary

Management
- Cholecystectomy, performed as an elective laparoscopic procedure, is the treatment of choice
- If US shows a dilated common bile duct, ERCP and sphincterotomy for stone removal may be indicated before surgery

4.7.5 Other presentations of gallstones
Silent stones
- Much more common than symptomatic gallstones
- Produce no symptoms
- Do not warrant surgical intervention

Mucocoele

- Follows an attack of biliary colic
- Stone impaction in neck of gallbladder causing an obstruction
- Mucus secretion continues after bile has absorbed
- Leads to a distended gallbladder filled with clear mucus
- Treat with aspiration and cholecystectomy

Empyema

- Follows an attack of acute cholecystitis
- Infection develops in the gallbladder after impaction of a stone in the neck
- Gallbladder fills with pus due to stasis and overgrowth of bacteria
- Patient may appear septic
- Treat as acute cholecystitis
- Perform urgent cholecystectomy if possible or drainage via cholecystostomy with delayed cholecystectomy

Acute cholangitis

- Bacterial infection of the biliary tract
- Untreated, can lead to septicaemia and death
- Aetiology
  - Gallstone is by far the commonest cause
  - Duct stricture
  - Tumour of the bile ducts or pancreatic head
  - Instrumentation, eg ERCP
- Usually caused by Gram-negative organisms
- Clinical features: 'Charcot's triad of
  - Right upper quadrant pain
  - Fever and rigors
  - Jaundice
- Management
  - IV antibiotics (eg cefuroxime and metronidazole ± gentamicin)
  - ERCP and stenting if cholangitis is suppurative with obstruction of the biliary tree

Gallstone ileus

- Gallstones occasionally erode the wall of the gallbladder and enter the duodenum, resulting in a cholecystoduodenal fistula
- Classic presentation – a patient with previous history of gallstones presents with a small-bowel obstruction with air in the biliary tree seen on X-ray
- Commonly the stone impacts at the terminal ileum as this is the narrowest part of the distal small bowel
- Treat with laparotomy for small-bowel obstruction. Future cholecystectomy if further symptoms occur

Others

- Acute and chronic pancreatitis (discussed in Section 4.8)
- Carcinoma of the gallbladder

4.7.6 Carcinoma of the gallbladder

Aetiology

- Mostly papillary adenocarcinomas
- Chronic irritation by gallstones in most cases
- Three times commoner in women
- Increased risk of carcinoma in porcelain gallbladders (calcified gallbladder due to chronic inflammatory scarring)

Clinical features

- Are similar to chronic cholecystitis
- Constant right upper quadrant pain
- Anorexia and weight loss
- Obstructive jaundice due to local spread into ducts and nodes
- Usually presents late with a poor prognosis (<10% survival at 1 year)

Management

- Often detected incidentally during cholecystectomy
- Cholecystectomy plus hepatic resection used for localised cancer

4.8 THE PANCREAS

4.8.1 Introduction to the pancreas

The pancreas is a large central gland extending retroperitoneally across the posterior abdominal wall from the second part of the duodenum (head) to the spleen (tail).

The pancreas consists of exocrine and endocrine cells. The **endocrine pancreas** consists of hormone-producing cells in islets (islets of Langerhans), comprising four main cell types:

- A (α) cells: synthesise, store and secrete glucagon
- B (β) cells: synthesise, store and secrete insulin
- D (δ) cells: secrete somatostatin
- F cells: secrete pancreatic polypeptide

The **exocrine pancreas** consists of acinar cells, which store digestive enzymes in secretory granules. These enzymes include amylase, lipase, colipase, phospholipase and the proteases. They are secreted as inactive precursors into the duodenum by exocytosis in response to hormonal stimulation.

4.8.2 Pancreatitis

Pancreatitis is inflammation of the pancreas that results from injury to acinar cells and can be acute or chronic. These are two clinically distinct entities. In acute pancreatitis, the gland is normal before the attack, and the patient presents with acute abdominal pain and nausea and vomiting with significantly elevated pancreatic enzymes. Most patients return to normal after resolution of the attack. However, acute pancreatitis varies in severity from mild to life-threatening. The recurrence of a severe (necrotising) attack may lead to irreversible damage to the pancreas, leading to a chronic pancreatitis with continued inflammatory disease. In contrast to acute pancreatitis, patients with chronic pancreatitis present with recurrent abdominal pains, mildly elevated pancreatic enzymes and evidence of exocrine failure of the pancreas (diabetes and steatorrhoea).

Acute pancreatitis

Aetiology

- Gallstones (commonest cause of acute pancreatitis)
- Alcohol
- Trauma
  - From accident
- Metabolic: $\uparrow Ca^{2+}$, $\uparrow$lipids
- Iatrogenic
  - Drug-induced, eg azathioprine, steroids, sulphonamides, thiazides, OCP, 5-aminosalicylic acid
  - Trauma from ERCP or surgery
- Infections
  - Viral, eg EBV, VZV, mumps, measles, coxsackievirus
  - Bacterial, eg *Mycoplasma pneumoniae, Salmonella, Campylobacter* and *Mycobacterium tuberculosis*
- Hypothermia
- Autoimmune disease (eg polyarteritis nodosa)
- Malignancy (eg pancreatic carcinoma)
- Idiopathic

Epidemiology

- Age: young/middle age
- Sex: M>F: in males, more often related to alcohol; in females, to biliary tract disease

Pathophysiology

Acinar cell or ductal cell injury (such as with the *CFTR* gene mutation) results in the release of protease and inflammatory cells into the pancreatic interstitium, leading to pancreatic autodigestion and hence acute pancreatitis.

Early mediators include tumour necrosis factor alpha (TNFα), and interleukins IL-6 and IL-8, which cause increased pancreatic vascular permeability, leading to local injury (haemorrhage, oedema and eventually pancreatic necrosis) and systemic complications (such as bacteraemia due to gut flora translocation, gastrointestinal haemorrhage, adult respiratory distress syndrome, pleural effusions and acute renal failure) resulting in haemodynamic instability and death.

> **Essential note**
>
> Acute pancreatitis occurs due to autodigestion of the pancreas by autoactivation of its own digestive enzymes

Clinical features

- **Symptoms**
  - Gradual-onset epigastric pain which gradually intensifies in severity, resulting in a constant ache
  - Characterised as dull and aching with radiation through to the back
  - Associated with nausea, vomiting, anorexia, shock
  - Duration of pain varies but typically lasts more than a day
  - Pain relieved by sitting forward/supine position
- **Signs**
  - May be shocked with tachycardia and hypotension (variable)
  - Patient looks unwell and has epigastric/central abdominal tenderness with guarding
  - Jaundice, ecchymoses due to haemorrhagic pancreatitis (Grey Turner's sign – flank bruising; and Cullen's sign – umbilical bruising), erythematous skin nodules (subcutaneous fat necrosis) may be present
  - There may be generalised peritonitis mimicking a perforated viscus
  - An ileus may be present with reduced bowel sounds

Differential diagnosis

- Hepatitis
- Cholecystitis
- Cholangitis
- Perforated ulcer
- Pyelonephritis

Investigations

- **Bloods** – FBC, U&E, Ca^{2+}, LFT, CRP, amylase, LDH, glucose
- **Urinalysis** – dipstick, MC+S
- **Radiology** – Erect CXR, AXR, USS, CT abdomen
- **Other** – Arterial blood gases

Severity

There are several scoring systems available to use, the most common of which are listed below:

- **Modified Glasgow score:** applied to alcohol-/gallstone-induced pancreatitis
  - PaO_2 <8 kPa (<60 mmHg)
  - Age >55 years
  - Neutrophils: WCC >15×10^9/l
  - Ca^{2+} <2 mmol/l
  - Renal function: urea >16 mmol/l
  - Enzymes: ALT >100 iu/l, LDH >600 iu/l
  - Albumin <32 g/l
  - Sugar: blood glucose >10 mmol/l

A score >3 indicates severe pancreatitis and the patient needs transferring to HDU/ITU.

- **Ranson criteria** (Box 4.10)
  - **Present on admission**
    - Age >55 years
    - WCC >16×10^9/l
    - Blood glucose >11 mmol/l
    - LDH >350 iu/l
    - AST >250 iu/l
  - **Developing during the first 48 hours**
    - Haematocrit fall >10%
    - Urea increase >1.8 mmol/l
    - Ca^{2+} < 2 mmol/l
    - PaO_2 < 8 kPa or 60 mmHg
    - Base deficit >4 mmol/l
    - Estimated fluid sequestration > 6l

- **APACHE II** score (acute physiology and chronic health evaluation)

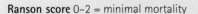

Box 4.10: Ranson criteria

Ranson score 0–2 = minimal mortality

Ranson score 3–5 = 10%–20% mortality

Ranson score >5 = 50% mortality and is associated with more systemic complications

Management

- **Conservative**
  - NBM + IV fluids
  - Oxygen as necessary
  - Nasogastric tube
  - Catheter to monitor urine output
  - Stepwise nutrition as pain settles
    - Enteral, eg Fortisips/Fortijuice, nasojejunal feeding
    - Parenteral, eg TPN
- **Medical**
  - **Antibiotics,** eg cefuroxime and metronidazole
  - **Analgesia,** eg paracetamol, opiates (avoidance of morphine due to sphincter of Oddi contractions is academic: it is given quite often in clinical practice)
  - **Antiemetic**
- **Surgical**
  - **Laparotomy** (may be performed to exclude other causes of peritonitis) or for complications which may develop such as abscess/pseudocyst drainage or removal of necrotic pancreatic tissue
- **Endoscopic**
  - **ERCP** (in severe acute gallstone pancreatitis not responding to supportive therapy or with ascending cholangitis with worsening signs and symptoms of obstruction)

Complications

- **Early**
  - Shock (IV fluids: crystalloids + colloids)
  - DIC (cryoprecipitate, fresh frozen plasma, RBC and platelet transfusion)
  - ARDS (O_2 + continuous positive airways pressure)
  - Respiratory failure (O_2)
  - Acute renal failure
  - Metabolic: hyperglycaemia (insulin), hypoalbuminaemia (human albumin solution), hypocalcaemia as Ca^{2+} is bound to albumin (calcium gluconate)
- **Late**
  - Pancreatic necrosis (parenteral nutrition ± laparotomy)
  - Pancreatic pseudocyst (percutaneous aspiration)
  - Abscess (percutaneous catheter drainage)
  - Thrombosis causing bowel ischaemia

Follow-up

Once the patient is discharged follow-up in the Outpatient department is indicated with a view to treating the cause if there is one (eg cholecystectomy for gallstones).

Prognosis

- **Mortality:** 10%–15%, whilst in severe pancreatitis can be up to 30%. Patients with biliary pancreatitis tend to have a higher mortality rate than patients with alcoholic pancreatitis.
- **Morbidity:** In the first week of illness, most deaths result from multiorgan system failure. In subsequent weeks, infection plays a more significant role, but organ failure still constitutes a major cause of mortality.

Chronic pancreatitis

Chronic pancreatitis is defined as continuous chronic inflammation of the pancreas characterised by remissions and relapses in the clinical course with irreversible changes in the structure of the gland and impairment of endocrine and exocrine function. As a result of recurrent inflammation, the pancreatic parenchyma undergoes progressive atrophy, fibrosis and calcification with dilatation of ducts. It presents a significant health burden with an increasing incidence, with 3000 new cases reported in the UK annually. The mean age of onset is 40 and the incidence is four times higher in men.

Aetiology

Excessive alcohol consumption is the main cause, accounting for up to 80% of cases of chronic pancreatitis. Other causes include:

- Hereditary: autosomal dominant with 80% penetrance – accounts for 1% of cases
- Cystic fibrosis
- Hyperlipidaemia
- Hypercalcaemia
- Idiopathic: subdivided into early-onset (peak incidence of 15–30 years) and late-onset forms (peak of 50–70 years)
- Obstruction of the pancreatic duct can impede flow of pancreatic juice and cause chronic pancreatitis. Obstructive forms may be congenital (eg pancreas divisum) or acquired due to abdominal trauma, duct sphincters, pseudocysts or periampullary tumours

Clinical features

- Persistent abdominal pain
  - Mostly in the epigastric area
  - Radiate to the back
  - Relieved by sitting forwards
  - May be intermittent (precipitated by alcohol) or continuous
  - May be very severe
- Diarrhoea and weight loss due to fear of eating (because of exacerbation of pain after eating) and steatorrhoea
- Features of exocrine pancreatic failure
  - Steatorrhoea: present in 50% of patients. Reduced in patients with a low-fat diet
  - Diabetes: present in about a third of patients. A late feature due to B-cell destruction
- Obstructive jaundice may be present if the common bile duct is obstructed. On examination there is usually epigastric tenderness

Differential diagnosis

The main differential diagnosis is pancreatic carcinoma, but it can be very difficult to distinguish between these. Imaging and endoscopy may help.

Investigations

- **Bloods**
  - Serum amylase is usually normal but may be slightly raised – insufficient pancreatic tissue to cause a large rise
  - Blood glucose may be increased, reflecting endocrine dysfunction
  - Serum calcium may be raised
- **Radiology**
  - Abdominal X-ray: may reveal calcification of the pancreas or calculi
  - US: performed percutaneously or endoscopically. May reveal gallstones, pancreatic morphology and duct dilatation
  - CT scan: reveals structural changes to the pancreas as well as cysts and is mainly used in looking for complications and planning surgical or endoscopic intervention
  - ERCP is the investigation of choice and may demonstrate dilatation of the pancreatic duct system in the early stages. Duct stricture and alternating dilatation with 'chain of lakes' appearance are found in late stages of the disease
  - MRCP helps with imaging of the pancreas and biliary tree

Management

Underlying cause (which in most cases is alcohol) should be identified. Complete alcohol abstinence is required. Conservative medical management is preferred, although surgical intervention is indicated in some instances, including for intractable pain. Surgery is inappropriate, however, in cases of necrotic pancreas and with continuing alcohol consumption.

- **Medical**
  - Analgesia: codeine and pethidine are often used, with steps taken to guard against narcotic habituation. Abstinence from alcohol is also important in pain relief, particularly in the initial stages of the disease
  - Supplements for endocrine insufficiency:
    - Oral supplements of fat-soluble vitamins (A, D, E, K) and vitamin B_{12}
    - Insulin or oral hypoglycaemic therapy
  - Supplements for exocrine insufficiency:
    - Diet: low in fat and high in protein and carbohydrate
    - Pancreatic enzyme supplements (Creon®)

- Surgical
  - Indications for surgery include:
    - o Pancreatic duct dilation: drainage by anastomosing a Roux loop of ileum to the distal end of the duct or longitudinal pancreatojejunostomy
    - o Localised inflammation of the pancreas (as determined by ERCP): partial resection
    - o Pseudocyst or abscess: percutaneous or surgical drainage
    - o Islet cell autotransplantation after pancreatectomy

Complications

May be divided into local and systemic (Box 4.11).

Box 4.11: Complications of chronic pancreatitis

Local	Systemic
Pancreatic pseudocyst	Diabetes mellitus
Pancreatic abscess	Steatorrhoea
Pancreatic ascites	Narcotic dependency
Pancreatic carcinoma	

4.8.3 Pancreatic pseudocyst

Aetiology

Pancreatic pseudocyst is a localised collection of pancreatic enzymes, inflammatory fluid and tissue debris enclosed in the lesser sac. It is therefore not a true cyst lined by epithelial tissue. Pseudocysts are formed by pancreatic secretions escaping from the damaged duct system and usually occur as a complication of pancreatitis. Continuing communication with the pancreatic duct results in persistence of the pseudocyst.

Clinical features

A pseudocyst is suspected when an acute attack of pancreatitis fails to resolve within 2 weeks, with one or more of the following features:

- Continuing epigastric pain and fullness
- Nausea and vomiting
- Weight loss
- Systemic evidence of cyst infection: fever, rigors, increased WCC
- Serum amylase or lipase remains elevated
- In cases of large cysts, a mass maybe palpable above the umbilicus that is classically:
  - Tender
  - Fixed
  - Tense

Investigations

- Bloods
  - WCC, amylase, CRP
- Imaging
  - Ideally CT, but also US can be used to confirm the presence, size and position of a pseudocyst

Management

Management depends on the size of the cyst. Those less than 5 cm may be managed expectantly with follow-up by serial ultrasounds for up to 6 months provided they are asymptomatic. If still unresolved, surgical intervention is undertaken.

For larger cysts, CT- or ultrasound-guided percutaneous drainage can be undertaken although reccurrence rates are high. More often, laparoscopic surgery consisting of internal drainage of the cyst into the stomach (cystogastrostomy) is undertaken at 6 weeks, by which time the wall of the cyst has thickened enough to hold sutures.

4.8.4 Carcinoma of the pancreas

Pathology

Histologically, pancreatic cancers mostly arise from the exocrine ductal epithelium lining the ductal system and are therefore adenocarcinomas. Some 70% arise in the head of the gland and 30% in the body or tail (in proportion to the tissue size of each part of the pancreas).

They are regarded as highly malignant, with:

- Direct invasion of
  - Pancreatic duct and common bile duct, causing obstructive jaundice
  - Duodenum, causing bleeding
  - Portal vein, causing portal vein thrombosis, portal hypertension and ascites
- Early metastases via:
  - Lymphatics: to adjacent and distant nodes, including nodes in the celiac axis and porta hepatis
  - Bloodstream: to the liver via the portal vein and then to the lungs
  - Trans-coelomic: to the peritoneum with peritoneal seeding

They are usually inoperable when the diagnosis is made.

Epidemiology

- Pancreatic cancer mainly affects the elderly, presenting at a mean age of 65 and is rare under the age of 50 years.

- It is third commonest cancer of the GI tract after colon and stomach cancers
- Sixth most common cause of cancer-related death
- Has an annual incidence of 1 in 10 000 in UK and is rising

Aetiology
Chronic pancreatitis is a substantial risk factor. Others include smoking, alcohol and diabetes mellitus.

Clinical features
Pancreatic cancer is usually asymptomatic in the initial stages; and inoperable at the time of diagnosis. Pain is often the first symptom in distal cancers (body and tail), while painless obstructive jaundice is classically seen in cancer of the head of pancreas.

- **Pain**
  - Mainly a feature of tumours in the body and tail
  - In the epigastrium
  - Dull in nature
  - Radiating to the back
  - Relieved by sitting forwards
  - Severe pain is indicative of retroperitoneal invasion with involvement of the splanchnic nerve plexus
- **Painless obstructive jaundice**
  - Mainly a feature of cancers of the head of the pancreas and ampulla of Vater
  - Due to obstruction of the head of the main pancreatic duct at the head of the pancreas
  - With dark urine, pale stools and pruritus
  - With tumour progression pain may become a feature

Other common features include:

- Anorexia and significant weight loss, which is partly due to early satiety and partly due to exocrine insufficiency caused by obstruction of the pancreatic duct
- Malaise, nausea, fatigue
- Pruritus
- Epigastric bloating and change in bowel habit
- Haematemesis and melaena indicate metastasis to the duodenal mucosa
- Steatorrhoea and diabetes in cases of pancreatic duct obstruction
- Recent-onset diabetes in the elderly should raise suspicion

Examination may reveal:

- Jaundiced and palpable gallbladder
  - According to Courvoisier's law, a palpable gallbladder in the presence of painless jaundice is unlikely to be caused by gallstones
- Epigastric mass (not gallbladder)

- Epigastric tenderness
- Hepatomegaly, splenomegaly, lymphadenopathy and ascites in late-stage disease
- Migratory thrombophlebitis (Trousseau's sign) characterised by recurrent superficial venous thrombosis and crops of tender nodules in the veins may also be present

Investigations
- **Bloods**
  - LFTs: evidence of obstructive jaundice with raised bilirubin and alkaline phosphatase
  - Tumour markers: CA 19-9 has a high sensitivity (80%) but low specificity
- **US:** detects dilated bile ducts and stones, as well as masses in the pancreas and liver
- **ERCP:** demonstrates biliary and pancreatic duct anatomy and sites of obstruction and may be used to obtain a sample for cytology when diagnosis is uncertain
- **CT:** Most reliable method of diagnosis and necessary before possible surgical intervention. Gives information on pancreatic structure, involvement of vasculature, lymph nodes and adjacent organs (eg liver)
- **MRI and MRCP:** used in a minority of patients to further define the tumour stage

Management
In the majority of patients, management is palliative and aimed at:

- Jaundice and pruritus: by placing a stent through the tumour trans-hepatically or via ERCP
- Vomiting (due to duodenal involvement): bypass surgery via gastrojejunostomy
- Pain control: upload analgesics, coeliac axis block, radiotherapy

Curative **surgical intervention** is only a possibility in those with an early resectable periampullary cancer with no local advancement. The procedure for cancer of the head of pancreas is a pancreaticoduodenectomy (Whipple's operation) as follows (Figure 4.11):

- Resection of:
  - Pancreatic head
  - Duodenum
  - Distal half of the stomach
  - Lower common bile duct
  - Gallbladder
  - Upper jejunum
  - Regional lymph nodes

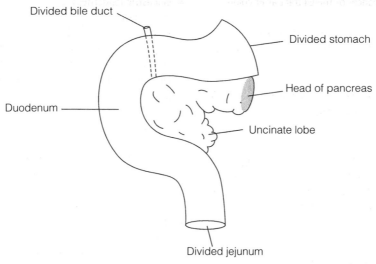

Divided bile duct

Divided stomach

Head of pancreas

Duodenum

Uncinate lobe

Divided jejunum

Resected specimen

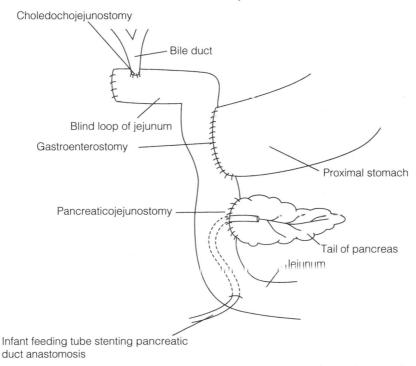

Choledochojejunostomy

Bile duct

Blind loop of jejunum

Gastroenterostomy

Proximal stomach

Pancreaticojejunostomy

Tail of pancreas

Jejunum

Infant feeding tube stenting pancreatic
duct anastomosis

Figure 4.11: Whipple's operation

- Anastomoses of the common bile duct
  (cholecystojejunostomy) and residual pancreas
  (pancreaticojejunostomy) to a segment of small bowel
- Gastrojejunostomy

In contrast, surgery of cancers of the tail of the pancreas
involves a pancreaticosplenectomy.

Only 20% of cancers are operable, and even after operation the
prognosis remains poor with a 5-year survival of around 15%.
Survival is improved with chemotherapy using 5-fluorouracil
and radiotherapy.

4.8.5 Endocrine tumours of the pancreas

Endocrine tumours of the pancreas are covered more extensively in Chapter 8.

They are touched on briefly in this section for the sake of completion of pancreatic disorders. In general, endocrine tumours of the pancreas are:

- Rare tumours (incidence of less than 1 in 100 000) that arise from the islet cells of the pancreas
- Capable of producing hormones and polypeptides according to their cell type of origin
- Since islet cells are all derived from APUD (amine precursor uptake and decarboxylation) cells, these tumours are often called 'APUDomas'
- Endocrine tumours can be benign or malignant. However, even when malignant these tumours are slow-growing and metastasise late in comparison with pancreatic adenocarcinomas; they are therefore usually amenable to curative surgical resection
- The most important clinical syndromes associated with these are insulinoma and gastrinoma (Zollinger–Ellison syndrome) associated with overproduction of insulin and gastrin respectively
- Around 25% are associated with other endocrine tumours as part of a multiple endocrine neoplasia type 1 (MEN1)

4.9 THE SPLEEN

The spleen deserves special mention as its disorders may fall within the realm of a general surgeon's practice. The spleen is an immunological organ and is the largest single lymphoid organ in the body. It sits tucked away within the left upper quadrant of the abdomen and can become enlarged due to a number of diseases.

4.9.1 Functions of the spleen

- Immune – antigen processing, IgM production
- Filtering – macrophages remove cellular and non-cellular material, including capsulated organisms
- Haemopoiesis – fetal haemopoiesis and also later in life if necessary
- Platelet pooling
- Iron reutilisation

There are four main topics to consider when learning about the spleen in relation to surgical practice. They include:

- Splenomegaly
- Splenic rupture
- Splenectomy
- Post-splenectomy features

4.9.2 Splenomegaly

The spleen must be enlarged to at least three times its normal size before it is clinically palpable. It normally descends towards the right iliac fossa as it enlarges. It is dull to percussion clinically, moves with respiration, and it may be possible to feel a notched edge in very large spleens.

Causes of splenomegaly are listed below by the initiating pathological process.

- Infection
  - Bacterial – TB, typhoid, typhus, septicaemia
  - Spirochaetal – syphilis, leptospirosis
  - Viral – glandular fever
  - Protozoal – malaria, kala-azar
- Cellular infiltration
  - Amyloidosis
  - Gaucher's disease
- Collagen disease
  - Felty's syndrome
  - Still's disease
- Autoimmune disorders
  - Rheumatoid arthritis
  - Systemic lupus erythematosus
- Cellular proliferation
  - Leukaemia
  - Pernicious anaemia
  - Polycythaemia rubra vera
  - Spherocytosis
  - Thrombocytopenic purpura
  - Myelofibrosis
- Congestion
  - Portal hypertension
  - Hepatic vein obstruction
  - Congestive cardiac failure
- Infarction
  - Emboli
  - Splenic vein or artery thrombosis
- Space-occupying lesions
  - Cysts
  - Lymphoma
  - Angioma
  - Lymphosarcoma

Essential note

Hypersplenism is defined as splenomegaly with associated anaemia, leukopenia, or thrombocytosis. There is compensatory hyperplasia of the bone-marrow

4.9.3 Splenic rupture

Splenic rupture usually occurs following blunt trauma to the abdomen. The risk is increased in any condition which results in splenomegaly. Spontaneous rupture or rupture with minimal trauma has been reported in cases of massive splenomegaly (including glandular fever).

Clinical features

Patients will often present with left upper quadrant, epigastric, or generalised abdominal pain. This will progress to peritonitis and shock with resulting blood loss. Diagnosis can be clinical or radiological if the patient manages to get a scan. In any patient with shock and peritonitis, an urgent laparotomy is required at which time the diagnosis is made.

Management

Initial treatment involves immediate resuscitation with fluids, oxygen, and blood in the presence of developing shock. Definitive treatment is with an urgent splenectomy in the operating theatre.

4.9.4 Splenectomy

A spleen will need to be removed for a variety of clinical reasons. Emergency splenectomy (unplanned) is usually performed for trauma, iatrogenic reasons, or spontaneous splenic rupture. The remaining indications are for elective splenectomy and can usually be performed via the open or laparoscopic approach depending on the size of the spleen and indication for removal.

Indications for splenectomy:

- Trauma
  - Blunt abdominal trauma
  - Operative trauma (eg colectomy)
  - Spontaneous rupture
- Neoplastic/staging
  - Lymphomas
  - Chronic leukaemias
  - With gastrectomy for stomach cancers
  - With distal pancreatectomy
  - Unexplained splenomegaly
- Hypersplenism
  - Haemolytic anaemias
  - Idiopathic thrombocytopenic purpura
  - Neutropenia
  - Tropical splenomegaly
  - Myelofibrosis
- Portal decompression
  - Bleeding varices with splenic vein thrombosis
  - Splenorenal shunt

- Infections
  - TB, hydatid cyst, splenic abscess
- Others
  - Splenic artery aneurysm
  - Splenic cyst

Post-splenectomy features

Although the spleen is not an essential organ, its removal results in notable features within the body.

The effects of splenectomy include:

- **Haematological**
  - Raised platelet count (thrombocytosis)
  - Raised white cell count (leucocytosis)
  - Blood film differences
    - Heinz bodies = denatured Hb
    - Howell–Jolly bodies = nucleus remnants
    - Pappenheimer bodies = iron granules
- **Immunological**
  - Reduced opsonisation and antibody production
  - Increased risk of malaria in endemic regions
  - Increased infections with capsulated organisms
    - *Streptococcus pneumoniae*
    - *Haemophilus influenzae*
    - *Neisseria* species

4.9.5 Management of patients after splenectomy

The effects above indicate that patients undergoing splenectomy are at risk of infections from capsulated organisms. Effort should be made to prevent infections from these organisms and to continue this prophylaxis in the long term.

In elective cases (especially young children), vaccination against pneumococcal infections should be given. Prophylactic penicillin or amoxicillin should also be given for at least 2 years or until the age of 15 and not lifelong. Vaccinations should also be given post-operatively with Pneumovax, Hib, and meningococcal vaccine, with boosters given every 5 years. Malaria prophylaxis is required. All patients should commence amoxicillin at the first sign of febrile illness. In cases of trauma, it is not usually possible to administer pre-operative vaccinations. Vaccinations should be given shortly after the operation. Long-term antibiotic prophylaxis post-splenectomy in older patients remains a debated topic and administration depends on local guidelines and clinical practice.

Abdominal surgery

4.10.1 Anatomy and physiology of the large bowel

Anatomy

The large bowel (colon and rectum) is approximately 1.5 metres in length. It is a continuous lumen connecting the small bowel to the anus. Its main function is the absorption of water.

It is subdivided as follows.

- **Caecum:** A pouch into which the small bowel plugs and from which the ascending colon emerges. At the junction of the small and large bowel is the ileocaecal valve. This is considered the start point of the large bowel. The blood supply is the ileocolic artery and branches of the right colic artery and vein. The appendix is attached to the caecum and supplied by the appendicular artery, which is a branch of the ileocolic artery from the superior mesenteric artery.
- **Ascending colon:** Arises from the caecum, although it is narrower in diameter. Typically it measures about 12–14 cm in length. The blood supply is mainly from the right colic artery and vein. It is fixed in the posterior abdominal wall by peritoneum in over 90% of people. It ascends to the liver and then turns sharply at the hepatic flexure where it becomes the transverse colon.
- **Transverse colon:** This is the longest, most mobile part of the colon. It hangs fixed at the hepatic and splenic flexures. It turns sharply at the underside of the spleen (splenic flexure) and becomes the descending colon. The blood supply is mainly by branches of the middle colic artery and vein. The watershed area at the distal part of the transverse colon is where the blood supply of the superior mesenteric artery ends and the inferior mesenteric artery begins. They do, however, anastomose via the marginal artery of Drummond.
- **Descending colon:** The descending colon is covered anteriorly by peritoneum and posteriorly attached to loose areolar tissue. It is retroperitoneal, like the ascending colon. The transverse colon and sigmoid colon are intraperitoneal structures. It turns medially at the inferior pole of the kidney and becomes the sigmoid at the level of the iliac crest.
- **Sigmoid colon:** This is another loose mobile section of large bowel held by its mesocolon. It averages about 40 cm in length. Due to its mobility it usually lies within the pelvis although it can deviate into the abdomen. It is roughly S-shaped (hence the name) and curves back on itself anterior to the sacrum before culminating in the rectum.
- **Rectum:** A fairly straight section of bowel, 15 cm in length, in the pelvis, terminating at the anus. It is the same calibre as the sigmoid at its commencement and dilates just above the anus (rectal ampulla). This acts as a reservoir for stool with receptors that are stimulated by stretch.
- **Anal canal:** Leads to the anus, the external opening of the bowel. It is 2.4–4 cm in length. Two sphincters prevent faecal leakage. The smooth muscle, which peristalses the faeces along, forms the internal sphincter and the external sphincter which is voluntary muscle. The dentate line (also referred to as the pectinate line) delineates the rectum from the anal canal. Above this line, stretch can be perceived but pain fibres end. The histology also changes from squamous epithelium below the line to mucosal glandular epithelium above the line.

Physiology

The colon has three main functions:

- The absorption of water and electrolytes
- Storing and controlling the excretion of faeces
- Further digestion and absorption of food

Its presence is not crucial to survival.

There are five main layers: the mucosa, submucosa, circular muscle and longitudinal muscle, and serosa.

The mucosa is a smooth surface compared with the villous covering on the small-bowel mucosa. There are numerous crypts containing goblet cells which secrete mucus into the lumen.

The haustrae denoted on radiographs result from circular muscle contractions. The haustrae are not circumferential like the valvulae conniventes on the small bowel due to the presence of the taeniae coli, which are the longitudinal muscles of the colon running from the caecum to the rectum where they fuse to form an outer muscular layer.

The colon is innervated by the autonomic nervous system (vagal) and the enteric nervous system. The nerves in these circuits modulate motility, secretion, blood flow and, indirectly, immune responses.

Colonic transit occurs via a combination of:

- Haustral churning – the longitudinal and transverse contraction help move the faecal matter forwards, creating larger masses and aiding fluid extraction
- Peristalsis – coordinated movements of the interior and exterior muscles produce a wave motion along the length of the colon
- Mass migratory reflex – food in the stomach initiates a reflex in the colon that propels faeces into the rectum

- Voluntary abdominal effort – coordinated contraction and relaxation of abdominal and pelvic floor muscles to allow defecation

Clinical features of colorectal disease

Colorectal disease may present with one of many features. A change in bowel habit with diarrhoea or constipation is the commonest symptom. Other common symptoms include rectal bleeding, abdominal pain, local anal symptoms, or systemic symptoms such as weight loss and anaemia. Recognition of symptom patterns in association with appropriate investigation will help lead to a diagnosis and initiate management. The next section on investigations allows a sensible approach to investigating the commonest and most alarming of colorectal complaints.

Investigations of rectal bleeding

After a thorough history and examination the most appropriate investigations must be chosen.

Blood tests

These include a full blood count to check for anaemia and neutrophilia, urea and electrolytes and liver function tests. An ESR and CRP are useful to check for inflammatory changes. Thyroid function tests and calcium may be checked if there is associated change in bowel habit.

Stool

Faecal occult blood (requires a stool sample) when looking for evidence of blood in the stool when not macroscopically evident.

Direct visualisation

Proctoscopy and rigid sigmoidoscopy can be performed in the Outpatient department. A **proctoscopy** allows visualisation of haemorrhoids, fissures, fistulas and polyps/low rectal tumours. This also allows haemorrhoids to be banded or injected. **Rigid sigmoidoscopy** can be used to assess the distal 20 cm of the bowel for inflammation or growths.

The following tests usually require booking and must be marked 'urgent' if cancer is suspected or if a quick result is required for any clinical reason:

- **Flexible sigmoidoscopy** – allows camera examination to the level of the splenic flexure. This can be combined with a barium enema to image the rest of the large bowel.
- **Colonoscopy** – allows full visualisation of the large bowel. This is a useful technique for detecting polyps, cancers, diverticular disease and inflammatory bowel disease. It also allows confirmation by biopsy of any pathology.

- Upper GI endoscopy (OGD) is important as upper GI bleeds may account for melaena or fresh rectal blood if the bleeding is torrential.

Scans

Barium enema is a useful tool for identifying papular lesions in the bowel and intimal thickening denoting inflammation as well as diverticular disease. In patients where the clinical suspicion of colorectal cancer is low it is a useful method of imaging the bowel. In those more at risk, a colonoscopy is more sensitive and also allows biopsies to be taken.

CT scans are useful for imaging pelvic and abdominal bowel pathology. Mucosal thickening denoting inflammation as well as fat streaking may be demonstrated. Masses can be identified as well as transition points in bowel obstruction.

MRI may be performed when looking at the extent of rectal tumours to determine the local invasion and to plan surgery.

Mesenteric angiography allows you to detect using contrast injection bleeds of a reasonable rate. It also allows for treatment via selective embolisation.

Plain abdominal X-ray would not normally be an investigation of choice in patients with PR bleeding but featureless inflamed bowel or toxic megacolon may be identified.

Positron emission tomography (PET) scans are the gold standard for looking for recurrence.

Capsule enteroscopy entails the patient being prepped and swallowing a capsule that transmits a video image as it passes through the GI tract.

Red cell scintigraphy allows detection of slower bleeds in the GI tract.

Investigation of diarrhoea

- A thorough history including recent travel and dietary intake and a clinical examination are required.
- The appropriate blood tests should be taken as above for rectal bleeding and a stool sample for microscopy, culture and sensitivity.
- Where there has been a history of bloody diarrhoea or diarrhoea with mucus, inflammatory bowel disease must be considered, especially in younger patients with a first episode or a relapsing remitting course of disease progression.
- With chronic change in bowel habit, towards diarrhoea or constipation, malignancy must be excluded, especially in those over 45 years of age. This would warrant a colonoscopy or at the very least a flexible sigmoidoscopy and barium enema.

- A strong family history of colorectal cancer also warrants colonoscopy. Current guidelines state that patients with first-degree relatives under the age of 60 or multiple relatives with colorectal cancer should be screened from 10 years prior to the age of diagnosis in their relatives.

Investigation of constipation

- A full history and examination must be performed.
- A faecal occult blood and blood tests such as FBC, electrolytes, Ca^{2+}, thyroid and liver function tests should be performed.
- If no cause is evident or the patient is over the age of 45, an initial colonoscopy or barium enema should be performed to exclude a cancer.
- The investigation of constipation can lead to complex electrophysiological tests and bowel transit studies if barium enemas and colonoscopy are normal. A malignancy must be excluded with confidence before entertaining other diagnoses in patients with chronic symptoms.

Investigation of faecal incontinence

- A careful history including an obstetrics and gynaecology history must be taken in women with faecal incontinence as well as a detailed sexual history.
- Barium enema is not likely to give much useful information as they will be unlikely to retain the barium.
- Colonoscopy may reveal the pathology.
- In those cases where it does not, the following investigations may be useful. It is not expected that you will need to know much about the following investigations as they are only carried out at specialist centres but it is always good to have an awareness that they exist:
  - Endoanal ultrasound – looks at both internal and external sphincters
  - Electrophysiology studies – looks at mucosal electrosensitivity and nerve conduction
  - Defecating scintography – barium is excreted under fluoroscopy and conditions such as a rectocoele or rectal prolapse may be detected.

4.10.2 Acute appendicitis

Acute appendicitis is one of the commonest surgical emergencies and affects 8.6% of males and 6.7% of females in a lifetime. Appendicitis is also one of the only inflammatory surgical conditions that requires an operation to treat it at the first time of presentation if the diagnosis is confirmed.

Anatomy

The appendix appears during the fifth month of gestation and runs into a serosal sheet of peritoneum (mesoappendix). Within the mesoappendix is the appendicular artery, which is derived from the ileocolic artery. Sometimes, an accessory appendicular artery (derived from the posterior caecal artery) may be found.

Macroscopically: wormlike extension of the caecum, approximately 8–10 cm. The course and position of the appendix may vary widely, accounting for non-specific signs and symptoms of appendicitis. Its locations include the retroperitoneal space; the pelvis; or behind the terminal ileum, caecum, ascending colon, or liver.

Microscopically: its wall has an inner mucosal layer, two muscular layers (an inner muscular layer which is circular, and an outer layer which is longitudinal and derives from the taeniae coli), and a serosa. Several lymphoid follicles are scattered in its mucosa, the number of which increases as individuals age from 8 to 20 years.

Aetiology

Obstruction of the appendiceal lumen.

- Lymphoid hyperplasia
  - Inflammatory bowel disease, eg Crohn's disease
  - Infections (more common during childhood and in young adults), eg measles, mononucleosis, GI and respiratory infections
  - Faecal stasis
- Faecalith (more common in elderly patients) – solid bodies within the appendix that form after precipitation of calcium salts and undigested fibre in a matrix of dehydrated faecal material
- Parasites (especially in Eastern countries, eg amoebiasis)
- Foreign bodies and neoplasms (increased incidence in elderly)

Epidemiology

- Incidence: 7% in European populations. Incidences lower in third-world countries because of their dietary fibre intake
- Age: highest incidence during second and third decades of life
- Sex: M/F 1.5/1

Pathophysiology

Obstruction is believed to cause increased luminal pressure resulting in a continuous secretion of fluids and mucus from the mucosa and stagnant material. The appendiceal bacteria multiply, leading to an inflammatory response.

Persisting obstruction causes venous congestion and, as a consequence, appendiceal wall ischaemia begins, resulting in a loss of epithelial integrity and allowing bacterial invasion of the appendiceal wall.

This localised condition can worsen as a result of thrombosis of the appendicular artery and veins, leading to perforation and gangrene of the appendix, such that a periappendicular abscess or peritonitis occurs.

Clinical features
- **Symptoms**
  - Site – initially periumbilical or epigastric
  - Onset – initially of gradual onset, but can occasionally be sudden
  - Character – dull pain later becoming sharp
  - Radiation – pain later migrating to the right iliac fossa (RIF)
  - Associated with nausea, vomiting, anorexia; change in bowel habit possible
  - Timing becomes constant as disease progresses
  - Usually patients are lying down, flexing their hips, and drawing their knees up to reduce movements and to avoid worsening the pain

In addition to recording the history of the abdominal pain, obtain a complete summary of the recent personal history surrounding gastroenterological, genitourinary and respiratory conditions. Also consider gynaecological history in female patients.

- **Signs**
  - **Observation:** ↑T, tachycardia, unwell
  - **Inspection:** positive cough test (increasing pain with cough), lying still, knees drawn up
  - **Palpation**
    - Guarding (may or may not be present)
    - Tenderness at McBurney's point (situated one-third of the way along a line drawn between the anterior superior iliac spine and the umbilicus)
    - Rebound tenderness related to peritoneal irritation elicited by deep palpation with quick release
    - Positive Rovsing's sign (when pressing LIF, pain in RIF > LIF)
  - **Percuss:** percussion tenderness (peritonitis)
  - **Auscultate:** bowel sounds normal/reduced
  - **DRE:** right-sided tenderness
  - **VE:** exclude salpingitis (positive cervical excitation)

Patients with atypical anatomy may not show this classic clinical picture of appendicitis. Patients with this condition usually have accessory signs:

- **Obturator sign:** internal rotation of the thigh elicits pain (pelvic appendicitis)
- **Psoas sign:** extension of the right thigh elicits pain (retroperitoneal or retrocaecal appendicitis)

Differential diagnosis

Males and females
- Any -itis, eg inflammatory bowel disease, Meckel's diverticulitis, mesenteric lymphadenitis, gastroenteritis, enterocolitis, pancreatitis
- UTI
- Aortic abdominal artery dissection

Females
- Salpingitis
- Ectopic pregnancy
- Ovarian cyst or torsion
- PID
- Torsion of pedunculated fibroid

Investigations
- **Bloods:** FBC, U&E, LFT, CRP
- **Urinalysis:** dipstick, MC+S, pregnancy test (βhCG)
- **Radiology:** USS (transabdominal ± transvaginal), AXR (plain), CT abdomen
- **Diagnostic laparoscopy:** to confirm the diagnosis in selected cases (eg infants, elderly patients, female patients) where clinical picture is not clear

Management
- **Conservative:** IV fluids + NBM
- **Medical:** appendicectomy remains the only curative treatment for appendicitis
  - **Antibiotics,** eg cefuroxime (aerobic cover) and metronidazole (anaerobic cover)
  - **Analgesic,** eg paracetamol, tramadol, Oramorph® (prn)
  - **Antiemetic,** eg cyclizine
- **Surgical**
  - Laparoscopic appendicectomy
  - Open appendicectomy
  - Midline laparotomy – in elderly patients in case of caecal pathology necessitating right hemicolectomy

Complications
- **Pre-operative**
  - **Appendix mass:** inflamed appendix covered by omentum
  - **Appendix abscess:** patient becomes more toxic (↑↑WCC), swinging pyrexia
  - **Appendiceal perforation:** features of peritonitis and shock
  - **Bowel obstruction** (from extrinsic mass compression)
- **Post-operative:** infection (pelvic or other abscess), bleeding, DVT/PE, wound infections and wound dehiscence

Follow-up

Usually no further follow-up after discharge, unless complicated post-operatively.

Prognosis

Prognosis is excellent provided treatment is given. Post-operative adhesions or adhesions from infections may cause future bowel obstruction.

- **Mortality**
  - No mortality has been reported in patients with a non-perforated appendix
  - Mortality rate is <1% if appendiceal perforation exists, except in elderly patients, who have a mortality rate that approaches 5%
  - Fetal mortality risk increases significantly in pregnant women with a perforated appendicitis
- **Morbidity:** complications account for an average morbidity near 10%

4.10.3 Inflammatory bowel disease

The aetiology of both Crohn's and ulcerative colitis (UC) is unknown (Table 4.5). There are several theories and there is some evidence that genetics may play a role as well as dietary, infective, environmental and immune factors. Unfortunately as we still know very little about the aetiology of these conditions most treatments are aimed at symptoms rather than cure.

Crohn's disease

Clinical features

- Crohn's is an autoimmune inflammatory condition mainly affecting the bowel.
- Most commonly found in the terminal ileum.
- Can affect anywhere in GI tract from mouth to anus.
- May be confined to the large bowel or the large and small bowel.
- Diarrhoea, malabsorption, rectal bleeding, mucus PR, weight loss, fever are common symptoms.
- Ulceration of the mouth, abdominal tenderness, anal/perianal lesions, clubbing and signs of weight loss/malabsorption are associated signs.
- Strictures can cause subacute/acute bowel obstruction.
- Abscesses and fistulation are a part of the disease process, especially in the perianal area, but these can be intra-abdominal as well.
- Extraintestinal/systemic manifestations include:
  - Erythema nodosum
  - Arthropathy
  - Conjunctivitis
  - Uveitis
  - Gallstones
  - Amyloidosis
  - Sacroiliitis.
- Perianal inflammation and multiple fistula-in-ano are also common.
- Surgery is often complicated by fistulas between bowel and skin/bladder/bowel/vagina.

Diagnosis

History and examination deliver clues to point towards inflammatory bowel disease but in order to diagnose the type, a biopsy is required of an inflamed area. These can be taken as rectal biopsies in clinic or more commonly when the patient undergoes flexible sigmoidoscopy or colonoscopy a series of biopsies may be made. Pathologists examine these for features of colitis and for features that point more towards a diagnosis of Crohn's, UC, infectious colitis or an indeterminate colitis. About 10% of patients never get a final diagnosis and are hence labelled as having an indeterminate colitis as many of the microscopic features of inflammation are common to both Crohn's and UC.

Features that point towards Crohn's include:

- Transmural inflammation of the bowel wall involving lymphocytes, macrophages and plasma cell invasion
- Skip lesions (unaffected areas between affected areas)
- Possible presence of granulomas and rose-thorn lesions

Treatment

- Sulfasalazine is often used to help maintain remission but is not curative.
- Azathioprine can also help maintain remission.
- Prednisolone foam enemas can help relieve local rectal symptoms.
- Oral prednisolone or budesonide may resolve flare-ups.
- If symptoms worsen, stronger immune suppressants are used and in the event of a severe flare-up IV hydrocortisone is administered and the patient is kept strictly nil by mouth.
- If there is no resolution on IV hydrocortisone and bowel rest or with toxic megacolon, a subtotal colectomy is performed and an end-ileostomy.
- Parks' pouch is not performed in Crohn's due to the significant risk of recurrence as well as sepsis and fistulation.
- In children there is a case for using enteral, elemental feeds or polymeric feeds instead of keeping them nil by mouth.
- There is no conclusive evidence that enteral feeds are as efficacious in bringing about remission in adults.

Ulcerative colitis

Clinical features

- UC is an inflammatory bowel disease.
- UC affects the large bowel with a relapsing and remitting pattern.
- The main features are abdominal pain, diarrhoea and bloody stools.
- UC also has systemic features such as: anaemia, jaundice, erythema nodosum (more common in Crohn's), clubbing, pyoderma gangrenosum, arthralgia and arthritis, episcleritis.
- Disease tends to start at the rectum.
- It affects a continuous area.
- It spreads contiguously and proximally.
- It is treated as though it is an autoimmune disease, though this is not necessarily the case.
- Dietary management has been shown to bring about some relief of symptoms but not to the extent of Crohn's disease.
- Histologically it has features of epithelial ulceration, oedema and bleeding as well as polymorphic neutrophils in the crypts.
- The condition predominantly affects caucasians though with a Western diet a greater number of Asians and Afro-Caribbeans are being diagnosed.
- There is no gender predisposition.
- Most present with symptoms aged 15–30 years, though there is a smaller peak in those aged 60–80 years.
- Most patients have mild disease (60%); moderate disease is found in about 30%; and 10% have severe disease involving more than six bloody stools per day, abdominal tenderness, fever, anaemia and leucocytosis.
- Complications may involve perforation, severe haemorrhage and toxic megacolon.

Diagnostic tests

Blood tests are useful in determining the disease activity. There are numerous scoring systems encompassing the patient's symptoms. The main tests are the Hb, which can drop due to blood loss or chronic disease, and the white cell count which tends to be elevated during flare-ups. The ESR and CRP also tend to be elevated during flare-ups. p-ANCA is positive in 80% of patients with UC and 20% of patients with Crohn's. This is of more use diagnostically than prognostically. Serum albumin may be low in colitic patients. Stool should be cultured to rule out infectious colitis and assayed for *Clostridium difficile* toxin. Micronutrients and vitamins may show low levels in both Crohn's and UC patients, particularly in Crohn's.

In terms of imaging:

- Plain abdominal X-ray may be useful to evaluate for obstruction or toxic megacolon.
- Barium enema may show strictures or mucosal abnormalities.
- Small-bowel follow through is useful for evaluating for small-bowel inflammation, which more supports a diagnosis of Crohn's than UC.
- CT scans of the abdomen and pelvis are useful for looking at mucosal thickening and mesenteric stranding implying inflammation, as well as signs of obstruction, abscesses or fistulas.
- MRI can be used to look for inflammatory changes.
- Radionuclide white cell scans can be used to demonstrate small-bowel inflammation to differentiate Crohn's from UC.
- The gold standard is colonoscopy with biopsy, which allows us to evaluate the extent and severity of the disease and diagnose the type of colitis.

Treatment

- For UC, sulfasalazine is often used to help maintain remission, but is not curative.
- Oral corticosteroids may resolve flare-ups.
- Immune-modulation agents such as azathioprine and 6-mercaptopurine can also help maintain remission.
- Prednisolone foam enemas can help relieve local rectal symptoms.
- If symptoms worsen, stronger immune suppressants are used and in the event of a severe flare-up IV hydrocortisone is administered and the patient is kept strictly nil by mouth.
- If there is no resolution on IV hydrocortisone and bowel rest or with toxic megacolon, a subtotal colectomy is performed and an end-ileostomy.
- Parks' pouch may be formed from the terminal ileum and a defunctioning ileostomy created as a second surgical stage.
- The final stage would be to close the ileostomy and continue to review the patient.
- Removal of the colon is seen as being almost curative. The rectum still needs surveillance as the risk of developing neoplasms is higher. Patients may also need a completion proctectomy if they develop pouchitis (a reasonably common problem) and if this cannot be controlled medically.
- Exclusion diets are less efficacious in ulcerative colitis than in Crohn's.

Table 4.5: Comparison of Crohn's and UC

	Crohn's	Ulcerative colitis
Histopathology	Granulomas	No granulomas
	Superficial ulcers	Deep ulcers
	Fibrosis	Crypt abscesses
	Involves full thickness of bowel wall	Involves mucosa only
Extraintestinal manifestations	Polyarthritis	Sacroiliitis
	Gallstones	Sclerosing cholangitis
Complications	Fistulas	Toxic megacolon
	Strictures = obstruction	Cancer
	Perianal disease	Strictures and fistulas rare
	Slightly increased risk of malignancy	Greatly increased risk of malignancy

4.10.4 Colorectal cancer

Colorectal cancer is the third most common cancer overall and the second most common cause of cancer-related death in the West. It is the commonest GI cancer in both men and women. It is thought to originate from a sequence of events which starts with inflammation, leading to dysplasia that can ultimately lead to neoplasm formation.

Epidemiology
- Second commonest cause of death from malignancy in the UK after lung cancer
- Third commonest cause of cancer overall
- Commonest GI cancer
- Geographic distribution
  - High incidence in Western Europe and America
  - Low incidence in Asia and Africa
- 95% of patients are over the age of 40
- Peak incidence in people aged 70–80
- Gender distribution is almost equal, with marginal F > M
- 75% of cases are sporadic and 24% of cases are genetic
- 1% of cases occur in patients with previous inflammatory bowel disease

Aetiology
Although the precise cause is unknown, several risk factors including genetic, environmental, and medical conditions are said to be associated with colorectal cancer.

Dietary risk factors
- Low-fibre diet
- High-fat diet
- High levels of bile acids (degraded into carcinogens)
- Previous cholecystectomy (not proved)

Medical risk factors
- Colonic polyps and villous adenomas
- Inflammatory bowel disease (UC >> Crohn's disease)
- Pelvic irradiation
- Ureterosigmoidostomy for urinary diversion

Genetic risk factors
- Familial adenomatous polyposis coli (FAP)
  - Autosomal dominant condition with *APC* gene on the long arm of chromosome 5 (5q21)
  - Characterised by multiple (hundreds to thousands) colonic adenomas and affects 1 in 10 000 births
  - Extracolonic manifestations include epidermoid cysts, retinal pigmentation, jaw osteomas, desmoid tumours and polyps within the stomach and duodenum
  - 100% of those affected will progress to colon cancer if left untreated within 20 years of adenomas developing
  - Treat with prophylactic colectomy
- Hereditary non-polyposis colon cancer (HNPCC)
  - Autosomal dominant inheritance due to mutation in repair genes
  - Associated with other cancers such as endometrial, ovarian, gastric, biliary, renal tract, brain and small-bowel cancer
  - Typically affects younger patients age <40 years and occurs with a very strong family history
- Other familial colon cancer

Colonic polyps
- Polyps are abnormal growths on the wall, usually of a mucous membrane.
- They tend to be either flat (sessile) or on a stalk (pedunculated).

- Polyps are extremely common and exist in as many as 15% of the adult population.
- They are usually asymptomatic but may present with rectal bleeding.
- They are usually discovered incidentally during endoscopic procedures or radiological investigations.
- Although they are usually benign below the size of 2.5 cm, they should be routinely removed as this reduces the risk of developing cancer in the future.
- Inherited polyposis syndromes include familial adenomatous polyposis, Peutz–Jeghers syndrome and familial polyposis coli.
- There are five main types of polyp:
  - Malignant polyps
  - Adenomatous polyps
  - Hamartomatous polyps
  - Hyperplastic polyps
  - Inflammatory polyps.
- The proposed theory for how polyps become malignant is called the adenoma–carcinoma sequence. It is a widely accepted theory for how adenomas, which are termed mild/moderate or severely dysplastic, may progress to carcinoma.

Distribution of cancer sites within the colon
According to figures published by Cancer Research UK (from 1997 to 2000):

- Rectum 29%
- Sigmoid 18%
- Caccum 13%
- Rectosigmoid junction 7%
- Ascending colon 5%
- Transverse colon 4%
- Hepatic flexure 2%
- Splenic flexure 2%
- Descending colon 2%
- Anus 2%
- Appendix 1%
- Unspecified 15%

Clinical features
- Change in bowel habit
  - Change in frequency
  - Change in stool consistency
  - Change in quality of stool
- PR bleeding (especially if the stool is mixed with blood or clots are present or blood is dark or altered, ie partly digested)
- Stools mixed with mucus
- Melaena (black tarry offensive stool)
- Tenesmus – feeling of incomplete evacuation
- Bowel obstruction (especially in left-sided colon cancers for large-bowel obstruction)

- Unexplained anaemia (especially in right-sided colon cancers)
- Abdominal mass (more in right-sided tumours)
- Weight loss
- Anorexia
- Weakness/asthenia
- Symptoms of secondary disease such as ascites, hepatomegaly, jaundice, effusions, bone pain
- Appendicitis (uncommon but caecal cancers can invade and obstruct the appendicular orifice)

Diagnosis
- A thorough history and examination is essential
- DRE – a good way to pick up large low rectal tumours or changes in stool with blood or mucus
- Faecal occult blood tests
- Endoscopy – flexible sigmoidoscopy can obtain views up to the splenic flexure and colonoscopy can intubate up to the caecum
- Double-contrast barium enema – a good method for polypoidal lesions but can miss flat tumours
- CT pneumocolon – alternative to colonoscopy or barium enema
- MRI is used in rectal cancers to evaluate the degree of tissue invasion (local metastases)
- Positron emission tomography (PET) is useful for looking for recurrent disease
- Transanal US – for staging rectal tumours, especially if being considered for local excision
- CT scan – for staging patients (chest, abdomen, and pelvis)

Complications of colorectal carcinomas
- Obstruction
  - Left-sided lesions >>> right-sided lesions
  - Left-sided lesions result in large bowel obstruction
  - Caecal lesions can cause small-bowel obstruction
- Perforation
  - May occur either through a carcinoma or proximal to it if there is obstruction
  - Occurs most commonly at the caecum if the ileocaecal valve is competent
- Fistula formation
  - Via direct invasion can result in colovesical, colo- or rectovaginal fistulas or others
- Haemorrhage
- Appendicitis
- Colo-colic intussusception

Abdominal surgery

Surgical management

For any cancer the aim is to resect the tumour fully and with a good clearance margin if possible. The aim is to remove the mesentery attached, along with the local lymph nodes and blood vessels. The tumour and nodes may then be examined microscopically to accurately grade and stage the tumour and determine the need for adjuvant therapy (radio/chemotherapy).

The types of surgery can be broadly classified (Figure 4.12) into:

- Right hemicolectomy – for right-sided cancers
- Extended right hemicolectomy – for transverse colon tumours up to the splenic flexure
- Left hemicolectomy – for left-sided tumours or high-sigmoid tumours

Right hemicolectomy

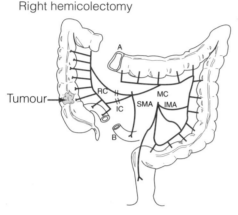

RC	Right colic artery
IC	Ileocolic artery
	Both divided for right hemicolectomy
	A is anastomosed to B
MC	Middle colic artery divided for extended right hemicolectomy
SMA	Superior mesenteric artery
IMA	Inferior mesenteric artery

Left hemicolectomy

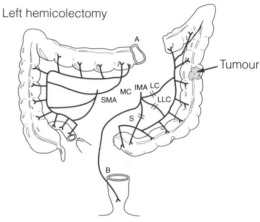

LC	Left colic artery
LLC	Lower left colic artery
S	Sigmoid artery
	All divided for left hemicolectomy
MC	Middle colic artery divided for extended left hemicolectomy

Sigmoid colectomy

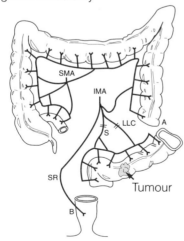

LLC	Lower left colic artery
S	Sigmoid artery
	Both usually divided for sigmoid colectomy
SR	Superior rectal artery
	Divided in anterior resection

Abdominoperineal excision of the rectum

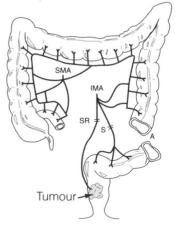

S	Sigmoid artery
SR	Superior rectal artery
	Divided for abdominoperineal exclusion of rectum

Figure 4.12: Large-bowel resection for cancer. A is anastomosed to B in each case.

- Sigmoid colectomy – for sigmoid tumours
- Anterior resection – for rectosigmoid to mid-rectal tumours
- Abdominoperineal excision (AP excision) – for low rectal and anal cancers

In each of these operations the affected bowel is removed and the remaining ends are brought together (anastomosed) either by sutures or staples. This is not possible in an AP excision however as the tumour is so low that the patient's rectum and anus are removed and sutured at the base. The patient is then left with an end-colostomy. In acute situations such as obstructing lesions or perforations, it may be necessary to perform the anastomosis as well as a defunctioning ileostomy. This is to protect the anastomosis from breaking down in the presence of oedema (in distended obstructed bowel) and infection (perforation).

Staging/grading

Duke's classification is one of the most commonly known staging methods. Duke originally described types A, B and C. D was later added, as were further subdivisions.

- **Duke A:** the cancer is confined to the bowel wall (83% 5-year survival rate)
- **Duke B:** the cancer has grown through the bowel wall (64% 5-year survival rate)
- **Duke C:** the cancer has spread to at least one lymph node (38% 5-year survival rate)
- **Duke D:** the cancer has spread with distant metastases (3% 5-year survival rate)

The other method of staging is the TNM system which has superseded Duke's system, but it is not necessary to learn its exact classification system at the undergraduate level.

Grading is performed by our pathologist colleagues when samples of tumour tissue are obtained by either biopsy or resection. This gives us further information on how aggressive the tumour is and helps guide our treatment of each individual.

Radiotherapy/chemotherapy

Radiotherapy and chemotherapy can be administered in many different ways.

The two main ways are as neoadjuvant for down-staging fixed and semi-fixed cancers pre-operatively and as adjuvant radiochemotherapy. Adjuvant therapy is usually given after surgery and after staging and grading have been done (if there is lymph node involvement or distant metastases).

Chemotherapy is indicated for Duke C tumours. The benefit in Duke B tumours is not clear yet. Chemotherapy consists of administering a 6-month course of 5-fluorouracil (5-FU) and folinic acid or a 1-week course of 5-FU administered by portal vein infusion.

Radiotherapy alone is usually used for rectal cancers rather than colon cancers as there is a well-defined anatomical location with less risk of bowel injury. It can reduce local recurrence rates by up to 40%, leading to a 6% improvement in 5-year survival rates. This may be given either pre- or post-operatively depending on the surgical and pathological indications.

Screening for cancers

Colonoscopy should be performed post-operatively in patients who have had colon cancers to screen for metachronous tumours. This should also be performed in patients with long-standing UC, patients with known adenomatous colonic polyps, and patients with familial cancer syndromes.

A strong family history of colorectal cancer also warrants colonoscopy. Current guidelines state that patients with first-degree relatives under the age of 60 or multiple relatives with colorectal cancer should be screened from 10 years prior to the age of diagnosis in their relatives.

Synchronicity

- **Synchronous** – two or more primary tumours diagnosed at the same time or within a defined period (usually 1–6 months) of each other. For this reason, the entire colon should be checked for synchronous tumours when resecting the primary lesion.
- **Metachronous** – a primary tumour diagnosed a defined period of time after another primary tumour was detected/resected.

Anal cancer

- Anal cancers are rare, with an incidence of 1 in 100 000, with 80% of them being squamous cell carcinomas.
- There is a strong association with human papillomavirus (HPV) and HIV.
- They are more commonly found in male homosexuals, people who practise anal sex and those with a history of genital warts.
- Patients are usually in their 50s or 60s and common presentations include bleeding, pain, swelling and ulceration. Occasionally, incontinence can occur if the sphincters are involved.
- Tumour spread occurs to the inguinal lymph nodes.
- Endoanal ultrasound and examination under anaesthesia may be required to assess the tumour, take biopsies, and plan for method of treatment.

- The mainstay of treatment is surgery and the results are very good, especially if detected early.
- Overall 5-year survival rate is 50%.
- Due to the location part of the anal sphincter often also needs to be removed, leading to faecal soiling. In order to avoid this, a colostomy may be needed for faecal diversion. Now, due to advances in radio/chemotherapy they can often be downsized to avoid the need for this and a local resection may be enough rather than an AP excision. Transanal resection and TEMS (transanal endoscopic microsurgery) has also played a role in reducing the extent of surgery. Chemotherapy mainly makes use of 5-FU and cisplatin in local disease and 5-FU, doxorubicin and capecitabine for metastatic disease.

Radiation proctitis

After radiotherapy for cervical, anal or prostate cancer, an inflammation of the bowel in the radiation field can ensue. This may occur in the acute or chronic phase and generally presents with diarrhoea or PR bleeding. The acute condition requires no treatment and usually settles over several months but the chronic form may require metronidazole, sucralfate or corticosteroids and may require surgery in the presence of obstructive or fistulating disease. Occasionally, a defunctioning stoma may be required to divert faeces from the inflamed area.

4.10.5 Benign anorectal disease

Anorectal fistulas

A fistula is an abnormal connection between two epithelial surfaces (usually lined by granulation tissue).

Fistulas can occur due to stand-alone conditions (such as inadequate or delayed treatment of abscesses) or due to systemic diseases such as Crohn's disease, TB, carcinomas and diverticular disease. Inflammatory bowel disease (especially Crohn's disease) is the most common cause of anorectal, entero-enteral and enterocutaneous fistulas. It is important in any fistula to treat the underlying condition to reduce the risk of recurrence.

Fistulas may occur as a result of infection. Abscesses can track through various planes, such as the intersphincteric plane or more commonly through the external sphincter to form an ischiorectal abscess.

SNAP is a useful acronym for remembering things that prevent fistulas from healing.

S – Sepsis: persistent infection may prevent healing

N – Nutrition: poorly nourished patients never heal as well as well-nourished ones

A – Anatomical obstruction: if there is a blockage of the fistula this predisposes to infection due to stasis and prevents healing

P – Persistent pathology: the underlying cause must be treated where possible to allow the best chance for healing and to reduce the risk of recurrence

Goodsall's rule (Fig 4.13a) is important in planning the management. Goodsall's rule states that if the external opening of a fistula is anterior to an imaginary transverse line between 3 o'clock and 9 o'clock it will communicate directly and radially to open internally in the nearest crypt. If the external opening is posterior to this line the internal opening is usually in the posterior midline via a curved tract. Exceptions exist when there are multiple openings and when the external opening is more than a few centimetres from the anal canal.

Stand-alone treatment of a fistula involves antibiotics and often surgical intervention. The type of surgery varies but the procedure would normally be to do an examination under anaesthetic first. If the fistula is a simple superficial fistula it can simply be laid open (a fistulotomy). If it is a deeper fistula involving the muscles of the sphincter a seton is placed to prevent closure, hence allowing pus to drain and preventing abscess formation (Fig 4.13b). Tight setons may also be placed and gradually tightened to cheese-wire through the sphincter and allow the sphincter to heal behind it, preventing faecal leakage.

Anal fissures

Anal fissures are tears which appear as cracks in the squamous layer of the anal canal. Fissures are a common cause of excruciating pain on defecation and rectal bleeding, especially in younger patients. They usually occur due to excessive straining and tend to heal spontaneously. However, constipated bowel habits and prolonged time straining on the toilet bowl do not help this occur. Conservative management, including an increase in fluid and fibre intake along with laxatives, aid healing and prevent recurrence. Most treatments for this are topical and there has been a move from using topical nitroglycerin to topical diltiazem cream in order to cause muscle relaxation and improve the local blood supply by inducing vasodilatation and hence improve healing times. A lateral sphincterotomy may be necessary after 3 months of twice-daily application if the fissure has not resolved (which approximately 80% have by this time). This usually involves a day-case procedure under general anaesthetic where a small cut is made in the internal sphincter on one side. The edges of the fissure can also be excised and freshened to allow healing. Deep fissures may involve the sphincters and care must be taken when operating in this area to be conservative as too large an incision may leave a patient with faecal incontinence.

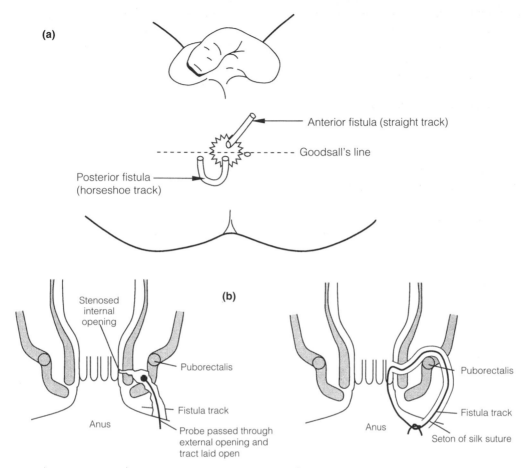

(a)

Anterior fistula (straight track)

Goodsall's line

Posterior fistula
(horseshoe track)

Stenosed
internal
opening

(b)

Puborectalis

Fistula track

Puborectalis

Anus

Fistula track

Anus

Seton of silk suture

Probe passed through
external opening and
tract laid open

Figure 4.13: a) Goodsall's rule b) Treatment of anorectal fistula with Seton

Ischiorectal/perianal abscess

Abscess – a localised collection of pus.

Abscesses in the perianal area are usually due to local infection of the epithelium of the anal canal, which can occur in a hair follicle or sebaceous gland. Normally the internal anal canal acts as a barrier to infection but this can be breached via the crypts of Morgagni. This way infection can enter the intersphincteric space and from here it can track out to adjacent spaces, including the ischiorectal, supralevator and the perianal spaces.

Patients present with perianal discomfort or pain exacerbated by movement, sitting and defecation. They also may present septic with a high temperature and tachycardia and neutrophilia. Examination reveals an erythematous, fluctuant, well-defined mass, sometimes indurated and pointing.

Treatment is by incision and drainage. Curettage and lavage are often performed before packing the wound. If the wound heals prematurely from above, an abscess will re-form. The packing allows the wound to heal from the bottom up. Antibiotics are required in severe cases where there may be a large area of surrounding cellulitis or in patients who are diabetic or immunosuppressed.

Pilonidal abscess/sinus

- Sinus – a blind-ending tract lined by epithelium.
- Pilonidal sinus is a chronic infection caused by ingrowth of hairs into the skin resulting in a sinus.
- Pilonidal literally means 'nest of hairs'.
- Pilonidal sinus disease is common in young adults aged 15–30.
- It is commonly found in hirsute people, truck drivers and those with a sedentary lifestyle (natal cleft) and hairdressers (between the fingers).
- Most commonly affects the area in the natal cleft about 5 cm above the anus (sacrococcygeal area).
- It is more common in this age category as after puberty sex hormones affect hair growth and the sebaceous glands.

- It is 3–4 times more common in males than females.
- The hair type is a known contributing factor, especially where it is a kinked hair type, with coarse growth and a fast rate of growth.
- The presumed aetiology is that keratin distends the hair follicle and occludes it causing oedema and stasis leading to folliculitis, which ruptures into the subcutaneous tissue forming a pilonidal abscess. This results in a sinus tract leading to a deep cavity.

Treatment

- For an abscess, incision and drainage with curetting to remove the debris and hair nests, followed by packing.
- If this is a recurrent problem many small pits will be visible for which an excision of the tracts is the most definitive procedure such as a Karydakis procedure. However, recurrence is still possible and patients are best advised to keep the area shaved.
- Complete en-bloc excision of the affected area with a local flap gives the best results.

Haemorrhoids

- Haemorrhoids are enlarged vascular cushions in the anorectal canal and **not** varicosities.
- About half the population has them at some time from mid-teens onwards.
- They are more common in pregnant women.
- They tend to bleed fresh bright-red blood, passed during defecation.
- They appear to be blue-red engorged swellings just inside the anus and are situated at the 3, 7, and 11 o'clock positions as related to the haemorrhoidal artery.
- They are not distinguishable by PR examination.
- External haemorrhoids are usually thrombosed piles, where a clot has formed inside one. These may be treated conservatively with ice packs and analgesia or by incision under local anaesthetic. They may eventually become external anal skin tags.
- Internal haemorrhoids are true haemorrhoids.
- They vary in grades of severity:
  - **Grade 1** – internal haemorrhoids are small swellings on the inside of the anal canal. They are not visible or palpable outside
  - **Grade 2** – visible on straining for defecation but reduce spontaneously
  - **Grade 3** – similar but larger and hang down but only return when introduced by a finger
  - **Grade 4** – permanently hang down and cannot be re-inserted.

Aetiology

The commonest cause is thought to be straining during bowel movements. Others include poor muscle synchronicity or tone and weak rectal vein walls or valves. Position may be a factor as the incidence is far lower in countries that use squat toilets rather than seated ones as this facilitates less straining. Portal hypertension can also be a factor.

Pregnancy, obesity and a sedentary lifestyle are also implicated as risk factors.

Poor diet can be a risk factor in terms of inadequate fibre and roughage intake, inadequate clear fluids or excessive coffee or alcohol. All of the above can lead to chronic diarrhoea or constipation, both of which are risk factors for haemorrhoid formation.

Prevention

Avoiding the modifiable risk factors above by means of reducing coffee and alcohol, increasing fibre and a good fluid intake help facilitate the easy passage of stool, reducing the risk of haemorrhoids. Limiting time on the toilet should be encouraged but the use of laxatives should not!

Examination

An abdominal examination and rectal examination should be performed. The digital rectal examination should aim to look for changes in stool consistency, rectal bulges or protruding haemorrhoids. A proctoscope should also be inserted to examine the anus and lower rectum. Other routes of examination include rigid sigmoidoscopy, which can get about 20 cm into the bowel, flexible sigmoidoscopy (about 60 cm) and colonoscopy, which can view the whole large bowel (about 1.5 m).

Treatment options

- Conservative measures are the same as the preventative measures but other local treatments such as sitz baths, cold compresses and topical analgesia may bring some relief.
- If haemorrhoids are noted to be grade 1, dietary advice and a topical gel such as Anusol® may be sufficient.
- At grade 2 (a common time for presentation) banding or sclerosing injections can be performed in the outpatient setting.
- At grade 3–4, surgical options may be discussed, which include haemorrhoidectomy.
- Newer methods of treatment such as stapled haemorrhoidectomy (PPH) and haemorrhoidal artery ligation operations (HALO) are also available depending on patient selection and indication.

Perianal haematoma

This results from straining to pass stool. It is due to a burst blood vessel near the anal verge. Conservative treatment involves leaving it to resolve. The pain normally settles over a few days and ice packs may help. If it is very painful it may be incised and drained under local anaesthetic.

Rectal prolapse

- Rectal prolapse is a condition where the wall or part of the wall of the rectum becomes detached from its normal attachments.
- This may lead to the subtypes:
  - Full-thickness prolapse
  - Mucosal prolapse
  - Internal intussusception.
- The main cause is thought to be straining to defecate, but penetrative anal sex may also be the reason in younger patients.
- The condition progresses from initial prolapse during bowel movements, to prolapse during increased intra-abdominal pressure and eventually it may remain outside.
- Medical management is aimed at reducing straining with stool softeners.
- There are abdominal and perineal options for surgical intervention.
  - The abdominal options are anterior resection and abdominal rectopexy, which can be done as an open or laparoscopic procedure
  - The perineal options are Delorme's procedure, where a sleeve resection is performed and the remaining mucosa is hitched up into place
  - Anal encirclement and haemorrhoidectomy are also options.

4.10.6 Bowel obstruction

Obstruction of the bowel can occur at any point from the pylorus to the anus. When presented with bowel obstruction, you should try to figure out whether the bowel obstruction is:

- Mechanical vs functional bowel obstruction
- Large-bowel obstruction (LBO) versus small-bowel obstruction (SBO)
- Complete vs partial bowel obstruction

Aetiology
- Mechanical
  - Extraluminal
    - Adhesions
    - Incarcerated/strangulated hernia
    - Volvulus (sigmoid, caecal)
    - Intra-abdominal abscess or inflammation

- In the wall
  - Bowel carcinoma
  - Diverticular disease
  - IBD, eg Crohn's disease
- Intraluminal
  - Gallstone ileus
  - Foreign body
  - Severe constipation/faecalith
- Functional (paralytic ileus)
  - Peritonitis
  - Iatrogenic
    - Drug-induced, eg analgesics such as opiates (especially codeine), anticholinergics, antacids, calcium supplements, loperamide
    - Surgery, eg major abdominal or peritoneal
  - Nerve lesion
  - Metabolic
    - Hypokalaemia
    - Hypercalcaemia
  - Muscular abnormalities, eg Guillain–Barré, motor neurone disease

Commonest causes of:

- Large-bowel obstruction: carcinoma, volvulus and diverticular disease
- Small-bowel obstruction: adhesions, incarcerated/strangulated hernia

Pathophysiology
- **Large-bowel obstruction:** Mechanical obstruction causes bowel dilatation proximal to the obstruction, causing mucosal oedema and venous congestion. Bowel oedema and ischemia increase mucosal permeability of the bowel, which can lead to bacterial translocation, systemic toxicity, dehydration and electrolyte abnormalities. Bowel ischaemia can lead to perforation and emptying of faeces into the peritoneal cavity, resulting in peritonitis. If the ileocaecal valve is competent, caecal perforation may occur.
- **Small-bowel obstruction:** proximal small-bowel dilatation results in the accumulation of GI secretions and swallowed air, which leads to increased peristalsis, causing loose stools and flatus early on. Early vomiting in bowel obstruction suggests the level of obstruction to be proximal.
- Small-bowel dilatation can lead to mucosal lymphoedema and increased hydrostatic pressure within the capillary beds. This results in third spacing of fluid, electrolytes and proteins, causing fluid loss and dehydration. Increased mucosal permeability leads to bacterial translocation, which can cause bacteraemia.

Abdominal surgery

Clinical features
- Symptoms: four cardinal symptoms
  - **Vomiting** (early in SBO and late in LBO)
    - **LBO:** faeculent and foul-smelling
    - **SBO:** bile-stained or non-bile-stained (gastric outflow obstruction)
  - **Abdominal colic**
    - Upper abdominal pain: foregut
    - Middle abdominal pain: midgut
    - Lower abdominal pain: hindgut
  - **Distension** (bloating)
  - **Absolute constipation** (bowels not opening and no flatus)
    - A late sign in proximal SBO
- Signs
  - **General:** dehydration ($\downarrow$JVP, hypotension, postural hypotension, thirsty, dry mucosa, tachycardia)
  - **Inspect:** distension, visible peristalsis, hernial swellings, scars (abdominal surgery vs virgin abdomen)
  - **Palpate:** tense abdomen, generalised tenderness with no guarding unless perforation has occurred (remember to palpate the hernial orifices!)
  - **Percuss:** hyper-resonant to percussion
  - **Auscultate:** bowel sounds hyperactive ('tinkling') or reduced/absent (ileus), succussion splash (gently shake abdomen)

Investigations
- **Bloods:** FBC, U&E, LFT, CRP, cross-match
- **Urinalysis:** dipstick, MC+S, pregnancy test (βhCG)
- **Radiology:**
  - **AXR** (Box 4.12)
    - Supine: dilated loops of bowel
    - Erect: air/fluid level, absence of air in the rectum with LBO
  - **CXR:** free air under the diaphragm (perforation)
  - **Barium or gastrografin enema/meal:** delayed transit or obstruction

Management
- Conservative
  - NBM
  - IV fluids ('drip') + NGT ('suck')
  - Urinary catheter to monitor hourly urine output
  - Non-operative decompression: watchful waiting for up to 3 days if partial obstruction, provided adequate fluid resuscitation and NG suctioning
  - Manual reduction: incarcerated hernia
  - Most obstructions as a result of adhesions resolve with conservative management
- Medical
  - **Antibiotics** not given unless perforation has occurred
  - **Analgesic**, eg paracetamol, opiates
  - **Antiemetic,** eg cyclizine (avoid anticholinergics as they worsen bowel obstruction)
  - **Therapeutic gastrografin:** SBO secondary to adhesions
- Surgical
  - **Laparoscopy or laparotomy**
    - **Adhesions:** adhesiolysis
    - **Bowel carcinoma:** resection with or without primary anastomosis
    - **Diverticulitis:** surgical resection follows the same principles as the treatment of carcinomas
    - **Volvulus**
      - Sigmoid: sigmoidoscopy (first choice), sigmoid colectomy (second choice)
      - Caecal: hemicolectomy (first choice) or colonoscopic reduction
    - **Incarcerated hernia:** hernia repair

Complications
- Pre-operative
  - Perforation
  - Bacteraemia and sepsis
- Post-operative
  - Intra-abdominal collections, eg abscess, fluid
  - Anastomotic leak
  - Peritonitis

- Infection
- Bleeding
- DVT/PE
- Wound dehiscence
- Future adhesions

Prognosis
Generally good prognosis. If secondary to bowel carcinoma, outcome is dependent on CT staging and histology.

Complete obstructions treated non-operatively have a higher incidence of recurrence than those treated surgically.

4.10.7 Bowel (mesenteric) ischaemia
Bowel ischaemia occurs due to occlusion of the mesenteric vessels causing hypoxic injury to the bowel.

Anatomy
- **Foregut:**
  - Coeliac artery
- **Midgut:**
  - Superior mesenteric artery (SMA)
- **Hindgut:**
  - Inferior mesenteric artery (IMA)
- **Distal rectum:**
  - Branches of internal iliac artery

Pathophysiology
Hypoperfusion of the small bowel and colon resulting in ischaemia. Potential areas of ischaemia are the watershed areas and include:

- **Splenic flexure:** where the SMA and IMA meet
  - The SMA is the visceral vessel most susceptible to emboli
- **Rectosigmoid junction:** where the IMA and branches of internal iliac artery meet

Classification
- Acute mesenteric ischaemia
  - Embolic
  - Thrombotic
    - Arterial
    - Venous
  - Non-occlusive
- Chronic mesenteric ischaemia
- Ischaemic colitis

Acute mesenteric ischaemia

Aetiology
Commonest cause is thromboembolic arterial disease.

- **Embolic (common):** cardiac origin
  - **Mural thrombi:** post-MI
  - **Atrial/auricular thrombi:** mitral stenosis, atrial fibrillation
  - **Septic emboli:** valvular endocarditis
- **Thrombotic**
  - **Arterial (most common):** usually have pre-existing **visceral atherosclerosis** and co-existing atherosclerosis, eg cardiovascular heart disease, stroke, peripheral vascular disease
  - **Venous (rare):** Virchow's triad (stasis, eg bowel obstruction; vessel wall damage, eg phlebitis; hypercoagulable state, eg combined oral contraceptive, factor V Leiden, protein C & S deficiency)
- **Non-occlusive:** massive hypoperfusion of mesenteric vessels secondary to shock

Clinical features
All types of acute mesenteric ischaemia have a similar presentation.

Cardinal features
1 Severe abdominal pain disproportionate to clinical signs
2 Shock

- Symptoms
  - Diffuse, non-localised, colicky abdominal pain
  - Sudden onset
  - Associated with diarrhoea (bloody), nausea, vomiting, anorexia, distension
  - Exacerbated by food intake
- Signs
  - **Observations:** ↑T, ↓BP, ↑HR (irregularly irregular in atrial fibrillation), ↑RR
  - **Inspect:** distension, patient looks unwell systemically, sweating
  - **Palpate:** variable tenderness; guarding may not be present until late
  - **Auscultate:** hyperactive to absent

Early in the course of the disease, in the absence of peritonitis, physical signs are few and non-specific. Tenderness is minimal. Peritoneal signs develop late, when infarction with necrosis or perforation occurs.

Investigations
- **Bloods:** FBC, U&E, LFT, CRP, cross-match
- **Urinalysis:** dipstick, MC+S, pregnancy test (βhCG)
- **Radiology**
  - AXR
  - Mesenteric angiography (invasive)
  - CTA/MRA (non-invasive)

- **Cardiac investigations** (should be done post-operatively)
  - **Echocardiography:** mural/atrial thrombi
  - **ECG:** atrial fibrillation

Management
- **Medical**
  - **NBM + IV fluids:** preparation for theatre and rehydration
  - **Nasogastric tube:** decompression
  - **Catheterisation:** monitoring urine output
  - **Antibiotics** if perforation suspected (cefuroxime and metronidazole)
  - **Analgesia** with morphine (also aids vasodilatation)
  - **Antiemetics** – cyclizine
  - **Anticoagulation** – heparin
  - **Antiarrhythmic** – digoxin if indicated
- **Surgical**
  - **Exploratory laparoscopy/laparotomy**
  - **Emergency laparotomy:** if signs of necrosis and peritonitis; bowel may have infarcted (black bowel) and appear pulseless .
    - ○ **Reversible:** revascularisation with embolectomy/bypass
    - ○ **Segmental ischaemia:** resection ± revascularisation
    - ○ **Complete (massive) ischaemia:** bowel resection with/without primary anastomosis
    - ○ **Open and close:** extensive infarction incompatible with life - palliative treatment only
- **Radiological**
  - **Angiographic thrombolysis ± angioplasty**

Complications
- **Pre-operative**
  - Bowel necrosis (requiring resection)
  - Septic shock
- **Post-operative**
  - Death
  - Short bowel syndrome (depending on resection length)
  - Malnutrition and lifelong TPN (if massive resection)
  - Dehydration
  - Infection
  - Bleeding
  - Perforation
  - DVT/PE
  - Wound dehiscence

Prognosis
Poor prognosis unless caught early with an adequate resection:

- **Mortality:** >70%

Chronic mesenteric ischaemia

Modifiable risk factors
- Hypertension
- Smoking
- Diabetes
- ↑Lipids
- Lack of exercise
- Obesity
- Diet (↑salt intake, ↑fat intake, ↑alcohol)

Pathophysiology
Diffuse atherosclerotic disease decreases blood flow to the bowel, typically progressing to involve all three mesenteric arteries, which become occluded or narrowed, causing symptoms to worsen.

Clinical features
Typically, pain starts after meals and is disproportionate to clinical findings. Mesenteric angina.

- **Symptoms**
  - Gradual epigastric/periumbilical dull pain
  - Associated with weight loss ('fear of food'), PR bleeding, nausea, vomiting, change in bowel habit, flatulence
  - Exacerbated by food and relieved by defecation/vomiting
- **Signs**
  - **Observations:** stable, apyrexial
  - **Inspect:** malnutrition, signs of peripheral vascular disease
  - **Palpate:** generalised mild abdominal tenderness
  - **Auscultate:** abdominal bruit may be present

Investigations
- Mesenteric angiography

Management
- Analgesia
- Modification of risk factors
- Surgical reconstruction of mesenteric vessels or resection as appropriate

4.10.8 Diverticular disease
Amongst clinicians there is confusion about the terms diverticulosis, diverticular disease and diverticulitis. **Diverticulosis** means the presence of diverticulae, which are pouches which form in the bowel. They are thought to be related to straining with bowel opening (raised intraluminal pressure) or to be related to weaknesses in the colon where the appendices epiploicae form (and nutrient vessels pass through the wall). This would account for their prevalence in the

sigmoid colon. Diverticulae can occur anywhere in the GI tract. They can be classified as true and false depending on whether they involve the entire wall or just the mucosa and submucosa. The diverticulae in the large bowel are false diverticulae.

Diverticular disease is where the presence of the diverticulae is symptomatic, causing abdominal pain or inflammation.

Diverticulitis is inflammation of the diverticulae, which may lead to many complaints such as PR bleeding, diarrhoea, fevers and abdominal pain.

Risk factors

- Diverticulosis is a common condition, especially in the Western world.
- It is strongly associated with age (one-third of people aged 45 and two-thirds of people aged 85 in the USA).
- It is rare in people under 40.
- It is not associated with gender.
- Low-fibre diet is the greatest modifiable risk factor.
- Genetics play a role and Westerners tend to have mostly left-sided disease whereas Asians have mainly right-sided disease.
- Colonic motility disorders are an uncommon cause.
- Long-term steroid use is thought to increase the risk of diverticulitis.

Signs and symptoms

- The most common presentation is diverticulitis causing low-grade fever, abdominal pain (usually left lower quadrant) and PR bleeding with diarrhoea.
- These pouches when inflamed can cause fistulation to other visceral surfaces within the abdomen. This in turn can account for vesicocolic, coloenteric, colovaginal fistulas.
- With diverticular disease the patient may complain of excessive flatulence and bloating.
- Most patients are asymptomatic from diverticulosis.
- In some cases diverticulitis may lead to a **diverticular abscess**, which requires radiological or surgical drainage and intravenous antibiotics or even a Hartmann's operation, where the diseased section is removed and the proximal bowel is brought out as a stoma and the distal end is either left as a mucous fistula or left as a rectal stump inside the abdomen, to be rejoined when the disease process has settled.
- It can also lead to **diverticular perforation**, which again may result in the need for an emergency Hartmann's.
- Colonic obstruction can occur and would also require a Hartmann's procedure.

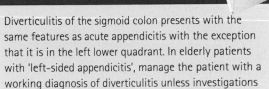

Essential note

Diverticulitis of the sigmoid colon presents with the same features as acute appendicitis with the exception that it is in the left lower quadrant. In elderly patients with 'left-sided appendicitis', manage the patient with a working diagnosis of diverticulitis unless investigations show otherwise

Diagnostic tests

History and examination again provide invaluable information when diagnosing this condition but because of the overlap of symptoms with colorectal cancer a barium enema or lower GI endoscopy is usually indicated and these both detect the presence of diverticulae quite easily.

Treatment

In general, diverticulosis requires no treatment

Diverticulitis requires that the patient is on a low-residue diet or nil by mouth, on IV fluids, antibiotics (usually a cephalosporin and metronidazole) and, once the condition has settled, an outpatient barium enema should be performed to confirm the cause, if this has not previously been done.

Diverticular abscess may settle with antibiotics if it discharges intraluminally. Otherwise, drainage will be necessary, either radiologically or surgically.

When **perforation** occurs the patient is likely to develop a faecal peritonitis and require urgent surgery. Where they are not fit for surgery they may be managed conservatively and patients sometimes settle where the omentum plugs the perforated area of bowel. However, this condition carries with it a high mortality (approximately 50%). When surgery is carried out a Hartmann's procedure is usually performed for sigmoid diverticulitis resulting in a sigmoid abscess, sigmoid obstruction or perforation that cannot be treated conservatively.

A Hartmann's procedure consists of:

- Resecting the diseased or inflamed sigmoid colon
- Stapling of the distal end of bowel
- The proximal end of healthy bowel (usually descending colon) is brought out through a left-sided end-colostomy
- The abdominal cavity is washed out and an abdominal drain inserted to allow any residual infection to drain out

Where a Hartmann's is performed only about 50% are deemed suitable for re-anastomosis and closure.

Fistulation to other organs may resolve with a defunctioning ileostomy and primary repair.

4.10.9 Stomas

- A stoma is a surgically created exteriorisation of an internal surface.
- The word stoma literally means 'mouth'.
- Within the topic of colorectal surgery, ileostomy and colostomy are the main two types, which are exteriorisation of the ileum and colon.
- They can be created when diversion, decompression or access to the bowel lumen are required.
- The main types of stoma you will be required to know about are end stomas and loop stomas:
  - **End stomas** are where the bowel is divided and the proximal end is brought out through the abdominal wall. The distal segment may be resected, it may be brought out through the same hole (as a double-barrelled stoma) or through another hole as a mucous fistula or it may be left in the abdomen as a stump once it has been stapled off across the open end.
  - A **loop stoma** has the advantage of being easier to close. They are good for decompression and reasonable for diversion, though not perfect as there is spillover from the afferent to the efferent limb of the stoma. They are fashioned by incompletely transecting the bowel wall and leaving a bridge. In loop ileostomies the proximal end is then spouted to avoid direct contamination of the skin by small-bowel contents as this is highly irritating. When forming colostomies spouting is not required.
- Both loop and end stomas may be created in the large and small bowel according to the cause.
- Very proximal stomas have more fluid output volume whereas more distal stomas show the opposite tendency.

- Positioning is important as care must be taken to avoid bony prominences, scars, the umbilicus, fat folds, and where clothes are worn, eg belt lines.
- Marking should ideally be done by a stoma nurse pre-operatively. **Ileostomies** tend to be sited in the right iliac fossa and come out though the rectus muscle. **Colostomies** tend to be in the left iliac fossa if done as part of an anterior resection, an abdominoperineal excision or for a Hartmann's but may be in the epigastrium if a transverse loop colostomy is done as a palliative procedure for a distal obstruction.

Complications

- Necrosis
- Retraction
- Stenosis
- Prolapse
- Ulceration
- High-output stomas leading to electrolyte abnormalities and dehydration
- Fistulation
- Parastomal hernias

Stomas can be reversed when the original indication for creating them no longer exists, eg a distal anastomosis has healed or the inflammatory mass has settled. It is usually wise to wait at least 6 weeks to allow inflammation to settle or the operation to reverse them may be more technically demanding. Most patients have them for a period of a few months at least. Some may be permanent, if the patient decides their quality of life is better with it or if they are not fit enough to undergo a general anaesthetic. After a Hartmann's procedure only 50% of patients undergo a reversal of the end-colostomy.

Orthopaedics and trauma surgery

CONTENTS

Orthopaedics and trauma surgery

EDITOR'S NOTE

Orthopaedics is concerned with the skeletal system and the structures that make it move. It should be studied in combination with its medical counterpart, rheumatology, to complete the disorders of the skeletal system. Although it is a large subject to cover in its entirety, it is not extensively examined in the undergraduate examinations. Learning the joint examinations are important, along with the most important topics as covered in this chapter. My personal recommendation is to read an orthopaedics examination textbook to learn the individual joint exams and the one I recommend is *Pocketbook of Orthopaedics and Fractures* by Ronald McRae. Some essential topics (including trauma) are covered and the pocketbook should remain with you during your orthopaedics rotation. This chapter on orthopaedics aims to revise the common and essential written examination topics as found in the final MBBS curriculum for orthopaedics and trauma.

Revision objectives

You should know:
- How to clinically assess a patient with an orthopaedic complaint, including taking a focused history and performing the relevant joint examination
- How to investigate a patient with an orthopaedic disorder or trauma to the skeletal system
- The main clinical features and epidemiology of benign and malignant orthopaedic conditions as applied to specific body regions
- The principles of managing fractures and the common complications which can occur in clinical practice
- The features of commonest fractures in clinical practice and how to assess and manage them briefly

5.1 GENERAL ORTHOPAEDICS

5.1.1 Introduction
The subject of orthopaedics deals with specific disorders of the skeletal system such as bone and joint abnormalities. Trauma, on the other hand, deals with injuries to the skeletal system such as fractures and dislocations and their subsequent management.

This chapter aims to cover the most commonly encountered conditions in orthopaedics and trauma surgery in an essential revision format. Theoretical orthopaedics does not usually carry much weight in the written examinations, but the OSCEs and clinical exams will almost always have at least one joint examination.

As with any subject, the clinical assessment with history, examination and investigations is essential in diagnosing and subsequently treating orthopaedic conditions. This next section introduces the orthopaedic assessment in general. It does not serve as a replacement for either clinical bedside learning of orthopaedic conditions or a good orthopaedics examination textbook.

Clinical assessment

Orthopaedic history (in addition to a full general history)
- **Pain:** location; nature; duration; radiation; relieving/exacerbating factors
- **Stiffness:** generalised/localised; locking; duration; relieving factors; morning/night
- **Instability:** previous trauma; recurrent; direction; ease of dislocation/reduction
- **Swelling:** location; tissue plane; post-trauma?; characteristics; painful; constant?
- **Deformity:** progressive; associated symptoms; correctable/fixed
- **Sensory changes/weakness:** distribution; deterioration; associated dysfunction

The above symptoms or their combination can lead to functional disability depending on their severity and the needs of the patient.

Examination
Observe from the moment the patient walks into the clinic to see if there is any:

- Syndrome
- Gait
- Deformity

When examining any particular joint always stick to the order of **Look**, **Feel** and **Move**. In some cases, it may be appropriate to measure the patient after inspection such as in hip examinations. Do not hurt the patient in your exams!

LOOK (and always compare the two sides)
- Joint swellings
  - Diffuse
  - Localised
- Bruising
- Skin discoloration or oedema

- Sinuses
- Scars
- Psoriasis
- Muscle wasting
- Alignment of the limb
- Position of the joint
- Shortening of the limb

FEEL (and always compare sides)
- Temperature (warmth)
  - Generalised
  - Localised
- Tenderness
- Lumps
- Joint effusions

MOVE (and compare with normal side or published figures on range of joint mobility)
- Active range of motion
- Passive range of motion
- Abnormal movements at specific sites
- Strength of movements
- Special tests of movement as applied to the joint (eg Apley's grind test or McMurray's test)

Always finish off a limb examination by checking the neurology and blood supply.

Always examine the joints proximal to and distal to the affected joint.

Radiographs
- Patient details
- Part being examined
- The orientation
- Systematically examine the radiographs: bones, joints, soft tissues
  - Bones: cortical abnormality, density (porosis/sclerosis) cysts, deformity
  - Joints: narrowing, osteophytes, erosions, sclerosis, loose bodies
  - Soft tissues: swelling, fat pad signs, blood/fat interface, calcification

Special investigations
- **Ultrasound:** useful for tendon rupture, abscesses, paediatric intraspinal disorders, haematomas, soft tissue masses, paediatric hip problems, rotator cuff pathology, image-guided injections
- **MRI:** uses radiofrequency pulses on tissues in a magnetic field and displays images in any required plane without using ionising radiation. Used to study soft tissues and bone marrow

- Examples: knee ligament/meniscal pathology, osteomyelitis, disc pathology, neoplasms
- **CT:** shows details of bony anatomy better than any other imaging
  - Examples: demonstrate anatomy pre-op (eg tibial plateau, os calcis, spine), accurate distance measurement (eg trochlear groove–tibial tubercle), malalignment post-arthroplasty
- **Bone scan:** technetium-99m is used to indicate blood flow in areas of pathology. Areas affected by infection, tumour and trauma will be highlighted. Does not show local anatomy well
- **Chest X-ray:** can be of value in rheumatoid arthritis when assessing for pulmonary nodules or fibrosis from other rheumatological diseases
- **Nerve conduction studies:** useful in peripheral nerve damage or compression, eg carpal tunnel
- **Blood tests:** full blood count (FBC), erythrocyte sedimentation rate (ESR), serum uric acid, calcium, phosphate and alkaline phosphatase (ALP), latex fixation text

5.1.2 Infection
Osteomyelitis is an infection of bone and bone marrow. It may be direct or indirect.

- **Direct:** open fracture, skin wound/infection over bone, iatrogenic (eg after fracture fixation)
- **Indirect:** via bloodstream from a distant site

Radiographic changes are visible usually after 10 days. Changes include:

- Tissue swelling
- Bone demineralisation
- Sequestra (necrotic bone with surrounding granulation tissue)
- Involucrum (periosteal new bone surrounding the sequestra)
- Brodie's abscess: a small oval cavity surrounded by sclerotic bone present usually in the metaphysis of long bones secondary to subacute osteomyelitis

Principles of treatment involve:

- Identification of the organism
  - Blood cultures
  - Deep tissue samples
  - Surface drainage samples not accurate
- Debridement/drainage of necrotic/infective material
- Treatment with empirical antibiotics followed by organism-specific antibiotics
- Making sure appropriate samples are taken before any antibiotics given

Acute haematogenous osteomyelitis

- Commoner in children, affecting the metaphysis and epiphysis of long bones
- Affects immunocompromised adults
- Discomfort, swelling and loss of function of the affected limb
- Blood cultures may be positive with an elevated white blood cell count (WBC) and ESR. C-reactive protein (CRP) is most sensitive
- MRI scan shows changes before X-rays
- Offending organisms:
  - Children up to 4 years: *Staphylococcus aureus*, *Haemophilus influenzae*, group B streptococcus
  - Children over 4 years: *S. aureus*, group A streptococcus, coliforms
  - Adults: *S. aureus*, various
  - Sickle cell anaemia: *Salmonella*
  - IV drug abusers and immunocompromised: *S. aureus*, *S. epidermidis*, *Pseudomonas*

Acute osteomyelitis

- Usually secondary to direct inoculation or post-operative procedure, eg open reduction with internal fixation (ORIF) or arthroplasty
- Correct management of open fractures is imperative to avoid infection
  - A&E
    - Remove visible foreign material
    - Wash wound and ends of exposed bone, cover with sterile dressings
    - Splint the injured limb
    - Prophylactic antibiotics and tetanus
  - Theatre
    - Thorough washout and debridement in theatre, do not close wound primarily
    - In the presence of infection leave metalwork holding a fracture in situ until the fracture has united; otherwise you will have to manage an unstable infected injury. If there is gross infection in the presence of internal fixation, then remove the metalwork and stabilise using an external fixator
- To avoid infection after joint arthroplasty
  - Scrub thoroughly, glove using non-touch technique
  - Aseptic preparation
  - Laminar flow theatres
  - Good surgical technique and meticulous dissection
  - Prophylactic antibiotics

Chronic osteomyelitis

- Secondary to inappropriate management of acute infection, post-trauma, or after arthroplasty

- Consists of sequestra of necrosed bone surrounded by sclerosed bone. Communicates to the surface via single or multiple sinuses
- The bacteria can remain quiescent for a long time and then present with recurrent flares
- Cultures for diagnosis and ESR/CRP for monitoring are most effective. WBC is usually normal
- Treatment involves removal of necrotic/infected material, debridement and antibiotics
- In the presence of an infected arthroplasty, if infection is detected within 3 weeks, then a washout, a change of the polyethylene liner and synovectomy may salvage the prosthesis
- In chronic cases of infected arthroplasty, a glycocalyx forms over the construct, making salvage difficult. The infected prosthesis has to be removed as part of a two-stage procedure

Septic arthritis

- One of the few orthopaedic emergencies in which urgent diagnosis and treatment are essential
- Delayed treatment can lead to life-threatening septic shock or irreversible joint destruction
- Bacteria acquire access via direct penetration, discharge of a bone abscess, or haematogenous spread
- Usual organism is *S. aureus*. In children below 4, *H. influenzae* is common
- Usually the hip is affected in children and the knee in adults
- Clinically the patient holds the joint in a fixed flexed position. The joint is swollen, warm, erythematous and globally tender
- Diagnosis is with joint aspiration, blood cultures, raised WBC, ESR and CRP
- Important to obtain samples for culture before any antibiotics are given
- Joint aspirate is sent for urgent microscopy, culture and sensitivity
- Treatment is in the form of joint washout and antibiotics
- Differential diagnosis for an acutely tender joint without trauma can include acute on chronic degenerative disease, gout, pseudogout, cellulitis and bursitis. It is therefore important that a good clinical diagnosis is established before the decision to introduce a needle into the joint is taken

5.1.3 Osteoarthritis

- Primary (intrinsic defect) or secondary (trauma, infection, haemophilic)
- Primary osteoarthritis (OA) commoner in the population with increasing age

- Pain and stiffness worsen gradually over months or years. Pain is increased by activity while stiffness is worse after periods of rest. As OA progresses symptoms are harder to control
- A good history, examination and X-rays usually give the diagnosis. All blood markers are normal
- In early disease:
  - Relieve pain: analgesics/anti-inflammatory agents, rest, change activities
  - Mobilise the joint: physiotherapy to improve power, stability, range of motion and function
  - Decrease loading: reduce weight, use a walking stick and stop exacerbating activity
- In intermediate disease:
  - Arthroscopic debridement of degenerative menisci and washout in the knee
  - Arthroscopic removal of anterior osteophytes causing impingement in the ankle or hip
  - In the young, realignment osteotomy where only part of the joint is affected
- In advanced disease:
  - Patient's sleep and level of activity are affected to the extent that the quality of life deteriorates
  - Several types of arthroplasties are available. Best used in the older patient as they only last approximately 15 years
- X-ray changes in osteoarthritis
  - Joint space narrowing
  - Osteophytes
  - Subchondral sclerosis
  - Subchondal cysts
- Complications after:
  - Knee replacement: infection, numbness around scar, deep vein thrombosis (DVT)/pulmonary embolism (PE), neurovascular (NV) damage
  - Hip replacement: infection, DVT/PE, leg length discrepancy, dislocation, NV damage

Charcot's disease

- Rapidly progressive degeneration in a joint lacking sensation
- Can occur in peripheral neuropathies (diabetes), tabes dorsalis and syringomyelia
- The patient has a deformed unstable joint in the absence of pain
- Treatment involves addressing the primary condition, protection of the affected limbs and splinting for stabilisation if necessary. Arthroplasty is not recommended

Haemophilic arthropathy

- Secondary to repeated haemarthrosis, causing chronic synovitis and cartilage destruction
- Patients with classic haemophilia (factor VIII) and Christmas disease (factor IX) are affected
- Prevention is by controlling bleeding. Aspiration in an acute bleed is avoided unless there is a very tense collection or suspicion of infection. The necessary clotting factor is given IV to help control bleeds

5.1.4 Rheumatic disorders

A group of systemic diseases affecting connective tissues, joints and viscera; commonly known for chronic joint pain and destruction leading to loss of function.

Rheumatoid arthritis

- Unknown initiating factor leading to abnormal production of antibodies against own IgG. These autoantibodies appear in the serum as rheumatoid factor in the majority of patients
- **Diagnostic criteria** include bilateral, symmetrical polyarthritis affecting the proximal joints of the hands or feet for at least 6 weeks
- A positive rheumatoid factor in the absence of symptoms does not confirm diagnosis while a negative rheumatoid factor in the presence of symptoms excludes diagnosis
- **Systemic manifestations** are vasculitis, lymphadenopathy, weakness and visceral disease affecting the lungs, kidneys, heart and brain. The synovium is most severely targeted
- Stages of the disease:
  - Stage 1: Synovitis
    - Gradual onset of polyarthritis affecting the extremities, early morning stiffness, malaise. Increased swelling, warmth and tenderness of metacarpophalangeal joints (MCPJs) and wrists. The disease spreads to other joints. The joints are still intact and the condition reversible
  - Stage 2: Destruction
    - Tissue damage because of continued inflammation
    - Reduced joint movement secondary to joint cartilage erosion. Tendon ruptures. Subcutaneous nodules [in 25% but pathognomonic of rheumatoid arthritis (RA)] over extensor surfaces
  - Stage 3: Deformity – capsular compromise, articular incongruity
    - Ulnar deviation of fingers, Boutonnière's and swan-neck deformities, Z thumb, fixed flexion deformity of the elbows, valgus deformities of the knees, clawed toes, atlantoaxial instability, vasculitis, sensory disturbance

- Muscle atrophy
- In 80%: intermittent flares, frequency decreasing with time, eventually subsiding. Unfortunately joints are permanently damaged by that stage
- In 5%: continued progression of the disease leading to visceral effects and complete joint damage
- In 10%: aggressive start to the disease followed by a mild course
- Rarely: no recurrence of the disease after the first few attacks
- **Investigations:** increased ESR and CRP during active phase. Rheumatoid factor positive in 80%
- **X-rays** show:
  - Reduced joint space
  - Thickened synovium
  - Periarticular osteoporosis
  - Marginal bony erosions
  - Joint deformity
- **Treatment** involves:
  - Controlling synovitis: anti-inflammatory analgesics, corticosteroids, gold/penicillamine/immunosuppressive drugs to control progression of the disease
  - Rest and splinting
  - Intra-articular injections
  - Synovectomy
  - Stop deformity: physiotherapy (joints rested during active disease but as flare diminishes physiotherapy is started to maintain mobility)
  - Operation to repair tendon rupture or improve correctable deformities
  - Reconstruction: when complete joint destruction has taken place the options are arthroplasty, arthrodesis and osteotomy
  - Rehabilitate: modelled to patient needs from start to finish
  - Occupational therapy: training to use adjuncts, psychological support
- **Disease monitoring** is done by observing symptoms and levels of ESR and CRP. Rheumatoid factor levels indicate prognosis
- **Differential diagnosis:**
  - Ankylosing spondylitis (AS): sacroiliac and intervertebral joints primarily affected
  - Reiter's disease: conjunctivitis, urethritis and large joints, including lumbosacral spine, affected
  - OA with interphalangeal joint (IPJ) osteophytes: Heberden nodes (distal IPJ) and Bouchard nodes (proximal IPJ)
  - Polyarticular gout: gouty tophi might be mistaken for rheumatoid nodules

- Connective tissue diseases: systemic lupus erythematosus (SLE), polymyalgia rheumatica
- Psoriatic arthritis: affects the IPJs in association with psoriasis. Back affected as in AS

Ankylosing spondylitis

- Chronic inflammatory disease primarily affecting the sacroiliac joints and back. Hips, shoulders and peripheral joints are also affected less commonly
- Runs in families, associated with HLA-B27
- **Pathological sequence:**
  - Inflammation
  - Granulation tissue
  - Damage to articular cartilage
  - Fibrous tissue
  - Ossification of fibrous tissue
  - Ankylosis
- Clinically, young men present with early morning stiffness of the lower back. Hips are often involved. Peripheral joints can also be swollen and tender, with the heels being tender. With progressive disease the entire spine can become rigid, giving the patient a 'question mark' appearance
- Visceral effects: ocular inflammation, aortic valve disease, pulmonary fibrosis and carditis
- **X-rays:**
  - Early on, erosion of the sacroiliac joints and squaring of the vertebrae
  - In late disease, bony bridges across intervertebral discs (syndesmophytes), across several levels (bamboo spine)
- **Treatment:**
  - Analgesia
  - Anti-inflammatory drugs
  - Physiotherapy
  - In advanced cases, arthroplasty

5.1.5 Osteonecrosis and osteochondritis

Ischaemic necrosis

- Avascular necrosis = bone death secondary to inadequate blood supply
- **Causes:**
  - Trauma
  - Sickle cell disease
  - Infection
  - Caisson disease
  - Steroids
  - Alcohol
- **Common sites:**
  - Femoral head and condyles
  - Scaphoid

- Lunate
- Talus
- Humeral head
- **Pathology:**
  - **Stage 1:** Bone death with intact structure
  - **Stage 2:** Repair around the necrosis (dense on X-ray), small fractures in dead bone
  - **Stage 3:** Collapse of necrotic portion
  - **Stage 4:** Distortion of the underlying surface leads to cartilage breakdown
- **Clinical presentation:**
  - Pain and stiffness in the joint. There can also be restriction of movement and swelling
- **Investigations:**
  - MRI: bone marrow ischaemia and oedema
  - X-ray:
    - Subarticular fracturing and deformity
    - Increased density due to reactive bone formation around the necrotic area
    - This sclerosis can appear up to 18 months after the necrosis has occurred
- **Treatment:**
  - Conservative
    - Analgesia and splinting
    - Weight relief
  - Surgical
    - Drilling of the affected area to improve vascularity
    - Re-alignment osteotomy to relieve stress from the affected area, arthroplasty and fusion

Osteochondritis

- Types:
  - Crushing: lunate (Kienböck), navicular (Kohler), metatarsal head (Freiberg)
  - Splitting: femoral condyle, talus, capitulum
  - Pulling: calcaneum (sever), tibial tuberosity (Osgood Schlatter)
- Symptoms: pain, limitation of movement, localised tenderness
- Investigations: X-rays, MRI or arthroscopy

- Treatment:
  - Conservative: rest, analgesia and splinting
  - Surgical: if the osteochondral fragment becomes detached it may cause locking and will either need to be removed or re-attached

5.1.6 Tumours

Classification of bone tumours, see Table 5.1.

- Metastatic bone tumours are commoner than primary bone tumours
- Common primaries for metastatic tumours are:
  - Kidney
  - Prostate (sclerotic)
  - Breast
  - Lung
  - Thyroid
- Primary bone tumours are classified by cell type
- Benign tumours can become malignant
- Symptoms: pain, swelling, tenderness, pathological fracture, warmth
- Signs: swelling, tenderness, ill-defined edge
- Investigations: X-ray, bone scan, MRI, CT, biopsy
- Treatment: if benign and asymptomatic then can be left alone. If doubt exists, biopsy can be taken without disturbing tissue planes and minimising spread of tumour. Biopsy should ideally be done by someone who may carry out definitive excision in a specialist centre

Osteoid osteoma

- Benign, consists of osteoid and new bone
- Affects patients below 30 years, presents with pain relived by aspirin but not rest
- X-rays show a small radiolucent area surrounded by dense sclerosis. Bone scan is positive
- Excision of the affected area is the treatment. No risk of recurrence

Osteochondroma

- Most common primary tumour of bone
- Exostosis capped by cartilage

Table 5.1: Classification of bone tumours		
Cell type	*Benign*	*Malignant*
Bone	Osteoid osteoma	Osteosarcoma
Cartilage	Chondroma, osteochondroma	Chondrosarcoma
Fibrous	Fibroma	Fibrosarcoma
Marrow	Eosinophilic granuloma	Ewing's sarcoma, myeloma
Vascular	Haemangioma	Angiosarcoma
Non-specific	Giant-cell tumour	Malignant giant-cell tumour

- The tumour starts off in adolescence and grows until the parent bone grows. Malignant change is thought to have occurred if the tumour continues to grow while bone growth has stopped
- Usually metaphysis of long bones is affected
- Treatment is by excision

Chondroma

- Single or multiple (Ollier's disease)
- Benign cartilaginous tumour
- Present in tubular bones
- Causes pain, swelling, or fracture after small injury
- Chondroma has calcification visible on X-rays (simple bone cyst does not)
- Lesion can be curetted and bone-grafted

Simple bone cyst

- Presents as a local ache or fracture
- Usually in children up to puberty
- Usually in upper humerus, femur and tibia
- X-rays show a translucent area on the shaft side of the physis
- If a fracture occurs through a cyst the cavity can spontaneously become obliterated
- Treatments include injection of corticosteroids or removal of the cyst wall followed by grafting

Aneurysmal bone cyst

- Expanded lesion, thinning the cortex, containing blood
- Affects young adults
- On X-rays: well-defined area, centrally placed, confined to metaphyseal side of growth plates
- Treat with curettage and grafting

Fibrous cortical defect

- Area resembling a cyst on X-rays but filled with translucent fibrous tissue
- Usually does not require treatment
- Can cause area of bone weakness and lead to pathological fracture

Giant-cell tumour

- Name derived from multinucleated giant cells, which are seen in large numbers
- The tumour occurs in subarticular cancellous bone
- Only bones with fused epiphysis are affected
- One-third remain benign, one-third become locally invasive and one-third metastasise
- Symptoms are usually pain near a joint with slight swelling
- Pathological fractures can be a presenting feature
- Patient age usually ranges between 20 and 40

- X-rays show a translucent area situated asymmetrically at the end of a long bone. The cortex can be very thin, ballooned and even perforated
- Treatment is with complete curettage and bone-grafting
- Lesions that have dramatically affected the joint may require excision followed by arthroplasty. Surgically inaccessible lesions are treated with radiotherapy

Osteosarcoma

- Primary malignant tumour arising from bone and producing osteoid
- Spreads directly to surrounding tissues and can also metastasise to the lungs
- Occurs between the ages of 10 and 20 and also after the age of 50 (bimodal distribution)
- Associated with Paget's disease in older patients
- Common site is metaphysis of long bones (eg knee and proximal humerus)
- Pain is the commonest symptom. It is usually constant and also present at night. Presence of a painful lump is also common. Patients can also present with a limping gait
- Examination findings can include a tender, diffuse mass with shiny and warm skin over it
- X-rays show that there is both bone destruction and formation:
  - Perforated cortex
  - Soft-tissue shadow
  - Sun-ray spicules: streaks of calcification in adjacent soft tissues
  - Codman's triangle: periosteum begins to be lifted away from the shaft
- MRI, CT and bone scan are required for staging
- Biopsy confirms the diagnosis
- Treatment consists of radical excision, which may lead to amputation or insertion of a prosthesis specially designed to be used for limb salvage. Recent improvement of chemo- and radiotherapy has improved survival

Chondrosarcoma

- Can occur primarily from the medullary canal or after malignant change in the cartilage cap of a osteochondroma
- Present with pain, swelling or a pathological fracture
- Investigations: X-rays, staging CTs, MRIs and bone scans
- As chondrosarcomas metastasise late, wide local excision may provide long-term relief

Metastatic tumours in bone

- Secondary tumours in bone are commoner than any of the other bone tumours
- Commonest primary sites are breast, prostate, thyroid, kidneys and lungs
- Metastases usually destroy and replace bone. These areas become weak and can lead to pathological fractures
- Can present with bone pain or pathological fracture
- Clinically one needs to examine all the areas for the primary source, eg breasts, thyroid
- Investigations: plain X-rays, FBC, ESR, CRP, protein electrophoresis, bone scan and CT
- X-rays: osteolytic lesions. If prostate is the primary, the deposits are sclerotic
- Pathological fractures or areas of impending fractures (eg femoral necks) can be internally fixed
- Radiotherapy and chemotherapy play an important role in treating multiple deposits

5.2 REGIONAL ORTHOPAEDICS

5.2.1 The shoulder

- Symptoms:
  - Pain, stiffness, deformity, reduced range of motion, instability
- Signs:
  - Look for scars and sinuses, muscle wastage, winging of scapula, swelling
  - The shoulder may be in an abnormal position (dislocation?)
  - Reduced/painful range of motion
  - Reduced power or sensation of instability on certain movements
  - Check passive and active motion in flexion, abduction, adduction, internal and external rotation. Stabilise the scapula with one hand when checking glenohumeral motion
- Investigations:
  - X-rays
  - Ultrasound
  - MRI
  - Arthroscopy

Rotator cuff disorders

The rotator cuff is a sheet of four tendons present over the shoulder joint capsule. It consists of:

- Anteriorly – subscapularis
- Superiorly – supraspinatus
- Posteriorly – infraspinatus and teres minor

Its purpose is to initiate movement and to hold the humeral head closely against the glenoid when the deltoid contracts.

Acute tendonitis

- Secondary to acute inflammation and calcification in the supraspinatus
- Usually a young adult complains of developing intense pain after a period of overuse
- Area of tenderness is mainly above the greater tuberosity and during the acute stage the arm is held immobile
- Treatment consists of resting the arm in a sling, non-steroidal analgesia and if necessary a injection of local anaesthetic and steroid. If pain still persists removing the area of calcification is helpful

Impingement syndrome

- Consists of inflammation and tears in the supraspinatus tendon
- Impingement of the cuff against the acromion and coracoacromial ligament is thought to play a role in the pathology
- Age range 40–60
- Pain in shoulder (tender under acromion) and over deltoid
- Pain is worse on abduction. There is a 'painful arc' of abduction between 60° and 120°. Repeating the abduction movement with the arm externally rotated takes the pain away
- Chronic cases show muscle wasting with reduced power
- In late disease X-rays can show upward migration of the humeral head
- USS and MRI scans will show any rotator cuff tears
- Treatment consists of anti-inflammatories, local anaesthetic and steroid injections, and, if symptoms are not settling, then acromioplasty is the preferred option

Rotator cuff tears

- Causes:
  - Tendinitis
  - Impingement
  - Trauma
  - Idiopathic
- Can be full-thickness or partial
- Partial usually heal with conservative methods
- Full-thickness tears do not heal spontaneously. They can retract further and become adherent to bone
- Age range 45–75
- History of overstressing the shoulder. Sudden pain after injury, difficulty in abduction
- If it is a full-thickness tear, weakness remains after the pain has subsided. In the acute stage, injecting local anaesthetic to abolish pain can distinguish between partial

and full-thickness tears. With partial tears the patient can still abduct; with full-thickness tears they are unable to fully abduct independently

- USS, MRI, or arthroscopy can confirm diagnosis
- Partial tears need only analgesic support and physiotherapy
- Full-thickness tears should be repaired in the young active patient. Repair can be open or arthroscopic

Frozen shoulder

- Inflammatory process involving the whole cuff and capsule
- Age range 40–60
- Sometimes follows minor trauma
- Increasing pain with difficulty in sleeping on the affected side. After 3–6 months pain decreases but the shoulder remains stiff. Stiffness persists for a further 6–12 months and then resolves
- Full movement may not be regained
- Treatment:
  - Analgesics
  - Anti-inflammatories
  - Local heat
  - Physiotherapy
  - If stiffness remains, a manipulation under anaesthetic can be beneficial

Shoulder instability

- Commonest joint to dislocate
- Dynamic and static stabilisers:
  - The rotator cuff, capsule, labrum and surrounding larger muscles all act to keep the humeral head articulating with the shallow glenoid cavity
- There are two main types of instability:
  - Traumatic unidirectional instability with a Bankart lesion requiring surgery (**TUBS**)
  - Atraumatic multidirectional bilateral instability requiring rehabilitation and inferior capsule plication (**AMBRI**)

TUBS

- Usually anterior dislocation
- Diagnosis with AP X-ray
- Needs to be reduced in Casualty under sedation
- 80% chance of recurrence after first dislocation in the young adult
- Surgery required for repetitive dislocations
- Anterior detachment of the labrum (Bankart lesion) usually needs repair in the young. Recurrent dislocations can produce a notch behind the humeral head (Hill–Sachs lesion)

- Posterior dislocation: rare. Usually following epileptic fit or electric shock. Light bulb appearance of humeral head on AP view

AMBRI

- Multidirectional in the young
- Can be habitual
- Do not reduce in Casualty as patient can usually reduce themselves
- Do not require surgery but need physiotherapy

5.2.2 The elbow

- **Symptoms:**
  - Pain
    - Medial (golfer's elbow)
    - Lateral epicondyle (tennis elbow)
    - Diffuse (OA, RA)
    - Posterior (bursitis)
  - Stiffness: OA, RA, post-immobilisation
  - Swelling: OA , RA, infection, bursitis
- **Signs:**
  - Varus or valgus deformity
  - Swellings, subcutaneous nodules, osteophytes, ulna nerve sensitivity behind medial epicondyle
  - Flexion, extension, pronation, supination, medial and lateral joint stability
  - Tenderness at epicondyles (tendinitis)
- **Investigations:**
  - AP/lateral X-rays
  - Arthroscopy

Cubitus varus/valgus

Cubitus varus

- Usually post-malunion of supracondylar fracture
- No functional deficit
- Osteotomy of the lower humerus can be performed for cosmetic reasons

Cubitus valgus

- Usually secondary to non-union of a lateral condyle fracture
- Patient may develop delayed ulnar nerve palsy
- Nerve will need to be transposed in front of the elbow joint

Olecranon bursitis

- Causes:
  - Repetitive friction (true bursitis)
  - Infection
  - Gout
  - RA

- Gout: previous history, tophi, bilateral, calcification in the bursa
- RA: polyarthritis, subcutaneous nodules
- Infection: warm, very tender, high blood markers, pus aspirated
- Treat underlying cause
- Drain any infection
- Excise chronically inflamed bursa

Tendinitis of the common extensor origin
- Also known as **tennis elbow** but not always due to tennis
- Excessive activity (eg DIY) can cause minor trauma to the insertion of the common extensors
- Pain is over the lateral epicondyle but can radiate down the arm
- Worse on certain activities such as pouring tea or turning door knobs
- Elbow flexion and extension are painless
- Pain can be reproduced by actively extending the wrist with the elbow straight
- Treatment includes rest and activity modification
- Injection of local anaesthetic and steroid
- In resistant cases, release the common extensor muscles from their origin
- In **golfer's elbow**, the flexor origin on the medial side is affected
  - It is less common
  - Management is same as above

5.2.3 The wrist and hand
- **Symptoms:**
  - Pain
  - Stiffness
  - Swelling
  - Deformity
- Also examine the hand, forearm and elbow
- Look for scars, deformities and swellings
- Feel for temperature changes, tenderness, sensory changes
- Check and compare palmar flexion, dorsiflexion, radial/ulnar deviation, pronation and supination. Check the movements passively and actively as well as grip strength
- Abnormalities may occur secondary to discomfort, tendon rupture, neurological abnormality or muscular problem
- **Investigate** with X-rays AP and lateral. Scaphoid views for wrist pain

Kienböck's disease
- Avascular necrosis of the lunate
- Usually occurs after injury or stress
- Young adult presenting with ache and stiffness
- Tenderness localised to centre of wrist dorsally

- Reduced wrist extension
- X-rays initially show increased density; later the bone looks deformed
- Treatments include osteotomy of the radius, prosthetic replacement or arthrodesis

Chronic carpal instability
- Post-trauma, avascular necrosis or arthritis
- Collapse occurs in the row of carpal bones. The scaphoid is the main pillar
- Pain, stiffness and clicking are the main symptoms
- Tenderness is usually non-specific
- X-rays, MRI and arthroscopy are useful
- The commonest type of instability is scapholunate dissociation
- Stress views are useful, showing an increased gap between the lunate and the scaphoid
- If diagnosed early, the bones are reduced and held in position by K-wires
- With chronic instability, treatment is with injections and splints; if very symptomatic, then arthrodesis

Arthritis
- Usually secondary to malunion following trauma
- The scaphoid can undergo avascular necrosis following a fracture and so collapses, predisposing to arthritis
- A common site for OA is at the carpometacarpal joint of the thumb
- Tenderness is directly over the joint
- Diagnosis is confirmed on X-rays
- Treatment involves analgesia, injections, trapeziectomy or arthrodesis

Ganglion
- Commonly present on the back of the wrist
- Cystic degeneration of joint capsule
- Usually firm, mobile; can increase and decrease in size; sometimes aches
- With time can resolve spontaneously; otherwise aspirate (high chance of recurrence) or excise

De Quervain's disease
- Inflammation and thickening of the sheath containing the extensor pollicis brevis and abductor pollicis longus tendons
- Occurs secondary to overactivity
- Common in women aged 30–50
- Pain is present over the radial styloid, a lump is also usually palpable (thickened sheath). Passive adduction of the thumb across the palm is painful (Finkelstein's test)
- Treatment involves rest (splint), injection, slitting of the sheath

Carpal tunnel syndrome

- Usually present with pain and paraesthesia in the median nerve distribution of the hand
- Symptoms are worse at night, and the patient has to shake the hand in the air to relieve the symptoms
- Occurs due to compression of the nerve by the flexor retinaculum
- Common during the menopause, pregnancy and in patients with rheumatoid arthritis (for list of common causes, see Section 6.5.1 Mononeuropathies)
- On examination there may be sensory changes in the median nerve distribution, wasting of the thenar muscles, weakness of thumb abduction and a positive Phalen's or Tinel's test
- LOAF muscles affected in hand
  - Lumbricals 1 and 2
  - Opponens pollicis
  - Abdomen pollicis brevis
  - Flexor pollicis brevis
- The treatment usually involves decompression, though steroid injections can be tried first

Dupuytren's contracture

- Nodular hypertrophy and contracture of palmar aponeurosis
- Causes: familial, diabetes, AIDS, phenytoin therapy, Peyronie's disease
- Presentation: middle-aged man, thickening extending from palm into ring and little fingers. Both hands can be involved. Flexion contractures of the MCPJ and proximal interphalangeal joints may occur
- Treatment: required if function affected by progressive deformity. The thickened part of the aponeurosis is excised. Careful dissection is performed to avoid damage to the digital nerves. Post-operative splinting and physiotherapy is required

Trigger finger

- Cause: thickening of the fibrous tendon sheath causing entrapment at the entrance to its sheath
- Symptom: finger gets stuck in flexion. Has to be extended passively with a sudden snap (triggering)
- Treatment: release of the tendon sheath

Tendon pathology

Mallet finger

- Disruption of the extensor tendon insertion on the terminal phalanx
- Usually after being hit on the finger by a ball
- Treatment: extension splint for 6 weeks

Boutonnière deformity

- A longitudinal gap in the extensor tendon central slip causes the proximal interphalangeal joint (PIPJ) to button-hole
- The PIPJ is flexed and the distal interphalangeal joint (DIPJ) extended
- Usually occurs in RA or post-trauma
- Post-traumatic deformities can be repaired

Swan–neck deformity

- Due to imbalance of finger extensor and flexors
- PIPJ is hyperextended and DIPJ is flexed (opposite of Boutonnière)
- If the joints are still mobile, then deformity can be corrected by tendon rebalancing

5.2.4 The back

- **Symptoms:**
  - Pain
  - Stiffness
  - Deformity
  - If the nerves are affected, then the patient may complain of shooting pain, paraesthesia and weakness down the legs. The symptoms can come on suddenly (prolapsed disc) or can be gradual (degenerative)
  - If the patient has continuous night pain, then tumour or infection need to be ruled out
- **On examination** look out for:
  - Scars (previous surgery)
  - Pigmentation (neurofibromatosis)
  - Abnormal hair (spina bifida occulta)
  - Unusual skin creases
  - Note the patient's shape and posture
  - Feel the spinous processes for tenderness, alignment, prominences or any gaps
  - Movement is checked in flexion, extension, lateral flexion and rotation
  - A lower limb neurological assessment is performed, including straight leg-raise testing
- AP and lateral X-rays are performed. MRI is useful to look at the soft tissues and nerves

Scoliosis

- Scoliosis = curved to the side ± twisted
- Postural = correctible or structural = fixed
- Postural deformity is compensatory (short leg or pelvic tilt). Self-corrects when the patient sits
- Structural is secondary to bony abnormality or rotation
- Secondary curves can appear to counterbalance
- Deformity can increase during growth period

- Spinal surgery is required to correct any structural deformity

Kyphosis

- Kyphosis is a dorsal curvature of the spine
- It is normal in the thoracic and sacral spine
- An excessive dorsal curvature is also described as kyphotic
- Structural kyphosis is due to the shape of the vertebrae and is fixed
- Causes:
  - Osteoporotic fractures in the elderly
  - Post-traumatic fracture
  - Congenital defect
  - Infection
  - Ankylosing spondylitis
  - Scheuermann's disease
- Treatment depends on the cause

Pyogenic infection

- Usually affects the vertebral body (pyogenic spondylitis) or the disc space (discitis)
- Symptoms:
  - Constant back pain
  - Muscle spasm
  - Reduced range of motion
  - Malaise
- Raised WBC, ESR, CRP
- Blood cultures may be positive
- X-rays may show narrowed disc space or bone destruction
- MRI will show signs of infection
- A biopsy should be taken for culture before antibiotics are given
- IV antibiotics are given for up to 6 weeks until blood markers of infection settle

Intervertebral disc prolapse

- Secondary to herniation of nucleus pulposus through the annulus fibrosis
- Symptoms depend on the structures compressed
- Swelling secondary to the herniation may cause increased symptoms
- History:
  - Young adult
  - Sudden onset of severe pain while lifting heavy object or stooping
  - Pain and paraesthesia down the leg (sciatica), made worse by coughing
  - There can be distal numbness and muscle weakness
  - Saddle anaesthesia and bowel/bladder disturbance are signs of cauda equina compression, a surgical emergency

- Examination:
  - Patient stands tilted sideways, away from the side of the disc prolapse
  - Range of motion is limited
  - There is midline tenderness and paravertebral muscle spasm
  - Straight leg-raise angle is reduced
  - According to the nerve roots affected, there can be reduced power, sensory changes and altered reflexes
- Investigations:
  - MRI is the best mode of imaging to identify the disc
- Treatment:
  - Initially conservative treatment is applied unless the symptoms are progressive or not settling for several weeks
  - Conservative treatment involves analgesics, heat and physiotherapy
  - Operation involves a posterior approach and removal of the extruded material. Cauda equina compression is one of the few orthopaedic surgical emergencies and once diagnosis is confirmed there should be no delay in operation

5.2.5 The hip

Slipped capital epiphysis

- Essentially, the upper femoral epiphysis slips with respect to the femur, usually in a posterior inferior direction
- Usually affects adolescents, more common in boys than girls
- Causes include:
  - Body habitus: obesity, thinness, tallness
  - Endocrinopathy: hypothyroidism, hypoparathyroidism, acromegaly, hypogonadism
  - Radiotherapy
  - Renal failure (or 2ry hyperparathyroidism
- Pathophysiology is due to a combination of both biomechanical (obesity, increased physeal slope, deeper acetabulum) and biochemical (growth, thyroid and sex hormones) factors, which contribute to the development of a slip
- Symptoms:
  - Pain: in acute slips, hip (groin) pain; in chronic slips, thigh or knee pain (referred)
  - Inability to weight-bear
  - Limp
  - History of irradiation, renal failure, endocrinopathy
- Signs:
  - Look:
    - Externally rotated and shortened
    - Wasting of the thigh in chronic slips

- o Trendelenburg gait
- o Antalgic gaits
- ■ Feel: tenderness on palpation of affected hip
- ■ Move:
  - o Reduced range of movement on flexion, abduction and internal rotation in varus slips
  - o Reduced range of movement on flexion, adduction and internal rotation in valgus slips
  - o Obligatory (gross) external rotation on flexion
  - o Trendelenburg sign
- Differential diagnosis includes:
  - ■ Trauma
  - ■ Infection
  - ■ Inflammation, eg synovitis, juvenile idiopathic arthritis (JIA)
  - ■ Idiopathic, eg Perthes' disease
  - ■ Neoplastic
- Investigations include:
  - ■ Bloods: FBC, U&E, full hormonal profile
  - ■ Radiology
    - o Hip radiography: AP, lateral, frog leg (contraindicated for unstable/acute slips)
    - o CT
    - o USS
    - o Bone scan
- Management is surgical: principles of treatment are stabilisation of the slip to prevent progression and promotion of closure of the upper femoral physis, by pinning the slipped head in position ± osteotomy
- Complications include:
  - ■ Avascular necrosis (AVN; occurs at reduction)
  - ■ Coxa vara (fusion of epiphysis in slipped position resulting in a painless deformity)
  - ■ Contralateral slip
  - ■ Secondary OA
  - ■ Chondrolysis

Perthes' disease

- Local self-healing disorder in which AVN of the proximal femoral head occurs secondary to changing vascularisation of the femoral head at early stage of development (5–10 years)
- Aetiology includes:
  - ■ Idiopathic
  - ■ Congenital: slipped capital epiphysis
  - ■ Infectious: septic arthritis
  - ■ Inflammatory: synovitis
  - ■ Haematological: sickle cell crisis
  - ■ Traumatic
- Principally affects boys aged between 5 and 10 years

- Rapid growth in relation to developing blood supply interrupts blood flow, causing AVN. Necrotic tissue is removed and replaced with new bone
- Symptoms:
  - ■ Pain: intermittent ache in the anterior portion of the thigh, may be referred to the knee
  - ■ Swelling
  - ■ Limping: intermittent
  - ■ Reduced range of movement
- Signs:
  - ■ Look: wasting, Trendelenburg sign positive, fixed flexion deformity
  - ■ Feel: Thomas test for fixed flexion deformity of hip
  - ■ Move: reduced range of movement (early), full range of movement (late)
- Differential diagnosis includes:
  - ■ Infection: septic arthritis, osteomyelitis
  - ■ Inflammation: synovitis
  - ■ Trauma: proximal femoral fracture
  - ■ Congenital: acute or chronic slipped capital epiphysis
- Investigation with AP and lateral view X-rays of the hip
- Management:
  - ■ Conservative: bracing
  - ■ Medical: analgesia
  - ■ Surgical: osteotomy
- Complications include:
  - ■ Secondary OA
  - ■ Premature fusion of the growth plates

Congenital dislocation of the hip (CDH) or developmental dysplasia of the hip (DDH)

- A condition in which one or both hips are dislocated at birth or within the first few weeks of life
- Incidence is 1.5 in 1000 live births
- Affects girls more than boys
- Higher incidence in breech presentations and is linked to hereditary factors
- Clinical presentation in neonates is with a dislocated hip on screening tests:
  - ■ Barlow's test dislocates the hip with the hip in adduction and 90° flexion
  - ■ Ortolani's test is positive as it relocates a dislocated hip
- Retest on second occasion at 3 weeks. If signs still persist or risk factors are present, then investigate with an ultrasound scan (2–4 weeks post-partum)
- Children in later life may present with a limp or waddling gait
- Treatment is with:
  - ■ Abduction splint or harness in infancy (held in 'frog' position)

- Children between 6 and 18 months require maintenance of reduction with
  - Hip spica
  - Hip traction
  - Plaster splinting
  - Open reduction at surgery
- Older children presenting may need treatment with
  - Acetabuloplasty
  - Osteotomy
- Complications include osteoarthritis in later life. This is linked to the length of delay in initiating treatment

5.2.6 The knee

Osgood–Schlatter's disease

- Traction apophysitis caused by repeated avulsion of the apophysis [protuberance of bone into which a tendon (in this case the patellar tendon) is inserted]
- Traction phenomenon is associated with physical exertion (ie repetitive quadriceps contraction through the patellar tendon at its insertion) before skeletal maturity of the tibial tubercle
- Clinical features:
  - Pain over tibial tubercle ± patellar tendon region, gradual onset, follows activity and may be bilateral
  - Tenderness of the patellar tendon and a lump over the tibial tubercle
  - Usually occurs around the pubertal growth spurt when the quadriceps is enlarged but the apophysis has not yet fused to the tibia
- Management may be:
  - Conservative: rest and avoidance of exercise for 6 months. Persistence of the condition may warrant immobilisation for up to 6–8 weeks in a cast
  - Surgical: continued pain despite conservative management and involves excision of all intratendinous ossicles, with or without removal of a portion of the prominent tibial tubercle

Chondromalacia patellae

- Abnormal softening of the articular cartilage of the patella
- Aetiology: indirect trauma
- Epidemiology: commonly seen in teenage girls, generally resolves by age of 30 years
- Clinical features:
  - Symptoms: retropatellar pain, exacerbated by rising from prolonged sitting, using stairs (especially when walking down), kneeling and squatting
  - Signs: crepitus, effusion, pain on movement of the patella sideways or if pressed against the femur and then moved
- Investigation: MRI

- Management:
  - Conservative:
    - Rest and avoidance of knee bending and exercise
    - Immobilisation in plaster cast
  - Medical: analgesia
  - Surgical:
    - In the presence of patellar misalignment
    - Patellectomy: in presence of severe softening and degeneration of the articular surface (reduces risk of future OA)
    - Arthroscopy

Meniscal tear

- Two semilunar wedges in the knee joint positioned between the tibia and the femur are the medial and lateral meniscus
- The superior surfaces are concave and in contact with the femoral condyles; the inferior surfaces are flat and conform to the tibial plateaux
- Aetiology of meniscal tears: twisting strain applied to a flexed, weight-bearing leg during sport
- Epidemiology: common in young adults, medial meniscus more commonly torn
- Pathophysiology: the meniscus is an avascular structure so spontaneous repair of a torn meniscus is unlikely. If left untreated, secondary OA and recurrent synovial effusions occur
- Symptoms:
  - Pain: attacks of severe pain, localised to the anteromedial joint line [medial meniscus tear (commoner)] or diffuse (lateral meniscus tear). Between attacks the knee may be asymptomatic
  - Swelling: appears some time after the injury (unlike ligamentous injury)
  - Mechanical complaints: locking, clicking, catching, giving way
- Signs:
  - Look: knee may be held slightly flexed, quadriceps muscle will be wasted in long-standing cases
  - Feel: effusion, localised tenderness over the medial joint line (typical of a medial meniscus tear) while tenderness on the lateral side is less well localised
  - Move: reduced extension, McMurray's or Apley's grinding tests may be positive, Thessaly test at 20° flexion
- Investigations:
  - MRI
  - Arthroscopy
- Treatment:
  - Conservative: post-op physiotherapy
  - Medical: analgesia, anti-inflammatories (NSAIDs)
  - Surgical: arthroscopy or open (less common) meniscectomy to reduce risk of secondary OA

Fat pad syndrome

- Aetiology: catching of the fat pad in the tibiofemoral joint; also associated with premenstrual fluid retention resulting in fat pad swelling
- Epidemiology: commoner in young women
- Pathophysiology: the infrapatellar fat pad becomes swollen and tender
- Clinical features: pain on knee extension
- Management:
  - Conservative: rest
  - Surgical: fat pad excision

Patella tendinitis

- Inflammation of the patella tendon
- Aetiology: small tendon tear
- Clinical features: patella tendon pain, swelling, redness and warmth
- This condition commonly occurs in sports players
- Management:
  - Conservative: rest
  - Medical: anti-inflammatory (NSAIDs, steroid injection around the tendon)

Ligamentous injury

- Aetiology: forceful angulation or rotation of the tibia and the femur on each other. The medial collateral ligament (MCL) is the most commonly injured knee ligament
  - Sports
  - Trauma
- Anatomy: essentially there are four ligaments of the knee that stabilise the joint:
  - **Anterior cruciate ligament (ACL):** prevents the tibia from sliding anteriorly, so a blow from behind, eg tackle, forces the femur forwards (anteriorly) on the tibia causing ACL injury
  - **Posterior cruciate ligament (PCL):** prevents the tibia from sliding posteriorly, so a blow from the front forces the femur backwards (posteriorly) on the tibia causing PCL injury
  - Collateral ligaments: provides side-to-side stability
    - **Medial collateral ligament (MCL):** injury results from valgus stress (bending the tibia laterally)
    - **Lateral collateral ligament (LCL):** injury results from varus stress (bending the tibia medially)
- Classification:
  - Partial tear
  - Complete tear
- Grading:
  - Grade I sprain: overall integrity of the ligament is preserved. Painful to stress but stable
  - Grade II sprain: partial tear. Painful to stress; there is detectable laxity but the ligament has an eventual endpoint
  - Grade III tear: complete tear. Minimal pain to stress (as nerves in ligament are torn), there is detectable laxity with no endpoint or stability to testing
- Symptoms include:
  - Pain: partial tear more than a complete tear (may have little or no pain)
  - Swelling: acute onset (in contrast to meniscal injuries where swelling appears some time after the injury). Partial tear more than complete tear
- Signs:
  - Look: swelling over the side of the torn ligament. Lag sign in ACL/PCL tears
  - Feel: tenderness is most acute over the side of the torn ligament
  - Move: stressing the joint exacerbates the pain in partial tears. Laxity to stress
- Management:
  - Partial tear:
    - Conservative: rest, ice, compression, elevation (RICE), non-weight-bearing status (NWB, ie crutches), bandaged dressings/posterior splint hinged bracing
    - Medical: analgesia
  - Complete tear:
    - MCL (commonest): conservative with hinged bracing and NWB 1–2 weeks
    - LCL: surgical
    - ACL: surgical (intra-articular reconstruction is gold standard). Conservative management may be considered in less active patients
    - PCL: surgical repair if displaced tibial avulsion fracture
- Complications:
  - Adhesions (local tenderness and pain present on medial and lateral rotation)
  - Instability

5.3 TRAUMA AND FRACTURES

5.3.1 Initial management of trauma

Trauma is the main cause of death in people under 40.

Trimodal mortality distribution:

1 Within first hour (golden hour): massive blood loss, head injury, airway compromise
2 Between 1 and 4 hours: uncontrolled blood loss, respiratory compromise
3 Several weeks later: infection, organ failure

The management is according to ATLS (Advanced Trauma Life Support) protocol:

1 airway and cervical spine (C-spine): management of airway with C-spine protection
2 breathing: make sure lungs are ventilated. CXR to exclude pneumothorax/haemothorax
3 circulation: stop haemorrhage, have good IV access and resuscitate with fluids
4 disability: assess neurology, signs of head injury, Glasgow Coma Scale (GCS)
5 exposure: make sure the whole body is inspected to rule out hidden injuries

The above sequence is called the 'primary survey', where the patient is stabilised. It is important to keep on repeatedly assessing the above modalities to make sure there is no deterioration.

The secondary survey consists of a detailed head-to-toe examination of the patient to make sure that no minor injuries are missed (for example finger dislocations).

The routine initial X-rays for a trauma patient consist of a CXR, AP pelvis and lateral C-spine.

Chest injuries
- Damage to rib cage or internal organs
- Inspect for respiratory distress, wounds, bruising. Palpate the trachea (tension pneumothorax) and chest wall (surgical emphysema). Auscultate for reduced air entry
- Chest X-ray will reveal a pneumothorax, haemothorax and lung collapse. A ruptured aortic arch will show as a widened mediastinum. Fractured ribs, sternum and vertebrae will also be picked up
- Adequate oxygen delivery is essential, so good airway maintenance and blood replacement are important

Rib fractures
- Painful condition, but the only treatment required is analgesia. Can cause complications such as a pneumothorax, atelectasis and lung infection. Infiltration with local anaesthesia may ease discomfort
- **Pneumothorax** = air in the pleural cavity

Tension pneumothorax
- Tension pneumothorax is a surgical emergency which causes rapid deterioration in the patient's condition
- Occurs when a tear in the pleura acts like a valve, allowing air into the pleural cavity during inspiration but trapping the air during expiration
- The patient deteriorates rapidly as the mediastinum is shifted towards the unaffected side, kinking the vena cava against the diaphragm and blocking the venous return to the heart

- Clinically, the patient is in respiratory distress, chest movements are reduced, there is reduced air entry (breath sounds) and increased percussion note on the affected side, and shift of the trachea to the unaffected side
- The patient only has minutes before arresting, so treatment should be started as soon as the diagnosis is made (do not wait for CXR!)
- Treatment involves insertion of a large-bore needle into the pleural cavity through the second intercostal space in the midclavicular line anteriorly
- Once the patient is stable a chest drain is inserted into the fourth intercostal space in the midaxillary line and connected to a underwater seal

Surgical emphysema
- Occurs secondary to air entry into the subcutaneous tissues
- On palpation there is a feeling of 'crackles' under the skin
- The primary cause should be treated

Flail chest
- Isolation of an entire section of the chest wall is a flail segment
- Rib fractures cause flail chests if they are broken in two different places in at least two different levels
- Occurs in high-energy trauma and is often associated with underlying lung contusion
- Clinically the flail segment gets sucked inwards during inspiration and blown outwards during expiration (paradoxical repiration)
- Treatment is strapping and positive-pressure ventilation

Abdominal injuries
- Can occur due to high-energy blunt trauma or sharp penetrating injury
- Clinically the patient may complain of severe abdominal pain or present with hypotensive shock
- On inspection there may be bruising or a puncture wound
- Clinically, the abdomen can be rigid with decreased bowel sounds
- Commonly injured organs are the spleen in blunt trauma and the bowel or liver in penetrating trauma
- An ultrasound scan will show intraperitoneal free fluid and this can be confirmed by abdominal paracentesis, diagnostic peritoneal lavage (DPL) or a laparoscopy
- A CT scan will show retroperitoneal and encapsulated splenic collections
- If a serious injury is suspected a laparotomy is indicated

Head injuries

This topic is covered extensively in Section 6.1.

5.3.2 General complications of trauma

Shock

- State of reduced tissue perfusion
- **Types:**
  - Hypovolaemic
  - Cardiogenic
  - Neurogenic
  - Pulmonary embolus
  - Tension pneumothorax
  - Septic
- Hypovolaemic commonest type after trauma
- **Signs and symptoms:** weakness, thirsty, rapid shallow breathing, pale, cold and clammy
  - As shock progresses, the pulse becomes rapid and thready, the blood pressure drops and the patient becomes confused secondary to reduced cerebral perfusion
  - The renal perfusion is reduced with a drop in urine output
- Treatment:
  - Oxygen supplementation
  - Control of haemorrhage and replacement of the blood loss. Treat the cause!
  - It is therefore important that trauma patients have good venous access via two large-bore cannulae, one in each antecubital fossa
- If long bone fractures are present their early reduction and stabilisation will reduce bleeding

Fat embolism

- Thought to occur secondary to circulating fat globules from bone marrow after closed long bone fractures
- The mechanism remains unclear
- Clinically the patient is usually young with multiple closed fractures
  - Symptoms develop within 72 hours: difficulty in breathing, restlessness, confusion, pyrexia and tachycardia
  - There can be petechiae in the conjunctival folds, arm-pits and chest
- There is no specific treatment other than to keep the patient oxygenated and well supported
- Aim to reduce intrapulmonary oedema and clotting; heparin and steroids can be given

Disseminated intravascular coagulation (DIC)

- Due to the release of tissue thromboplastins, endothelial damage and platelet activation

- A complex mixture of coagulation, fibrinolysis, thrombocytopenia and depletion of clotting factors occurs. Microvascular occlusions lead to infarctions while depletion of clotting factors leads to bleeding
- The best treatment is prevention by early control of shock
- Once DIC is established, clotting factors, platelets and ITU support is required

Adult respiratory distress syndrome (ARDS)

- Shock leads to endothelial cell damage and increased permeability of the capillaries
- Extravasation of protein-rich fluid into the pulmonary interstitial tissue and alveoli leads to congestion and eventual destruction
- If progressive, severe hypoxia, multiple organ failure and death occur
- Symptoms start to develop 48–72 hours after injury with a reduction in arterial oxygen and shortness of breath
- Chest X-rays show diffuse infiltrates
- Treatment involves maintenance of oxygenation via artificial support
- The best method of prevention is early control of shock and stabilisation of fractures

5.3.3 Basics of fractures

- Fracture = break in the structural continuity of bone with a soft tissue injury
- Remember the soft tissue damage with the bony injury, as bone receives its nutrients from the blood! Vascular compromise? Periosteal stripping? Massive soft tissue loss?
- Remember to treat the patient using the ATLS protocol (ABCDE)
- Fracture causes (Box 5.1).

> **Box 5.1: Fracture causes**
>
> - Trauma
>   - Direct: usually transverse fractures, eg ulna
>   - Indirect: usually spiral fractures, eg tibia
> - Pathological
>   - Osteoporotic
>   - Malignant: primary or secondary (lung, renal, breast, prostate, thyroid)
>   - Infective: usually *Staphylococcus aureus*
>   - Metabolic: osteomalacia, Paget's disease, renal osteodystrophy
> - Stress fractures
>   - Repetitive loading
>   - Sites: metatarsals, tibia, pubic rami

- Fracture configuration: transverse, oblique, spiral, impacted, comminuted, segmental
- Closed or open (communicating skin laceration over fracture)
- Complete (both cortices involved), incomplete (one cortex involved, eg greenstick)
- When describing X-rays with fractures use the following terms to describe displacement:
  - Translation: relationship of fragment ends to each other
  - Length: shortened (usually) or lengthened
  - Rotation: fragments rotated in long axis
  - Angulation: is the alignment altered?
- When describing the fracture it is the position of the distal fragment which determines the direction of fracture
- Bones in children are relatively soft and so can buckle or break with the fracture involving only one cortex (greenstick)
- Bones heal faster in children than in adults and have a greater potential for remodelling, so more often can be treated non-operatively without anatomical reduction
- The Salter and Harris classification (Table 5.2) is used to describe physeal injuries

Table 5.2: Salter and Harris classification

Type 1: Separation of epiphysis

Type 2: Fracture along physis and through metaphysis

Type 3: Fracture is along the physis then cuts across the epiphysis into the joint

Type 4: Vertical fracture through the metaphysis, physis and epiphysis, going into the joint

Type 5: No fracture visible but the physis is crushed

- History: mechanism of trauma and associated injuries
- Past medical history (could it be pathological?)
- Current medication (eg steroids or warfarin)
- On examination:
  - Look for bruising, swelling, deformity, lacerations, skin colour
  - Feel for tenderness, bony incongruity, skin temperature and pulses (vascular injury)
  - Move if patient is unconscious or a dislocation/subluxation is suspected
- X-rays are obtained in at least two views showing the joint above and joint below the site of injury
- CT scans are useful for showing fracture configurations in difficult areas such as the calcaneum or pelvis

5.3.4 Basics of fracture treatment

The aim of fracture treatment is fracture union, so that the patient is left with normal function and preferably normal appearance after treatment.

The treatment of fractures usually involves three stages:

- **Reduction** of the fracture
- **Immobilisation** until the fracture unites
- **Rehabilitation** to regain normal function

Reduction

Aim: normal alignment, rotation, length and apposition.

Sometimes reduction is not required depending on the extent of displacement and site.

Intra-articular fractures require perfect reduction to avoid post-traumatic arthritis.

Methods of reduction are:

1 **Manipulation** – fragments easily reduced without needing 100% accuracy and are relatively stable
2 **Skin or skeletal traction** – once reduced force needs to be kept applied to counteract a deforming force, eg femoral fractures
3 **Open reduction** – interposition of soft tissue, needed for perfect reduction, an unstable fracture and when needing to internally fix it

Immobilisation

Methods of immobilisation are:

1 **Cast** – plaster of Paris (POP) or synthetic:
   - POP: usually used in the acute setting, back-slabs, etc. Easy and safe to handle. Can be cut and removed more easily than synthetic casts (important: if patient is complaining of increasing pain under a plaster, then split the cast as it may be too tight; look out for compartment syndrome). Relatively cheap and easy to mould
   - Synthetic: stronger/durable, lighter and more expensive than POP
   - Complications: displacement of fracture, compartment syndrome, pressure sores, skin damage when removing cast
2 **Internal fixation** – usually for unstable fractures or where accurate reduction is required. Also used for multiple fractures, pathological fractures and non-union:
   - Kirschner wires (K-wires): holds fracture fragments together. Inserted percutaneously with the end exposed (can be removed in clinic). Usually used with cast, for example in distal radius fractures

- Intra-fragmentary screws: hold fragments together, for example tibial plateau in knees or medial malleolus in ankles
- Plates and screws: can be used in bridging (connecting two fragments together), compressing (compressing fragments together) and neutralisation (stops twisting action on long bones) modes
- Intramedullary nailing: used for long bone fractures, for example tibia or femur. Useful as provides rigid fixation, with small incision sites and because the patient can start full weight-bearing straightaway
- Complications: infection, breakage of metalwork, nerve or vascular injury, fracture around prosthesis (metal is hard while bone is soft so a stress riser is created), prominence of metalwork

3 **Continued traction** – presently used mainly for paediatric long bone fractures, for example paediatric femoral fractures. Elderly patients can be treated in skeletal traction as a last resort if unfit for surgery
- Complications: pressure sores, malunion, DVT/PE

4 **External fixation** – used as an alternative to internal fixation where infection may be risk, for example in grossly contaminated open fractures

Rehabilitation

- Reduce swelling by elevation
- Exercise the uninjured joints
- Start active mobilisation as soon as possible (prevents adhesions, keeps muscles strong, encourages callus formation)
- Physiotherapy to strengthen muscles and regain independence

Complications of fractures

See Box 5.2.

Box 5.2: Complications of fractures

- **Early**
    - Nerve/vascular injury
    - Direct visceral/soft tissue injury
    - Infection
    - Bleeding/haematoma
    - Compartment syndrome
    - Ligament/tendon injury
    - Pressure/plaster sores
- **Late**
    - Mal/non-union
    - Post-traumatic arthritis
    - Avascular necrosis
    - Myositis ossificans

Compartment syndrome

Compartment – closed anatomical space within a limb, which is bound by bone and fascia and enclosed by soft tissue, eg muscles.

Anatomy

Upper limb compartments (forearm)
- Ventral:
    - Nerves: median and ulnar
    - Arteries: radial and ulnar
- Dorsal:
    - Nerves: posterior interosseous
    - Arteries: no major vessels

Lower limb compartments
- **Anterior tibial:**
    - Nerves: deep peroneal
    - Arteries: anterior tibial
- **Superficial posterior:** no major nerves or vessels
- **Deep posterior:**
    - Nerves: posterior tibial nerves
    - Arteries: posterior tibial and peroneal
- **Peroneal:**
    - Nerves: deep and superficial peroneal

Aetiology
- **External restriction**
    - Tight splints, casts, dressings
    - Burns
    - Localised external pressure
- **Internal restriction**
    - Haemorrhage
    - Fractures
    - Reperfusion oedema
    - Oedema
    - Rhabdomyolysis

Pathophysiology
Essentially in a closed anatomical space elevated intrafascial compartment pressure (tissue pressure) causes reduced tissue perfusion causing muscle and nerve ischaemia. Therefore management involves prompt diagnosis and early decompression before irreversible tissue necrosis occurs.

Clinical features
- **Symptoms:**
    - Gradual onset of dull pain localised to a compartment
    - Associated with swelling (tense feeling); others (late, ie 5 P's: pallor, pulsless, paralysis, poikilothermia, paraesthesia)
    - Timing – crescendo of pain despite immobilisation
    - Exacerbated by passive extension of muscles within compartment

- Severity out of proportion with injury
- **Signs:**
  - Look: swelling, pale
  - Feel: poikilothermia and pulseless (late). Tense, tender compartment
  - Move: **pain on passive stretching** of muscles within the compartment, eg passive extension of the toes or fingers causes increased pain in the calf or the forearm respectively

Differential diagnosis
- DVT
- **Normal post-op/fracture pain:** remember crescendo and out of proportion!

Investigations
- **Bloods:**
  - FBC: anaemia
  - U&E: hyperuricaemia, acute renal failure
  - ↑CK: rhabdomyolysis
  - Coagulation screen (INR, aPTT, TT): DIC
- **Urinalysis:** dipstick, myoglobinuria
- **Radiology:** CT, MRI
- **Direct pressure measurement:** intracompartmental pressure measurement is diagnostic (>40 mmHg)

Management
Essentially you aim to decompress, therefore reducing any restrictions on affected limb(s).

- **Conservative:**
  - Elevation of affected limb(s) to level of heart (elevation above this is contraindicated because it decreases arterial flow and narrows the arterial-venous pressure gradient)
  - Reduce external restrictions
    - Release one/both sides of a plaster cast
    - Reduce dressings
    - Remove TEDS or compression stockings
- **Surgical:** fasciotomy

Essential note

Do not delay any treatment in compartment syndrome. Seek senior help immediately if compartment syndrome is suspected. Always start by removing any plaster or restricting cast. Treat urgently if pain continues and do not wait for compartment pressures if the clinical diagnosis is straightforward. Fasciotomies can save limbs from future disabling contractures

Complications
- Tissue ischaemia and/or necrosis
- Volkmann contracture
- Recurrent exertional compartment syndrome

5.3.5 Examples of common fractures
Some common fracture examples are included here for completeness of this section on fractures. For the written examinations, very few fractures are examined in the syllabus. The five commonest fractures are mentioned here very briefly, but they should be covered more extensively in an orthopaedics and trauma textbook and during the orthopaedics rotation. It is much more important to retain the principles of fracture management and have knowledge of complications such as compartment syndrome than it is to know specific fracture details. Only pelvic fractures are covered in a little more detail as they can be life-threatening injuries causing huge amounts of blood loss.

Neck of femur
- Intra- (within) or extra- (outside) capsular
- Important to distinguish as outcome and treatment differ
- Femoral head receives most of the blood supply from vessels in the capsule, so when intracapsular fracture occurs the blood supply is disrupted, leading to avascular necrosis of femoral head
- Grading is by Garden's classification grades I–IV
- Intracapsular fractures are treated with a hemiarthroplasty (half a hip replacement, where the acetabulum is not resurfaced but the head is replaced)
- Extracapsular fractures (blood supply not disrupted) are fixed with a dynamic hip screw

Distal radial fractures
- If dorsally angulated and within 2.5 cm of the articular surface, they are known as Colles' fractures
- Extra-articular fractures with a volar tilt are known as a Smith's fracture (important to distinguish Colles' from Smith's when manipulating and putting a slab on in Casualty, as a Colles' back-slab goes on dorsally and a Smith's on the volar side)
- Minimally displaced Colles' fractures can be manipulated and treated in a cast
- Unstable fractures can be held with K-wires under a cast
- Comminuted fractures or intra-articular fractures in the young can be openly reduced and fixed with locking plates
- Smith's fractures are usually treated with a volar buttress plate

Ankle fractures

- Can involve only the lateral malleolus, medial and lateral malleolus or medial, lateral and posterior malleolus
- Usually if only the lateral malleolus is involved then the injury is stable, ie the ankle does not dislocate and the fracture can be treated in a cast
- If both malleoli are fractured it is usually an unstable injury and can cause dislocation of the ankle. Usually requires an open reduction and internal fixation. A fracture dislocation of the ankle should be reduced in Casualty under sedation until definitive fixation can be performed. This is done to reduce any inflammation and oedema that may result from the unreduced injury, which would make operative reduction more difficult

Fractured tibia or femur

- Long bone fractures are best treated with an intramedullary nail. This allows small incisions and early mobilisation of patients. If the tibial fractures are stable and minimally displaced then they can be treated in plaster
- Femoral fractures are always unstable because of the pull on the distal fragment from the quadriceps. In adults they are usually treated with nailing. In children they can be treated in traction

Pelvic fractures

Anatomy

The pelvis is formed by two hip bones (innominate bones, connected anteriorly at the symphysis pubis and posteriorly to the sacrum at the sacroiliac joints), sacrum and coccyx. The sacrum and the two innominate bones form a ring. The pelvis is divided anatomically into the false pelvis (iliac crests superiorly to the pelvic brim inferiorly) and the true pelvis (pelvic brim inferiorly to the pelvic floor).

Its contents include the neurovascular bundle, which includes the common iliac vessels and its branches, and the lumbosacral plexus.

Aetiology

Low- and high-energy trauma, eg road traffic accident

Clinical features

- Pain and tenderness: pelvic, axial and abdominal
- Soft tissue: swelling, bruising (inguinal, perineal, scrotal/labial), lacerations, abrasions, degloving
- Muscle: rupture and hernia
- Bone: deformity, crepitus (instability)
- Pelvic organs: urethral tear (blood at external urethral meatus, high-riding prostate on digital rectal examination), bladder disruption (gross haematuria), rectal, perineal and genital lacerations
- Neurovascular: haemorrhagic shock (visceral damage or associated injuries), motor and sensory loss, sphincter dysfunction (bladder and anus), erectile dysfunction

Investigations

- **Bloods:** FBC, U&E, LFT, coagulation screen, G+S, cross-match 6 units
- **Radiology**
  - Pelvic radiographs
    - AP view: demonstrates major pelvic disruptions
    - Lateral view: demonstrates AP and mediolateral translations, and internal/external rotatory deformities
    - Inlet view: demonstrates AP and mediolateral translations, and internal/external rotatory deformities
    - Outlet view: demonstrates superior and inferior translations, abduction ± adduction, and flexion ± extension rotational deformities
    - Sacral view: demonstrates transverse fracture of sacral body ± kyphosis of sacrum
  - Pelvic CT: for operative planning
- Others: CXR and ECG if high-energy trauma or pre-op assessment, angiogram if suspected pelvic haemorrhage, cystogram/urethrogram if damage to urinary tract suspected

Management

- ATLS
- Depends on site and stability of fracture
  - Immobilise: canvas sling, bedrest 6–8 weeks
  - Reduce: skin/leg traction up to 12 weeks
  - Fixation: internal (plates and screws) or external fixation

Complications

- VTE (DVT/PE)
- Infection
- Muscle rupture and hernia
- Injury to pelvic organs, eg bladder, urethra, ureters, kidneys, genital organs
- Injury to neurovascular bundle

BIBLIOGRAPHY

McRae R. 2006. *Pocketbook of Orthopaedics and Fractures.* London: Churchill Livingstone.

Head, neck and neurosurgery

CONTENTS

Head, neck and neurosurgery

EDITOR'S NOTE

Head, neck and neurosurgery are regarded as specialist topics in the general undergraduate curriculum. Not much time will be allocated in the clinical years on these firms compared with general surgery and medicine, yet knowledge of the topics required in the syllabus is still essential.

Many of the topics covered in this chapter represent important clinical conditions which will be encountered in a variety of settings, regardless of specialty. There is considerable overlap between neurosurgery, spinal orthopaedics and neurology in terms of clinical presentation of conditions such as stroke, tumours and other lesions of the brain and spinal cord. Virtually every A&E doctor, radiologist and member of the trauma team will be involved at some stage in their careers with managing head injuries. GPs see patients with headaches on a daily basis.

The important features of learning topics in this chapter concentrate more on diagnosis and clinical features than on specific management. It is more important for a junior doctor to know how and when to appropriately refer a specialist patient, than to know which particular treatment a patient should receive.

The last section of this chapter completes the 'head and neck' section by dealing with lumps in the neck which have not been covered elsewhere, and cervical lymphadenopathy.

Intracranial mass lesions, strokes, haemorrhages, injuries, spinal cord lesions and compression, mononeuropathies and neck lumps are all commonly examined topics in undergraduate exams.

It is these topics that should be revised with greater emphasis than ear, nose and throat or ophthalmology when covering the head and neck region.

Revision objectives

You should know:

- The causes, clinical assessment, investigation and basic management of head injuries
- How and when to refer patients to a neurosurgeon appropriately
- Briefly about the different brain tumours and their effects, such as hydrocephalus, mass compression and clinical course
- Indications, contradictions and complications in performing a lumber puncture
- The features of the different types of cerebrovascular diseases that present
- The clinical features of trauma and lesions affecting the spinal cord and how they are managed on a basic level
- The clinical features of the common mononeuropathies and the causes and management of carpal tunnel syndrome in particular detail
- The causes and clinical features of the common lumps in the neck
- The clinical examination of the neck for OSCE and clinical exams

6.1 HEAD INJURIES

Head injury is defined as head trauma leading to any alteration in mental or physical status in which loss of consciousness is not necessary.

6.1.1 Head injury assessment (Figure 6.1)

The severity of head injuries is most commonly classified by the initial post-resuscitation Glasgow Coma Scale (GCS) score (Box 6.1), which generates a numerical summed score for eye, motor and verbal abilities.

The general approach to history taking is almost universal to all complaints. The neurological history can be divided up as follows:

- Age, gender, hand dominance, occupation
- Presenting complaint
- History of presenting complaint
- Screening questions
- Past medical history
- Drug history and allergies
- Family history
- Social history

Resuscitate with Airway, Breathing and Circulation (ABC)

GSC ≤ 8	GSC 9–14	GSC 15
Involve anaesthetist/intensivist early to provide adequate airway management and assist with resuscitation	Immediately	Within 15 minutes of arrival

Assess risk of clinically important brain injury/cervical spine injury

High risk
Extend assessment to full clinical examination to establish need for imaging of head and/or cervical spine

Low risk
Re-examine within a further hour – part of assessment should establish need for CT imaging of head and/or cervical spine

Figure 6.1: Assessment in the Emergency department

Essential note

Exclude significant brain injury before ascribing depressed conscious level to intoxication

Screening questions include:

- Headaches
- Memory disturbance
- Dizziness, blackouts and loss of consciousness
- Sensory changes, eg sight, smell, taste, numbness
- Speech disturbance
- Difficulty swallowing
- Weakness, eg in upper and/or lower limbs

Need for spinal immobilisation:

- GCS <15
- Neck pain or tenderness
- Focal neurological deficit
- Paraesthesiae
- Any clinical suspicion of C-spine injury

Primary investigation of choice: CT scan of head (Figure 6.2).

Glasgow Coma Scale

The severity of head injuries is most commonly classified by the initial post-resuscitation GCS score (Figure 6.1).

Box 6.1: Glasgow Coma Scale (GCS)

Best motor response
6 Obeys commands
5 Localising response to pain
4 Withdraws to pain
3 Flexion response to pain (decorticate posturing)
2 Extension response to pain (decerebrate posturing)
1 None

Best verbal response
5 Oriented (time, person, place)
4 Confused conversation, but able to answer questions
3 Inappropriate words
2 Incomprehensible speech, eg moaning sounds
1 None

Best eye-opening response
4 Spontaneous eye opening
3 Eye opening in response verbal stimuli, command, speech
2 Eye opening in response to pain only (not applied to face)
1 None

Overall score: sum of the best scores in three assessed areas

Range: 3 (lowest) to 15 (highest)

NB If a patient exhibits asymmetrical response, you are to take the higher one, eg right hand withdraws to pain (4) but left hand localises pain (5), therefore the best motor response is taken (5)

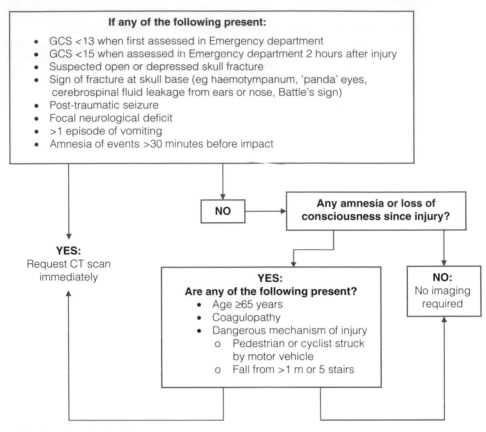

If any of the following present:

- GCS <13 when first assessed in Emergency department
- GCS <15 when assessed in Emergency department 2 hours after injury
- Suspected open or depressed skull fracture
- Sign of fracture at skull base (eg haemotympanum, 'panda' eyes, cerebrospinal fluid leakage from ears or nose, Battle's sign)
- Post-traumatic seizure
- Focal neurological deficit
- >1 episode of vomiting
- Amnesia of events >30 minutes before impact

NO

Any amnesia or loss of consciousness since injury?

YES:
Request CT scan immediately

YES:
Are any of the following present?
- Age ≥65 years
- Coagulopathy
- Dangerous mechanism of injury
  - Pedestrian or cyclist struck by motor vehicle
  - Fall from >1 m or 5 stairs

NO:
No imaging required

Figure 6.2: Selection of adults for CT scan

Head injury is classified according to the following scores:

- Coma: 3–8
- Severe: ≤8 (unable to maintain airway)
- Moderate: 9–12
- Mild: 13–15, eg concussion

Neurological assessment

A good neurological history is a key feature of the neurological examination. Neurologists/neurosurgeons learn most from the history when identifying the cause of the symptoms and arriving at a diagnosis.

The general approach to history taking is almost universal to all complaints. In addition to the normal full history, the following screening questions should be taken as part of a focused neurological history.

Screening questions

- Headaches
- Memory disturbance
- Dizziness, blackouts and loss of consciousness
- Sensory changes, eg sight, smell, taste, numbness
- Speech disturbance [abnormalities can be due to: different language spoken by patient; deafness, dysphasia (disorder in speech)/aphasia (absence of speech), dysphonia (impaired ability to produce normal volume of sound); or dysarthria (impaired ability to articulate words)]
- Difficulty swallowing
- Weakness, eg in upper and/or lower limbs

Higher mental function assessment

- Level of consciousness
- Attention and orientation
- Memory (short term and long term)
- Calculation
- Registration
- Language

Methods of higher mental function assessment:

- **GCS:** ascertains the level of consciousness
- **Mini Mental State Examination (MMSE)** (Box 6.2) measures the remaining areas of higher mental functions. A shorter, **Abbreviated Mental Test (AMT)** (Box 6.3), is sometimes used to screen for disorientation and cognitive impairment, but it does not test all areas of cognition

Box 6.2: Mini Mental State Examination

Temporal orientation

What year is it? ☐

Season? ☐

Month? ☐

Date? ☐

Day of the week? ☐

_____ /5

Spatial orientation

What country are we in? ☐

County? ☐

City/town? ☐

Hospital? ☐

Ward? ☐

_____ /5

Registration

'I am going to say three words. I want you to say them out loud after me.'

Apple ☐

Table ☐

Penny ☐

_____ /3

Allow 1 second between each word. Score 1 point for each correct word. The order does not matter. This score is based on this first trial only. If the patient is unable to repeat all three words, allow further attempts and prompting up to a maximum of five times until the patient is able to repeat all three back to you. Ask the patient to keep these words in their mind to test for recall later.

Attention and calculation

Ask the patient, 'Subtract 7 from 100, and then keep subtracting 7 from each answer until I tell you to stop.' Score 1 point for each correct answer, up to a maximum of five subtractions. The answer is correct if it is exactly 7 less than the previous answer, regardless of whether the previous answer was correct.

Patient's answer

93 _____

86 _____

79 _____

72 _____

65 _____

_____ /5

171

Recall

Ask patient to recall the objects repeated in the registration test.

Apple ☐

Table ☐

Penny ☐

_____

/3

Naming

Show the patient a pen and then a watch and ask him or her to name them. Score 1 point for each object (or part of object) correctly identified.

Pen ☐

Watch ☐

_____

/2

Repetition

Ask the patient to repeat the following phrase, 'no ifs, ands or buts'. Score 1 point if the patient repeats the entire phrase correctly, on the first attempt.

_____

/1

Comprehension

Have a piece of paper ready and give the following three-stage command to the patient:

'Take this paper in your right hand, fold it in half and put it on the floor/your lap.' (Use the left hand if the right is impaired.) Score 1 point for each stage.

Taking paper in right hand ☐

Folding paper in half ☐

Putting paper on the floor/lap ☐

_____

/3

Reading

On a blank piece of paper write 'CLOSE YOUR EYES' in large print and ask the patient to obey what is written. Score 1 mark if the patient closes their eyes

_____

/1

Writing

Give the patient a blank piece of paper and ask them to write a sentence. Score 1 point if the sentence is sensible and has a verb and a subject.

_____

/1

Drawing

Ask the patient if they can copy the intersecting pentagons below. Score 1 point if this is correctly copied

_____

/1

_____**Total**

/30

Borderline: 25–27

Dementia: <25 (also consider acute confusional state and depression)

Score 1 point for each correct response:

Age ☐

Time to the nearest hour (make sure the patient does not look at their watch or a clock) ☐

Year ☐

Name of the **institution** (eg hospital) ☐

Ask the patient to memorise the following address for recall later: 42 West Street

Date of birth ☐

The year the **First World War** began ☐

The name of the **monarch** ☐

Recognise two people, eg doctor and nurse ☐

Count backwards from 20 to 1 ☐

Recall the address they were asked to memorise ☐

Total /10

Normal: 8–10

Mild to moderate dementia: 4–7

Severe dementia: 0–3

Imaging

Types of imaging (Box 6.4) include:

- Skull X-ray
  - Indications:
    - Skull X-rays have become largely redundant due to the introduction of CT and MRI imaging.
    - They are most commonly performed for identification of skull fractures, if CT is not available.
- Computer tomography (CT) a collimated X-ray source moves synchronously with photon detectors placed in a gantry to produce a series of slice images of the brain

tissue, between 2 mm and 13 mm thick. The difference in X-ray attenuation of materials, measured in Hounsfield Units (HU), enables identification of abnormalities (Table 6.1). Iodine-containing contrast agents may be used to enhance areas of oedema and increased blood supply and delineate areas of blood–brain barrier breakdown, eg around infarctions and tumours.

- **Indications:** areas in which CT is either approximately equivalent or superior to MRI
  - Exclusion of intracerebral haemorrhage in acute stroke
  - Acute subarachnoid haemorrhage
  - Acute head injury
  - Exclusion of neurosurgical emergencies in critically ill patients
  - Lesions of orbits and paranasal sinuses.
- **Magnetic resonance imaging (MRI):** MRI utilises the phenomenon of nuclear magnetic resonance, in which an image is created by upsetting protons (usually hydrogen) aligned by a strong magnetic impulse, using radiofrequency waves at right angles to their alignment. Detecting the signal at different stages of relaxation, as the protons return to equilibrium, produces images in different sequences, known as T1- and T2-weighted images. The promagnetic agent, gadolinium, is the contrast agent used.
  - **Indications:** MRI effectively demonstrates
    - Intracranial tumours, particularly tumours in areas prone to bony artefact on CT, eg posterior fossa
    - Precise staging of malignancy, eg involvement of bone marrow
    - Arteriovenous malformations
    - Disorders of myelination, eg multiple sclerosis
    - Dementia: can demonstrate multi-infarct dementia
    - Intracranial and spinal cord infections
    - Various spinal cord conditions, eg syringomyella

Table 6.1: X-ray attenuation of materials (Hounsfield units)			
	Attenuation (HU)	Examples	
	+1000	Bone	White
Biological soft tissues	+80	Blood and muscle	⬍
	0	Water and CSF	
	−100	Fat	
	−1000	Air	Black

Box 6.4: MRI vs CT

	MRI	CT
Radiation	No exposure to radiation	Small exposure to radiation
Shape	Tubal	Doughnut
Magnetic field	Contraindicated in patients with internal metallic bodies, eg pacemakers, mechanical heart valves and vascular clips	No exposure to magnetic fields
Resolution	Resolution > CT	Relatively poor resolution
Vasculature	Without contrast	Contrast
Spinal cord	Without contrast	Contrast necessary to image spinal cord
Bony artefact	Enable imaging of areas prone to bony artefact on CT, eg posterior fossa	Sometimes misses lesions in posterior fossa

Criteria for hospital admission

- New, clinically significant abnormalities on imaging
- Not returned to GCS 15 after imaging, regardless of the imaging results
- Criteria for CT fulfilled, but scan not done within appropriate period
- Persistent worrying signs (eg vomiting, severe headaches)
- Other sources of concern (eg intoxication, other injuries, shock, suspected non-accidental injury, meningism, cerebrospinal fluid leak)

Criteria for neurosurgical referral

Care of all patients with new, surgically significant abnormalities on imaging should be discussed with a neurosurgeon.

Irrespective of imaging, other criteria for neurosurgical referral include:

- Persisting coma (GCS ≤8) after initial resuscitation
- Unexplained confusion >4 hours or other neurological disturbance
- Deterioration in GCS after admission, especially motor response deterioration
- Progressive focal neurological signs
- Seizure without full recovery
- Definite or suspected penetrating injury
  - Depressed fracture of skull vault
  - Suspected fracture of skull base
- Cerebrospinal fluid (CSF) leak
- Skull fracture plus any of
  - Confusion or greater impairment of consciousness
  - One or more seizures
  - Neurological signs

6.1.2 Types of head injuries

Head injuries include:

- External injury to the scalp
- Skull fractures
- Concussions
- Contusions (bruises)
- Lacerations (tears)
- Intracranial haematoma

Risk factors/causes

- Road traffic accidents (RTAs)
- Physical assaults
- Sports-related accidents
- Falls (especially in elderly and children)
- Alcohol-related accidents
- Drug-related haemorrhage: anticoagulants and anti-platelet medication increasing risk of intracranial haemorrhage
- Liver disease: reduced ability to synthesise proteins and clotting factors, increasing risk of intracranial haemorrhage

6.1.3 Intracranial haemorrhage

Definition: pathological accumulation of blood within the cranial vault.

Types:

- **Spontaneous**
  - Intracerebral haemorrhage: mostly hypertensive
  - Subarachnoid haemorrhage: mostly aneurysmal
  - Mixed intracerebral and subarachnoid haemorrhage: typically associated with arteriovenous malformations

- **Traumatic**
  - Extradural haemorrhage: arterial, typically the middle meningeal artery
  - Subdural haemorrhage: venous, typically cortical bridging veins

(Refer to Section 6.3 for an in-depth look at types of intracranial haemorrhage.)

6.1.4 Management of head injuries

Management geared towards prevention of secondary causes of brain damage.

- ATLS
  - If GCS ≤8: early involvement of an anaesthetist/intensivist for appropriate airway management (see Box 6.5)
- Assess:
  - Severity of injury
  - Need for imaging
  - Need for admission
  - Need for neurological referral
- Observations:
  - GCS
    - GCS =15
      - Every 30 minutes for 2 hours
      - Hourly for 2 hours
      - Two hourly
    - GCS <15
      - Every 30 minutes
  - Pupil size and reactivity
  - Limb movements
  - Vital signs
    - Respiratory rate
    - Pulse rate
    - Blood pressure
    - Temperature
    - Oxygen saturation

Transfer from secondary setting to neurosurgical unit: if possible, all patients with serious head injuries (GCS ≤8) should be transferred, regardless of need for neurosurgery. If not possible, ongoing advice from the neurosurgeons is essential for clinical management.

Management of raised intracranial pressure (ICP)

Raised ICP is caused by intracranial lesions causing an increased volume of blood, CSF or parenchymal tissue.

Box 6.5: Intubation and ventilation

Circumstances	Action
<ul><li>Coma: GCS ≤8</li><li>Loss of protective laryngeal reflexes</li><li>Ventilatory insufficiency:<ul><li>Hypoxaemia (PaO_2 <13 kPa on oxygen)</li><li>Hypercapnia ($PaCO_2$ >6 kPa)</li></ul></li><li>Spontaneous hyperventilation causing $PaCO_2$ <4 kPa</li><li>Irregular respirations</li></ul>	Intubate and ventilate immediately
<ul><li>Significantly deteriorating conscious level (1 or more points on motor score), even if not coma</li><li>Unstable fractures of facial skeleton</li><li>Copious bleeding into mouth</li><li>Seizures</li></ul>	Intubate and ventilate before transfer to neuroscience unit

- Muscle relaxation and short-acting sedation
- Analgesia
- Aim for:
  - PaO_2 >13 kPa
  - $PaCO_2$ 4.5–5.0 kPa
  - Mean arterial pressure ≥80 mmHg (infuse fluid and vasopressors)
- If clinical or radiological evidence of raised intracranial pressure (ICP), aggressive hyperventilation indicated and increase inspired oxygen concentration

Causes of raised ICP

Numerous causes, including:

- Expanding mass:
  - Tumour
  - Haemorrhage
  - Abscess
- Increased cerebral blood volume:
  - Vasodilation
    - Hypercapnia
  - Venous outflow obstruction
  - Venous sinus thrombosis
- Increased CSF:
  - Impaired absorption
    - Hydrocephalus
    - Benign intracranial hypertension
  - Excessive secretion
  - Choroid plexus papilloma
- Cerebral oedema:
  - Chronic meningitis
  - Hypertensive encephalopathy
  - Head injury

Pathophysiology

Cerebral blood flow (CBF) = cerebral perfusion pressure (CPP)/ cerebral vascular resistance (CVR)

$$CPP = BP - ICP$$

Factors affecting CVR:

- **Chemoregulation:** accumulation of metabolic by-products such as H^+, which is formed when CO_2 passes across the blood–brain barrier according to the Henderson–Hasselbach equation
- **Autoregulation:** maintains cerebral blood flow (CBF) over CPP by vasoconstriction and vasodilatation

Clinical features

- Headache – typical of raised ICP
- Vomiting
- Visual disturbances:
  - Blurring
  - Obscurations – transient blindness
  - Papilloedema in some patients
  - Retinal haemorrhages if the rise in ICP has been rapid
- Brain shifts – often with depression of conscious level
- Cushing's (stress) peptic ulceration
- In infants, slowly increasing ICP may present as slowly increasing head size
- Brief depression of conscious level after an insult, followed by improvement then progressive drowsiness (acute medical emergency)

- Gradual dilation of one pupil and a decreasing responsiveness to light
  - Indicates expansion of a clot over ipsilateral hemisphere

Management

Raised ICP is monitored with a ventricular catheter or surface pressure recording device.

Management depends on the source of the raised pressure:

- **Medical**
  - Steroids
  - Barbiturates
  - Hyperventilation
  - Osmotic diuretics, eg mannitol
- **Surgical**
  - Surgical excision of space-occupying lesion (SOL)
  - Burr hole with an external drain or shunt if increased CSF

6.1.5 Complications of head injuries

- Cranium
  - Intracranial bleeding
  - Fracture
- Cerebrum
  - Headache
  - Concussion
  - Cerebral oedema
  - Raised ICP
  - Infection, eg meningitis
  - Hypopituitarism
  - Diabetes insipidus (cerebrogenic)
  - Acute confusional state
  - Vegetative state
- Cranial nerves
  - Palsy
- Cerebellum
  - Cerebellar syndrome
- Ears
  - Tinnitus
  - Hearing loss
  - Ear pain
- Nose
  - Epistaxis
  - Rhinorrhoea
- Eyes
  - Visual disturbances

Long-term complications include:

- Hemisphere syndromes – hemiplegia; aphasia – dominant hemisphere; spatial neglect – non-dominant hemisphere; visual field defects; rarely, dystonia, resulting from damage to deep basal ganglia

- Brainstem syndromes – limb tremor, unsteadiness of gait
- Cranial nerve syndromes
- Post-traumatic epilepsy
- Meningitis – associated with CSF leakage through nose and/or ear
- Cerebral atrophy
- Communicating hydrocephalus
- Post-concussion syndromes
- Caroticocavernous fistulas (rare)
- Neuropsychological

6.1.6 Brain death

Defined as irreversible damage of the ascending reticular activating system (ARAS).

- Pre-conditions
  - **Comatose (GCS 3)**
  - **Cause compatible with irreversible brain damage**
  - **Absent**
    - **Respiration:** on ventilator
    - **Drugs:** CNS depressants, neuromuscular junction blocking agents, and any overdosage
    - **↓Temperature (T⁰):** must be >35°C
    - **Metabolic and endocrine abnormalities:** ↓blood glucose, ↑H⁺, U&E imbalance
  - **Doctor**
    - Qualified >5 years
    - Two sets of tests must be compatible and performed by different senior doctors within 12–24 hours
    - Should not be part of the transplant team
- Diagnostic tests
  - **Brainstem reflexes (absence of all)**
    - **Midbrain:** fixed (unreactive to light), dilated pupils
    - **Midbrain and pons:** absent oculocephalic (doll's head movements) and vestibulo-ocular (caloric test) reflexes
    - **Pons:** absent corneal, gag and cough reflexes
    - **Midbrain, pons and medulla:** no motor response to pain, spinal reflexes may be present; no respiration if ventilator stopped and $PaCO_2$ allowed to rise >6.7 kPa

Note:
- **Spinal reflexes are not relevant to diagnosis**
- **EEG or neurologists are not essential**
- **Differential diagnosis of fixed dilated pupils:**
  - Parasympathetic paralysis
    - Iatrogenic: atropine
    - Neuropathy (CN III palsy): multiple sclerosis, Guillain–Barré syndrome, cerebrovascular accident
    - Trauma
    - Intracranial mass compression

- Sympathetic stimulation
  - Iatrogenic: sympathomimetics (ephedrine, noradrenaline, etc)
  - Phaeochromocytoma
- **Miscellaneous:** cardiac arrest, ↓T⁰

6.2.1 Space-occupying lesions (SOL)

Causes
- Neoplastic
  - **Secondary (30%; commonest cause of SOL):** breast, lung, melanoma
  - **Primary:** gliomas (43%), pituitary adenoma (20%), meningioma (10%; 2F:1M), astrocytoma and glioblastoma
- **Infectious:** cerebral abscess, cyst
- **Vascular:** haematoma, aneurysm, chronic subdural haematoma
- **Inflammatory:** granuloma, eg tuberculoma

Pathophysiology (brain functions)
- **Frontal lobe:** pre-motor cortex, and primary motor cortex (pre-central gyrus)
- **Parietal lobe:** primary somatosensory cortex (post-central gyrus)
- **Temporal lobe:** auditory cortex
- **Occipital lobe:** visual cortex

Clinical features
- **↑ICP:** confusion, headache, drowsiness, coma, nausea and vomiting, seizures, papilloedema (50% of tumours), ↑BP, ↓PR, irregular RR
- **Seizures:** <50% of tumours
- **Personality changes:** irritable, socially inappropriate behaviour, lack of initiative and application to tasks
- **False localising signs:** due to ↑ICP – abducens (VI) nerve palsy (commonest, due to its long intracranial course)
- **Evolving localising signs** (Table 6.2):
  - Partial seizures
    - **Simple partial** – paroxysmal attacks of abnormal movements/sensations
    - **Complex partial** – brief alterations in mood, perception, behaviour
  - Sensory/motor deficit
  - **Psychological deficit:** language, memory, perception, personality

Table 6.2: Signs of space-occupying lesions

Site	Signs
Temporal lobe	• **Complex partial seizures:** absences, disturbances of mood (fear/rage), hallucinations (olfactory, visual, auditory), déjà vu, automatism (purposeless behaviour), hypersexuality • **Sensory/motor deficit:** contralateral *upper* quadrantanopia • **Psychological deficit:** dysphasia [Wernicke's (receptive) aphasia], disturbances of memory (forgetfulness)
Frontal lobe	• **Simple partial seizures:** Jacksonian seizures (focal motor seizures) • **Sensory/motor deficit:** contralateral hemiplegia, +positive grasp reflex (significant if unilateral), urinary incontinence • **Psychological deficit:** dysphasia (Broca's 'expressive' aphasia), alexia (impaired reading), agraphia (impaired writing), personality changes (indecent, indolent, indiscreet)
Parietal lobe	**Left** • **Simple partial seizures:** sensory seizures (contralateral sensory abnormality) • **Sensory/motor deficit:** contralateral hemisensory loss, contralateral *lower* quadrantanopia, ↓ two-point discrimination, sensory inattention • **Psychological deficit:** anomia (inability to name objects), alexia, agraphia, acalculi (inability to calculate), astereognosis (inability to recognise objects by touch alone) **Right** • **Psychological deficit:** constructional apraxia (difficulty assembling objects/drawing, eg 5-point star)
Occipital lobe	• **Simple partial seizures:** visual hallucinations, eg palinopsia • **Sensory/motor deficit:** contralateral homonymous hemianopia
Cerebellum (DASHING)	Dysdiadochokinesia / Ataxia (truncal) / Slurred speech / Hypotonia / Intention tremor / Nystagmus / Gait abnormality
Corpus callosum	**Rare:** severe rapid intellectual deterioration; focal neurological signs; signs of loss of communication between lobes, eg hand unable to carry out verbal response
Cerebello-pontine angle	**Usually vestibular schwannoma:** ipsilateral deafness and tinnitus, ipsilateral cerebellar signs, nystagmus, VI nerve palsy, papilloedema, ↓corneal reflex, facial weakness

Differential diagnosis
- Stroke
- Epilepsy
- Benign intracranial hypertension
- Colloid cyst of third ventricle
- Multiple sclerosis
- Todd's palsy
- Vasculitis, eg panarteritis nodosa, systemic lupus erythematosus, giant-cell arteritis, syphilis
- Metabolic, or electrolyte imbalance

Investigations
- **Imaging:** CT all patients; skull X-ray, chest X-ray, others (if indicated), eg MRI, magnetic resonance angiography
- **Biochemistry:** ESR, tumour markers (AFP, human chorionic gonadotropin)

- **Procedures:** LP contraindicated due to ↑ICP in the presence of SOL

Management
- **Tumour:**
  - Surgical excision:
    - Benign
    - Malignant: gliomas
  - Radiotherapy: gliomas post-op, tumour inaccessible for surgery, or metastases
  - Chemotherapy: gliomas
- **Hydrocephalus:** ventriculoperitoneal shunt if tumour inaccessible for surgery
- **Headache:** codeine (opiate analgesic)
- **Epilepsy:** antiepileptic prophylaxis, eg phenytoin (unreliable)

- **Cerebral oedema:** steroid (dexamethasone)
- **↑ICP:** intubation and hyperventilation at head-up tilt ± osmotic agent (mannitol IVI), loop diuretic, steroids IV

Complications
- **↑ICP and midline shift** due to SOL or obstructive hydrocephalus lead to:
  - Supratentorial: tentorial herniation
  - Infratentorial: tonsillar herniation
- **Disturbed function:**
  - Supratentorial (cerebral): CN I–VI damage
  - Infratentorial (cerebellar): CN III–XII damage
- **Epilepsy:** infrequent with tumours of the posterior fossa or brainstem

Prognosis
- **Benign:** total cure if complete resection
- **Malignant:** poor prognosis (<50% 5-year survival)

6.2.2 Intracranial tumours
Commonest intracranial tumours are **secondary metastases**.

Epidemiology
- **Incidence:** 5–15 per 100 000 per year; account for 2% of UK deaths
- **Prevalence:**
  - **Children:** medulloblastomas of the posterior fossa are most common
  - **Adults:** gliomas, meningiomas and metastases are most common
- **Age:** bimodal distribution, 5–9 years old and in late middle age

Pathophysiology
Secondary metastases (20%): spreading through the bloodstream or by direct invasion, these are the most common types of intracranial SOL.

- Lung (33% of all intracranial tumours; 25% of lung tumours metastasise to brain)
- Breast (20% of all intracranial tumours; 25% of breast tumours metastasise to brain)
- Kidney

Primary brain tumours: rarely metastasise outside the brain

- Gliomas (43%) – 90% occur in frontal, parietal or temporal lobes; poor prognosis
  - Astrocytoma
  - Glioblastoma multiforme
  - Oligodendroglioma
  - Ependymoma
- Meningiomas (10%)

- Pituitary adenomas (10%) – adenoma, adenocarcinoma
- Others are comparatively rare

Sites
It is possible for any type of cell within the brain or spinal cord to undergo neoplastic change.

- **Cerebral hemispheres**
  - **Extrinsic**
    - Meningioma
    - Cysts (dermoid, epidermoid, arachnoid)
  - **Intrinsic**
    - Astrocytoma
    - Glioblastoma
    - Oligodendroglioma
    - Primary lymphoma
    - Metastasis
- **Hypothalamus**
  - Astrocytoma
- **Sellar/suprasellar region**
  - Pituitary
    - Benign (adenoma)
      - Microadenoma (<1 cm – common)
      - Macroadenoma (>1 cm)
    - Malignant
      - Primary (rare)
      - Secondary (metastatic)
  - Craniopharyngioma
  - Meningioma
  - Optic nerve glioma
  - Cysts (dermoid, epidermoid)
- **Skull base and sinuses**
  - Carcinomatous meningitis
  - Chordoma
  - Glomus
  - Osteoma
- **Ventricular system**
  - Colloid cyst
  - Choroid plexus papilloma
  - Ependymoma
  - Germinoma
  - Teratoma
  - Meningioma
- **Pineal region**
  - Pineal cytoma
  - Pineal blastoma
  - Astrocytoma
  - Ependymoma
  - Germinoma
  - Teratoma
  - Meningioma

- Posterior fossa
  - Extrinsic
    - Neuroma
    - Meningioma
    - Cysts (dermoid, epidermoid, arachnoid)
    - Metastasis
  - Intrinsic
    - Metastases
    - Haemangioblastoma
    - Medulloblastoma
    - Astrocytoma

Clinical features

- Symptoms
  - Insidious onset (weeks or years) with often only minor intellectual and emotional impairment; more rarely, they may present acutely due to haemorrhage or the development of hydrocephalus
- Signs
  - Mass effects
    - ↑ICP and midline shift due to SOL or obstructive hydrocephalus
      - Supratentorial: causes tentorial herniation
      - Infratentorial: causes tonsillar herniation
  - Focal damage
    - Seizures: >one-third of patients with intrinsic tumours of the cerebral hemispheres
      - Epileptiform convulsions are more frequent with slow-growing than rapidly growing tumours
      - Epilepsy is infrequent with tumours of the posterior fossa or brainstem
    - Disturbed function
      - Supratentorial (cerebral): CN I–VI damage
      - Infratentorial (cerebellar): CN III–XII damage

Differential diagnosis

- Vascular: stroke, haematoma, CVT, giant aneurysm, AVM, migraine
- Infection: abscess, tuberculoma, sarcoidosis, encephalitis
- Cysts

Investigations

- Imaging
  - CT: all patients
  - Skull X-ray
    - ↑ICP, eg suture separation
    - Calcification, eg hyperostosis of adjacent bone in meningioma
    - Erosion of posterior clinoids, eg craniopharyngioma
    - Osteolytic lesions, eg dermoid, epidermoid, meningiomas
  - MRI: if atypical, or for visualisation of posterior fossa or skull base
  - MRA: to differentiate tumours (eg meningiomas, secondary tumours and gliomas); also to exclude arteriovenous malformation and aneurysms
  - Chest X-ray: establish whether primary tumour
- Biochemistry: ESR (establish whether metastasis), tumour markers (AFP and human chorionic gonadotropin, especially for germinomas)
- Procedures
  - LP contraindicated due to ↑ICP, but CSF may be obtained from other sources (eg ventricular drainage on shunt insertion)
  - Biopsy: tumours by burr hole, stereotactic, open with decompression

Management

Depends on: grade (benign or malignant), site (accessibility) and type of tumour. In general, conservative therapy is the treatment of choice.

- Benign tumours: best treated by excision, except if inaccessible or are attached to adjacent structures, ie non-excisable benign lesions
- Malignant tumours or non-excisable benign lesions
  - Treatment: aim to reduce raised ICP – intubate and hyperventilate, nurse at head-up tilt (30°), osmotic agent (mannitol IVI), loop diuretic (furosemide), steroids IV
  - Monitor small, asymptomatic tumours: serial CT; initial CT provides baseline to assess the progress of the tumour
  - Surgical excision: partial or complete excision; depends on histology (burr hole or stereotactic biopsy) and site of lesion (imaging)
  - Radiotherapy: often used either alone or post-op. Many but not all intracranial tumours are radiosensitive
  - Chemotherapy: may be used depending on tumour type, but results are disappointing

Referral to neurologist

Urgent referral

- Suspected brain tumour + CNS symptoms
  - Progressive neurological deficit
  - New-onset seizures
  - Headaches
  - Mental changes
  - CN palsy
  - Unilateral sensorineural deafness, or tinnitus

- Headache (recent-onset), and features of ↑ICP
  - Confusion, drowsiness/coma, vomiting, posture-related headache, pulse-synchronous tinnitus, papilloedema, focal (eg seizure) CN III palsy or non-focal neurological signs (eg blackout) change in personality or memory loss; Cushing's reflex (late) – ↑BP, ↓PR, irregular RR
- Headache: new, unexplained, qualitatively different and progressively severe
- Seizure: recent-onset
- Previous medical history of any cancer and CNS symptoms
  - Seizure of recent onset
  - Progressive neurological deficit
  - Persistent headaches
  - New mental or cognitive disturbance
  - New neurological signs

Consider urgent referral

Rapid progression of:

- Subacute focal neurological deficit
- Unexplained cognitive impairment, behavioural disturbance or slowness, or a combination of these
- Personality changes in the absence of the other symptoms and signs of a brain tumour

Consider non-urgent referral

Unexplained headaches of recent onset:

- Present for at least 1 month
- Not accompanied by features of ↑ICP

6.2.3 Pituitary tumours

Anatomy
- Two lobes
  - Anterior:
    - Luteinising hormone (LH)/follicle-stimulating hormone (FSH) (Figure 6.3)
    - Growth hormone (GH) (Figure 6.4)
    - Thyroid-stimulating hormone (TSH) (Figure 6.5)
    - Adrenocorticotropin (ACTH) (Figure 6.6)
    - Prolactin (PRL) (Figure 6.7)
  - Posterior: does not produce hormones, only releases them
    - Antidiuretic hormone (ADH; also known as vasopressin)
    - Oxytocin
- Site: lies in the sella turcica (Turkish saddle)
  - Superior: optic chiasm (hence bitemporal hemianopia)
  - Lateral: cavernous sinus (contains anterior branch of internal carotids, cranial nerves III, IV, V1,2, VI)

Classification
- Benign (adenoma)
  - Non-functional
  - Functional
- Malignant
  - Primary (rare)
  - Secondary (metastatic)

Clinical features
- Compression effects
  - Bitemporal hemianopia
  - Headaches

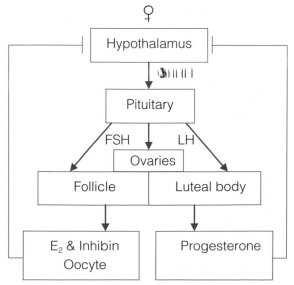

Figure 6.3: Actions of LH and FSH in men and women. DHT = dihydrotestosterone; E_2 = oestradiol; GnRH = gonadotropin-releasing hormone

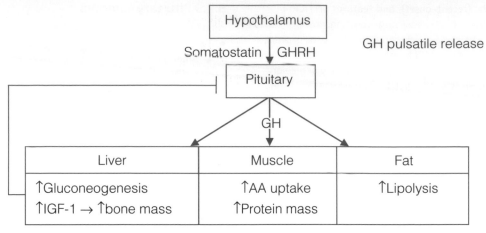

Figure 6.4: Actions of GH. GHRH = growth hormone-releasing hormone; IGF = insulin-like growth hormone

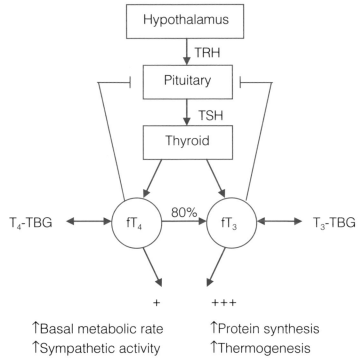

Figure 6.5: Actions of TSH. fT_3 = free triiodothyronine; fT_4 = free thyroxine; TBG = T_4-binding globulin; TRH = thyrotropin-releasing hormone

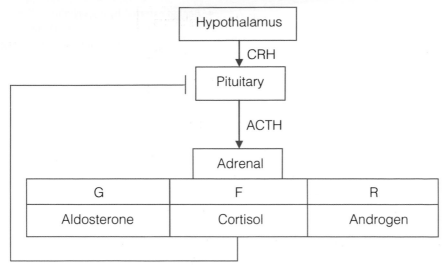

Figure 6.6: Actions of ACTH. CRH = corticotropin-releasing hormone; F = zona fasciculata; G = zona glomerulosa; R = zona reticularis

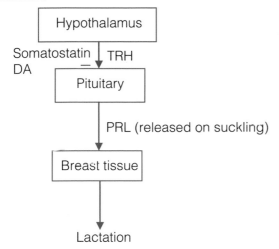

Figure 6.7: Actions of PRL. DA = dopamine

- **Hypopituitarism:** hormonal underproduction; loss of hormones in the following order
  - ↓LH/FSH
    - ○ ↓Libido, infertility (erectile dysfunction, amenorrhoea), hypogonadism (♂ hair loss, small testicular volume, ↓spermatogenesis; ♀ breast atrophy, osteoporosis, dyspareunia)
  - ↓GH
    - ○ ↓Lipolysis (atherosclerosis, central obesity), ↓muscle bulk, ↓strength and exercise ability, ↓cardiac output, ↓hypoglycaemia, osteoporosis (↓IGF-1)
  - ↓TSH
    - ○ Hypothyroidism: weight gain, ↓appetite, constipation, menorrhagia, feels the cold

- ↓ACTH
  - ○ Addisonian crisis: hypotension (dizziness, syncope, collapse, shock), pain (arthralgia, myalgia, abdominal pain, cramps, headaches), GI features (nausea and vomiting, diarrhoea, constipation, weight loss), metabolic derangement (hypoglycaemia)
- ↓PRL
  - ○ Inability to lactate post-partum
- **Hyperpituitarism:** hormonal overproduction
  - ↑GH
    - ○ Acromegaly: carpal tunnel syndrome, hypertension, obstructive sleep apnoea
  - ↑TSH
    - ○ Hyperthyroidism: weight loss, ↑appetite, diarrhoea, oligomenorrhoea, heat intolerance
  - ↑ACTH
    - ○ Cushing's disease
  - ↑PRL: hyperprolactinaemia causing galactorrhoea

Investigation
- **Bloods**
  - FBC, U&E, LFT, lipids, blood glucose
  - **Full hormonal profile:** LH/FSH, testosterone, E_2, progesterone, GnRH, PRL, ACTH, thyroid function tests, short Synacthen test® (synthetic ACTH), cortisol
  - **Dexamethasone suppression test (low- and high-dose)**
- **Urinalysis:** 24-hour cortisol
- **Radiology**
  - CT
  - MRI
- **Petrosal sinus sampling:** ACTH- or TSH-producing adenomas; in selected cases

Management
- **Medical**
  - **Hypopituitarism**
    - ↓LH/FSH
      - ♂ – testosterone IM/patch
      - ♀ – oestrogen ± testosterone (improvement of libido)
    - ↓GH: GH, GHRH, IGF-1, oxandrolone
    - ↓TSH: thyroxine, liothyronine
    - ↓ACTH: hydrocortisone
  - **Hyperpituitarism**
    - ↑TSH
      - **Symptomatic:** propranolol
      - **Suppression:** carbimazole, propylthiouracil
    - ↑GH: octreotide (somatostatin analogue), dopamine agonist, eg bromocriptine/cabergoline, GH-receptor antagonist, eg pegvisomant
    - ↑ACTH: metyrapone, ketoconazole, aminoglutethimide
  - ↑PRL: dopamine agonists, eg bromocriptine/cabergoline
- **Surgical**
  - Hypophysectomy
  - Adrenalectomy (↑ACTH)
- **Radiological**
  - DXT (deep X-ray therapy)
  - Cranial irradiation

6.2.4 Hydrocephalus

Increased volume of CSF within the ventricles of the CNS.

Anatomy

CSF is produced by the choroid plexus located within the ventricular system of the CNS. It flows from the lateral ventricles to the third ventricle via the interventricular foramen of Monro. Then it passes to the fourth ventricle via the cerebral aqueduct of Sylvius, after which it passes through the two lateral foramina of Luschka and one medial foramen of Magendie to the subarachnoid space. From there it flows to the arachnoid granulations, the dural sinus and finally enters the venous drainage system.

Classification

- **Non-communicating:** obstruction to CSF flow within the ventricular system (the ventricular system does not communicate with the subarachnoid space)
- **Communicating:** obstruction to CSF flow outside the ventricular system (the ventricular system communicates with the subarachnoid space)
- **Normal–pressure hydrocephalus (NPH):** form of communicating hydrocephalus in which the ICP measured by lumbar puncture is normal or intermittently raised

- **Benign external hydrocephalus:** self-limiting absorption deficiency of infancy and early childhood with raised ICP and enlarged subarachnoid spaces (prognosis: resolution within 1 year)
- **Obstructive hydrocephalus:** obstruction of the flow of CSF, intraventricular or extraventricular. Most hydrocephalus is obstructive
- **Arrested hydrocephalus:** stabilisation of known ventricular enlargement, most likely secondary to compensatory mechanisms

Aetiology

- **Congenital:** stenosis of aqueduct of Sylvius, Dandy–Walker and Arnold–Chiari malformations
- **Acquired:** SOL, subarachnoid haemorrhage, intraventricular haemorrhage, infections, trauma
- **NPH**
  - Infection: meningitis
  - Iatrogenic: radiotherapy, posterior fossa surgery
  - Idiopathic
  - Vascular: subarachnoid haemorrhage
  - Traumatic: severe head injury
  - Neoplastic: tumours

Clinical features

- Acute onset
  - ↑ICP: headache, vomiting, papilloedema and impaired conscious level
  - Impaired upward gaze
- Gradual onset
  - Confusion
  - Upper motor neurone lesion and gait apraxia
  - Sphincter dysfunction
  - Hypopituitarism

Investigations

- **Radiology:**
  - Skull X-ray
  - CT head (contrast)
  - USS (anterior fontanelle – infants)

Management

- **General**
  - Intracranial shunt
    - Ventricular
      - Ventriculoatrial
      - Ventriculoperitoneal
    - Lumbar
      - Lumboperitoneal
  - Ventriculostomy
  - Lumbar puncture (contraindicated in the presence of SOL)

- **Specific**
  - Treat underlying cause

Complications
- Shunt failure
- Cognitive function: infants/children – poor development; adults – loss of cognitive function
- Visual loss
- Tonsillar herniation

Prognosis
Untreated hydrocephalus: death can occur by tonsillar herniation secondary to raised ICP with compression of brainstem followed by respiratory arrest.

6.2.5 Lumbar puncture
Spinal needle punctures into subarachnoid space of the lumbar region to obtain CSF for diagnostic or therapeutic purposes.

The adult spinal cord ends at the level of L1–2. The plane of the iliac crests runs through L4, so this level can be used to define the L3/4 or L4/5 interspace for use in lumbar punctures.

Indications
- **Diagnostic**
  - **Infection:** meningitis
  - **Vascular:** subarachnoid haemorrhage
  - **Inflammatory:** Guillain–Barré syndrome, systemic lupus erythematosus, sarcoidosis, Beçhet's syndrome
  - **Autoimmune:** multiple sclerosis
  - **Neoplastic:** lymphoma, leukaemia, paraneoplastic disorders
- **Therapeutic**
  - Relief of pseudotumour cerebri (benign intracranial hypertension)
  - Relief of raised ICP due to communicating hydrocephalus
  - Intrathecal drugs, eg antibiotics, antifungals, cytotoxics

Indications for brain CT prior to LP:

- >60 years old
- Immunocompromised
- Known or suspected CNS lesion
- Seizure within 1 week
- Impaired conscious level (GCS)
- Focal neurological signs, eg CN III or VI palsy
- Features of ↑ICP

Contraindications
- **↑ICP in presence of an SOL:** headache, confusion, drowsiness, ↓conscious level, nausea and vomiting, seizures, focal neurological signs (eg CN III palsy), papilloedema (50%); Cushing's reflex – ↓PR, ↑BP, Cheyne–Stokes respiration – ↓RR
- **Bleeding disorders:** coagulopathy (eg haemophilia, thrombocytopenia), bleeding diathesis (eg anticoagulation therapy)
- **Cerebral abscess**
- **Infection at site of needle entry**
- **Cardiorespiratory compromise**
- **CT features**
  - Midline shift
  - Posterior fossa mass
  - Loss of suprachiasmatic and basilar cisterns
  - Loss of the superior cerebellar cistern
  - Loss of the quadrigeminal plate cistern

Complications
- **Headache (up to 70%)**
  - **Site:** bilateral fronto-occipital
  - **Onset:** occurs within 24–48 hours of lumbar puncture
  - **Character:** constant, dull, ache
  - **Time:** self-limiting, usually resolves over hours (up to 7 days)
  - **Exacerbation:** exacerbated when upright, relieved when supine (positional exacerbation)
  - **Aetiology:** continued CSF leak from the puncture site and intracranial hypotension
  - **Prevention:** use smallest needle gauge, or blunt needle
  - **Treatment:** responds to analgesia; if severe or prolonged treat with epidural blood patch (anaesthetist); if persistent CT may be needed to exclude subdural haematoma
- **Bloody tap (50%):** microtrauma gives rise to false-positive RBC in CSF. To exclude collect CSF ×3 bottles
- **Infection (rare; immunocompromised):** cellulitis, skin/epidural/spinal abscesses
- **Haemorrhage (rare):** epidural haematoma, subdural haematoma, subarachnoid haemorrhage
- **Coning (very rare):** cerebral or cerebellar tonsil herniation

6.3.1 Stroke

Definitions

Stroke/cerebrovascular accident (CVA)
Clinical term used to describe acute loss of circulation to an area of the brain resulting in ischaemia and corresponding **sudden neurological deficit**.

Reversible ischaemic neurological deficit (RIND)

Neurological deficit (stroke) that **lasts >24 hours to 1 week**, without interruption, and that resolves with complete recovery.

Transient ischaemic attack (TIA)

Sudden onset of focal **neurological deficit lasting <24 hours**; ('minor stroke').

Epidemiology

- **Incidence:** increases with age
- **Prevalence:** 8/1000 (0.8%) >25 years old
- **Third commonest cause of death in UK** (12%)

Categories

- Complete/partial infarction
- TIA
- RIND

Pathophysiology

- Stroke classification is shown in Table 6.3
- Two circulations supply the brain (Tables 6.4, 6.5; Figure 6.8)

Causes

- **Ischaemic (85%)**
  - **Thrombosis–in–situ (53%)**
    - **Intracranial atherosclerosis – thrombogenic factors:** stasis, vessel wall damage, hypercoagulable state (Virchow's triad)
    - **Others** – coagulopathies, haemoglobinopathies (eg sickle cell disorder) drug abuse (cocaine)
  - **Embolism (31%)**
    - **Cardiac source – atrial fibrillation** (commonest cause), acute myocardial infarct, valvular heart disease, prosthetic heart valves, congestive heart failure, patent foramen ovale, atrial septal defect, ventricular septal defect
    - **Arterial source** – commonly **carotids**
  - **Hypoperfusion (rare):** sudden drop in BP >40 mmHg
- **Haemorrhagic (15%)**
  - **Intraparenchymal (10%) – hypertension** (commonest cause), trauma, long-term anticoagulation therapy, drug abuse (cocaine), vasculitis (rare; eg giant-cell arteritis)
  - **Subarachnoid (atraumatic; 5%) – ruptured aneurysm** (80%), atrioventricular malformation (15%), idiopathic (15%)

Table 6.3: Classification of stroke

Stroke	
Ischaemic (85%)	*Haemorrhagic (15%)*
<ul><li>**Thrombosis–in–situ (53%)**</li><li>**Large vessel (70%):** ICA, ACA, MCA, PCA, VBS</li><li>**Small-vessel and lacunar strokes (30%)**</li><li>**Embolism (31%)**</li><li>Cardiac</li><li>Arterial</li><li>**Hypoperfusion (rare)**</li></ul>	<ul><li>Intraparenchymal (10%)</li><li>Subarachnoid (5%)</li></ul>

ACA = anterior cerebral artery; ICA = internal carotid artery; MCA = middle cerebral artery; PCA = posterior cerebral artery; VBS = vertebrobasilar system.

Table 6.4: Cerebral arterial circulation

Cerebral arterial circulation	
Anterior circulation	*Posterior circulation*
Composition: ACA, anterior communicating artery, ICA, MCA, posterior communicating artery	**Composition:** PCA, VBS (BA and VA)
Supply: majority of cerebral hemispheres except occipital and medial temporal lobes	**Supply:** occipital lobes, medial temporal lobes, brainstem and cerebellum
Occlusion: commonest cause of AIS (70%)	

AIS = acute ischaemic stroke; BA = basilar artery; VA = vertebral artery.

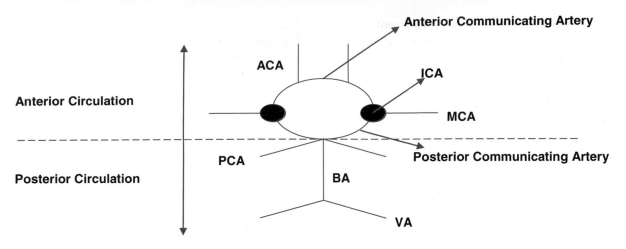

Figure 6.8: Cerebral artery territories (CVA). ACA = anterior cerebral artery, BA = basilar artery, ICA = internal carotid artery, MCA = middle cerebral artery, PCA = posterior cerebral artery, VA = vertebral artery

Table 6.5: Cerebral arteries – areas of perfusion and clinical effects of occlusion

	ACA (uncommon)	ACA (60% of CVA)	PCA	VBS	ICA
Supply	Frontomedial surfaces of cerebral hemispheres	Lateral surfaces of cerebral hemispheres	Occipital lobe	Occipital lobe, brainstem and cerebellum	Anterior two-thirds and basal ganglia
Occlusion effects	**Unilateral:** Contralateral leg monoparesis and numbness with facial sparing **Bilateral:** Akinetic mute state (damaged cingulate gyrus); paraplegia (a rare cause), incontinence and hemisensory loss	Contralateral hemiplegia, hemisensory loss (mostly face and arm), homonymous hemianopia, ipsilateral gaze palsy, dysphasia (dominant affected) and visuospatial disturbance (non-dominant, eg neglect of contralateral limbs, dressing difficulties)	Homonymous hemianopia **Most common cause: cardioembolism**	**Occipital lobe:** Cortical blindness, hemianopia **Brainstem:** Quadriplegia (usually asymmetric >70%); disturbances of gaze and vision (ischaemia of abducens nucleus, PPRF, MLF causing ipsilateral CN VI palsy, ipsilateral conjugate gaze palsy, INO, (ocular bobbing); locked-in syndrome (aware but unable to respond) **Cerebellum (DASHING):** **D**ysdiadochokinesia **A**taxia (truncal) **S**lurred speech **H**ypotonia **I**ntention tremor **N**ystagmus **G**ait disturbance	**Partial:** Similar to MCA occlusion; prodromal symptoms prior to occlusion include amaurosis fugax (sudden monocular blindness), transient hemisensory/hemimotor disturbance **Total:** Fatal

CVA = cerebrovascular accident; INO = internuclear ophthalmoplegia; MLF = medial longitudinal fasciculus; PPRF = parapontine reticular formation.

Head, neck and neurosurgery

Risk factors
- **Modifiable:** hypertension (most important), smoking, diabetes mellitus, ↑lipids, lack of exercise, obesity, diet (↑NaCl intake, ↑fat intake, ↑alcohol, ↓K$^+$ intake, ↓vitamin intake), combined oral contraceptive pill + smoking, previous medical history of TIAs or cardiovascular disease (ischaemic heart disease, atrial fibrillation, valvular heart disease)
- **Non-modifiable:** age (↑), sex (M), race (Afro-Caribbean), genetics (positive family history)

Clinical features
See Table 6.6.

Commonest clinical features
- **Sudden onset**
  - Weakness/numbness of: limb/face, usually unilateral
  - Disturbance of: vision; speech/understanding; balance/coordination
  - Confusion
  - Dizziness
  - Severe headache (unknown cause)
- **Accompanied by**
  - Nausea
  - Vomiting
  - Fever
  - Transient loss of consciousness

Differential diagnosis
- Hypoglycaemia (commonest cause of stroke-like features)
- Subarachnoid haemorrhage
- Subdural haemorrhage
- Migraine
- Todd's palsy: post-ictal paralysis lasting <24 hours
- Drug overdose
- Tumour

Investigation
All patients should have:

- **CT (non-contrast):** preferred method of imaging for both ischaemia and haemorrhage
  - **Uses:**
    - Confirm diagnosis of cerebrovascular accident
    - Distinguish acute ischaemic stroke from intracerebral haemorrhage
    - Exclude non-vascular cause, eg tumour, cerebral abscess
    - Identify patients requiring urgent neurosurgical referral
    - Confirm safety of lumbar puncture (ie excludes haemorrhage)
  - **Advantage:**
    - Exclude intracerebral haemorrhage, subdural haemorrhage, and other intracerebral pathology prior to administration of thrombolytic therapy in ischaemia
  - **Disadvantage:**
    - Poor visualisation of posterior fossa due to bony artefacts
- **Haematology**
  - FBC: ↑PCV (Hct) – polycythaemia, ↓ platelet (thrombocytopenia)
  - Blood glucose: hypoglycaemia or hyperglycaemia
  - ESR: giant-cell arteritis

Table 6.6: Clinical features and prognosis of stroke		
Territories	*Clinical features*	*Prognosis*
Anterior circulation infarction (total)	• Contralateral hemiplegia, contralateral hemisensory loss, dysphasia (dominant) and • Contralateral homonymous hemianopia, and • Disturbance of higher cerebral function	Poor
Anterior circulation infarction (partial)	• Any two above; or • Isolated disturbance of higher cerebral function	Variable
Posterior circulation infarction	• Brainstem dysfunction (quadriplegia, disturbance of gaze and vision, locked-in syndrome); or • Cerebellar dysfunction ('**DASHING**'); or • Isolated homonymous hemianopia	Variable
Lacunar infarction	• Pure motor signs (contralateral); or • Pure sensory signs (contralateral); or • Sensorimotor signs (contralateral); or • Ataxia	Good – out of all types of strokes, lacunar infarcts have best prognosis

- Coagulation studies (INR and activated partial thromboplastin time)
- Biochemistry
- U&E: electrolyte imbalance
- Blood lipids: ↑lipids
- ECG
- Chest X-ray

Other investigations, if indicated include:

- **MRI:** preferred method of imaging for posterior circulation (posterior cerebral artery and vertebrobasilar system) strokes, lacunar strokes, central venous thrombosis, carotid dissection
- **Cerebral angiography:** first-line diagnostic test to exclude haemorrhage after CT if thrombolysis indicated

Indications for MRI/angiography:

- Subarachnoid haemorrhage (angiography)
- Intracerebral haemorrhage (angiography)
- Carotid artery stenosis (MRI)
- Brainstem/cerebellar strokes (MRI)
- Any patient <50 years old (MRI)

If intracerebral haemorrhage:

- Clotting screen

If acute ischaemic stroke (<60 years old):

- **Thrombophilia screen** (protein C, protein S, activated protein C resistance, angiotensin III, lupus anticoagulant)
- Autoantibody screen
- Anticardiolipin antibodies

If carotid territory or suspected:

- **Carotid duplex USS ± magnetic resonance angiography (if USS positive):** to exclude carotid artery stenosis that may require carotid endarterectomy

If significant cardiac abnormality in past medical history or ECG, or patients <65 years old:

- **Echo** to investigate possible cardiac sources of emboli, eg patent foramen ovale, including aortic arch
- **Transoesophageal echocardiography** if <50 years, or recurrent unexplained stroke

Practical procedure:

- **Lumbar puncture:** only if CT negative (no haemorrhage) and high clinical suspicion of meningitis or subarachnoid haemorrhage, as lumbar puncture is a contraindication to thrombolysis

Management

Acute stroke

- **Admit to stroke unit** (reduces mortality)
- **Aspirin (first-line treatment):** ↓recurrence of acute ischaemic stroke if given within 48 hours; if intolerance/GI bleed, give clopidogrel; if recurrent stroke while on aspirin, give dipyridamole
- **Urgent neurosurgical opinion if indicated**
- **Maintain airway:** intubate (Guedel airway) if ↓consciousness/comatose/↑ICP
- **Monitor:** BP, PR, RR, pulse oximetry, urine output, CNS examination and GCS regularly
- **General management**
  - **Prevent:**
    - **Hypoxia:** O_2 if hypoxic, intubate if ↓conscious level or poor airway protection
    - **Incontinence:** catheterise
    - Pressure sores: regular turning, DeCube® mattress, etc
    - **Pneumonia:** assess swallowing, nil by mouth, early mobilisation
    - **Fever:** paracetamol (acetaminophen)
    - **Asphyxia:** nil by mouth if dysphagia, head-up tilt
    - **Thromboembolic prophylaxis:** TED stockings, aspirin and/or low-molecular-weight heparin (if haemorrhage excluded by CT or MRI, or no excessive risk of haemorrhagic transformation)
    - **Frozen shoulder/contractures:** physiotherapy and early mobiliation
  - **Treatment**
    - **↑BP:** acutely elevated BP is common in stroke due to loss of cerebral perfusion autoregulation mechanisms, so aggressive reduction can worsen prognosis. Indications:
      - □ Patients already on antihypertensives should continue treatment
      - □ Systolic BP ≥220 mmHg or diastolic BP >110 mmHg, gradually reducing BP using β-blocker (first-line; eg labetalol – combined α- and β-blocker) or nitrates (eg IV nitroprusside). This prevents exacerbation of intracerebral haemorrhage
    - **↑ICP:** intubate and hyperventilate, head-up tilt (30°), osmotic agent (mannitol), loop diuretic (furosemide), steroids
    - **↑Glucose:** insulin should be considered, as constant hyperglycaemia >10 mmol/l can worsen ischaemic damage
  - **Ensure**
    - **Hydration:** oral, or IV fluids to maintain cerebral perfusion (caution: cerebral oedema)

- o **Nutrition:** blend food; if nil by mouth then nasogastric tube, percutaneous endoscopic gastrostomy tube (PEG), or IV feeds
- **Specific management**
  - ■ **Ischaemic stroke**
    - o **Medical therapy**
      - □ **Antiplatelet agents:** give aspirin (first-line treatment) to all patients; ↓recurrence of acute ischaemic stroke within 14 days, but small improvement in outcome
      - □ **Thrombolytic therapy (rt-PA):** within 3 hours of signs' onset can improve outcome
      - □ **Absolute contraindication:** haemorrhage. Urgent CT (non-contrast) to exclude haemorrhage
  - ■ **Intracranial haemorrhage**
    - o **Surgical therapy:** urgent neurosurgical opinion if
      - □ Subarachnoid haemorrhage
      - □ **Cerebellar haematoma – urgent evacuation** as mass effect can be rapidly fatal
      - □ Invasive ICP monitoring
      - □ Urgent cerebral angiography
    - o **Medical therapy**
      - □ **Treatment:** coagulopathies – vitamin K, protamine, fresh frozen plasma, or platelet transfusion
      - □ **Prophylaxis of seizures:** may be induced by cortical damage; antiepileptic, eg phenytoin
      - □ **Prophylaxis of peptic ulcer disease:** associated with intracerebral haemorrhage; antacids (H_2-receptor antagonists)
  - ■ **Carotid dissection**
    - o High risk of recurrent stroke within first 4 weeks
    - o **Investigations:** MRI and carotid magnetic resonance angiography
    - o **Treatment:**
      - □ **Referral** to neurology registrar
      - □ **Anticoagulation:** heparin then warfarin
- **Chronic management (neurorehabilitation)**
  - ■ **Aim:** promote cerebral reorganisation
  - ■ **Multidisciplinary team approach:** including physiotherapist, speech and language therapist, occupational therapist, social services, dietician
  - ■ **Assess independence:** Barthel's index of activities of daily living (BAI)
  - ■ **Treat co-morbidities:** depression (50%) with selective serotonin reuptake inhibitors, eg fluoxetine (Prozac®)

Prevention
- **Primary:** includes approaches to **reduce stroke risk in patients without previous stroke**

- ■ **Anticoagulation therapy:** warfarin if cardioembolic stroke risk, eg atrial fibrillation
- ■ **Antiplatelet agents:** aspirin (first-line) if estimated 10-year coronary heart disease risk ≥15% with BP controlled
- ■ **Antihypertensives:** angiotensin-converting enzyme inhibitor, β-blockers, calcium blockers, diuretic (thiazide)
- ■ **Statins (HMG–CoA reductase inhibitor):** eg simvastatin for all patients with ischaemic stroke/transient ischaemic attack
- ■ **Exercise, stop smoking, diabetes mellitus control**
- **Secondary:** include approaches to **reduce recurrence of stroke in previous stroke patients**
  - ■ **Anticoagulation therapy:** warfarin if cardioembolic stroke risk and venous thromboembolism
  - ■ **Antiplatelet agents**
    - o **Aspirin:** first-line treatment to ↓risk of ischaemic stroke recurrence
    - o **Dipyridamole:** only if recurrent strokes (acute ischaemic stroke/transient ischaemic attack) while on aspirin
    - o **Clopidogrel:** only if proved tolerance or allergy to aspirin
  - ■ **Antihypertensives:** angiotensin-converting enzyme inhibitor, eg ramipril and thiazide diuretic
  - ■ **Statins (HMG–CoA reductase inhibitor)**
  - ■ **Carotid endarterectomy or angioplasty:** if >70% internal carotid stenosis
  - ■ **Vitamins:** folic acid, pyridoxine (B_6), and cobalamin (B_{12}) may help ↓serum homocysteine levels (risk factor for all atherosclerotic diseases)
  - ■ **Exercise, stop smoking, diabetes mellitus control**

Complications
- **Cerebral**
  - ■ **Cerebral oedema (41%):** may lead to ↑ICP and cerebral herniation. Earlier (24 hours) in intracerebral haemorrhage than in acute ischaemic stroke (4–5 days)
  - ■ **Haemorrhagic transformation (74% of cardioembolic and 30% of ischaemic strokes)** may result in acute hydrocephalus or focal neurological deterioration
  - ■ **Seizures (11%):** usually single and focal; one-third occur within first 2 weeks, of which 90% occur within first day
  - ■ **Depression (50%)**
- **Systemic**
  - ■ **Hypertension (84%):** can develop in the absence of herniation. Will worsen a pre-existing hypertension or initiate hypertension

- Endocrine abnormalities
  - **Hyperglycaemia (28%)**
  - **Syndrome of inappropriate antidiuretic hormone (SIADH) (10%)**
- **Fever (44%):** a direct result of stroke or more usually a result of other complication, eg pulmonary infection, urinary tract infection or deep vein thrombosis
- **Venous thromboembolism (>50%)**
- **Pressure sores:** especially if patient unconscious
- **Painful limbs:** post-stroke thalamic pain
- **Dysphagia**
- **Frozen shoulder**
- **Contractures**
- Cardiac
  - **Ischaemic heart disease/myocardial infarction:** common cause of sudden death, especially in days 1–2
  - **Arrhythmias (31%)**
  - **Myocytolysis**

Driving (DVLA)
Patients with **visual field defects** including partial or complete homonymous hemianopia/quadrantanopia or complete bitemporal hemianopia are **not allowed to drive**.

Prognosis
- 20% mortality at 1 month (females more likely to die from stroke); 5%–10% per year thereafter
- 40% complete recovery rate; majority recover function within first week, eg hemiplegia; any deficit remaining at 1 month is likely to be permanent
- ↑Recurrence risk: 50% survivors are likely to experience a second stroke within 5 years

6.3.2 Subarachnoid haemorrhage
Bleeding beneath the subarachnoid mater (within the subarachnoid space), spontaneously (atraumatic), or following head injury (traumatic).

NB Atraumatic subarachnoid haemorrhage + sudden neurological deficit = haemorrhagic stroke.

Incidence: 8/100 000 per year.

Pathophysiology
- Subarachnoid space lies between the pia mater and arachnoid mater, and it contains the internal carotids.
- It is suggested that aneurysms rupture during times of stressful or exertional events (eg defecation, urination, sexual intercourse, heavy work, exercise and emotional stress).
- Bleeding into this space results in ↑ICP and ↓cerebral perfusion, hence ↓GCS.

- Delayed effects result in vasospasm which can lead to infarction and communicating hydrocephalus.
- Common sites of berry aneurysms include junction of posterior communicating with internal carotid artery, anterior communicating with anterior cerebral artery, or bifurcation of middle cerebral artery; 15% of berry aneurysms occur in multiple sites.

Causes
- **Traumatic:** head injury
- **Atraumatic:**
  - **Ruptured intracranial aneurysm** (75% of atraumatic subarachnoid haemorrhage): associated with adult polycystic kidney disease, connective tissue disorder, eg Marfan's and Ehlers–Danlos syndromes, and coarctation
  - Arteriovenous malformations (10% of atraumatic subarachnoid haemorrhage)
  - Idiopathic (15% of atraumatic subarachnoid haemorrhage)

Risk factors
- **Smoking**
- **Hypertension**
- Bleeding disorders (coagulopathies, haemoglobinopathies)
- Genetics: positive family history of aneurysm (↑×3–5)
- Alcohol abuse
- Age: 5th and 6th decades of life
- Intracranial tumours
- Mycotic aneurysm post-subacute bacterial endocarditis/infectious endocarditis
- Post-menopausal females (F:M>1 due to lack of oestrogen)

Clinical features

Symptoms: SOCRATES
- **Site:** often occipital
- **Onset:** sudden onset
- **Character: severe 'thunderclap' headache** (25% are subarachnoid haemorrhage)
- **Associations:** nausea and vomiting, altered conscious level
- **Time:** maximal intensity within seconds
- **Severity:** often described as 'worst headache in my life'

Signs
- **Altered conscious level**
- **Meningism:** neck stiffness (positive Kernig's sign), photophobia
- ↑**ICP:** confusion, drowsiness/coma, nausea and vomiting, seizure, papilloedema; ↑BP, ↓PR, irregular RR (Cushing's reflex)
- **Retinal and subhyaloid haemorrhage (fundoscopy)**

- Focal neurological signs (?site of subarachnoid haemorrhage/haematoma)
  - Cranial nerve palsies
    - Oculomotor (III) nerve palsy: posterior cerebral artery aneurysm rupture
    - Abducens (VI) nerve palsy: ↑ICP (false localising sign)
    - Monocular blindness: ophthalmic artery aneurysm rupture
  - Hemiparesis ± dysphasia
    - Middle cerebral artery aneurysm rupture
  - Leg monoparesis or paraparesis ± akinetic mute state
    - Anterior cerebral artery aneurysm rupture

Differential diagnosis
- Stroke
- Cerebral venous thrombosis (thunderclap headache)
- Meningitis
- Migraine

Investigations
- Bloods: FBC, U&E, blood lipids, blood glucose, ESR, coagulation studies [prothrombin time (INR), activated partial thromboplastin time, thrombin time], group and save
- Radiology (Table 6.7)
  - CT: always indicated; most sensitive within 24 hours after subarachnoid haemorrhage.
    - Acute subarachnoid haemorrhage (2–3 days): non-contrast CT
    - Chronic subarachnoid haemorrhage (days to weeks): contrast CT
  - Cerebral angiography: always indicated; however, negative angiogram does not rule out aneurysm
  - CT angiography: if patient unstable and cannot undergo angiography, or prior to urgent operative intervention for clot evacuation
- Practical procedure
  - Lumbar puncture ×3 CSF: indicated if CT negative (xanthochromia and RBCs). Most sensitive 12 hours after onset of symptoms

- Echo: more sensitive than ECG in detecting myocardial infarction, and more useful in setting of subarachnoid haemorrhage
- ECG

Complications
- Ischaemia as a result of
  - Vasospasm (70%)
    - Symptoms vary with arterial territory involved; often the internal, anterior or middle cerebral arteries
    - Distinguished from rebleed by cerebral angiography or transcranial Doppler
  - Rebleeding (30%)
- Cardiac arrhythmias (90%): ↑levels of circulating catecholamines, and neurogenic sympathetic hyperactivity, patient can develop premature ventricular contractions, bradyarrhythmia, supraventricular tachycardia, or myocardial infarction
- Seizures (25%): ↑risk of rebleed and neurological deterioration by causing ↑cerebral blood flow, hypertension and ↑ICP
- Hydrocephalus (20%): distinguished from rebleeding by CT ('Mickey-mouse' appearance of ventricles); associated with poorer prognosis
- Hyponatraemia (10%)
- Pulmonary oedema: almost universal in severe subarachnoid haemorrhage

Management
- Urgent neurosurgical opinion: all cases of suspected subarachnoid haemorrhage
- Medical therapy
  - Basic life support and assess GCS: intubate if coma, ↓conscious level, ↑ICP
  - IV access and sedation: short-acting benzodiazepine, eg midazolam prior to all procedures
  - Monitor: BP, CVP, PR, RR, pulse oximetry, urine output, CNS examination (regularly), GCS, repeat CT if deteriorating
  - Antihypertensive: only if systolic BP >220 mmHg and diastolic BP >110 mmHg; first-line agent if no contraindications is β-blockers; avoid nitrates (↑ICP)

Table 6.7: Radiological findings in subarachnoid haemorrhage (SAH)

Time	CT: subarachnoid cisterns and sulci
Normal (CSF)	Hypoattenuating (black)
SAH 2–3 days (acute)	Hyperattenuating (white)
SAH several days to weeks (chronic)	Isoattenuating (relative to brain parenchyma); evidence of SAH: • ↓Visualisation of normally hypoattenuating CSF in basal cisterns and sulci • Enlargement of ventricles due to communicating hydrocephalus

and angiotensin-converting enzyme inhibitors (slow onset)

- ◼ **↑ICP/coning:** intubation and hyperventilation at head-up tilt; others – osmotic agent (IVI mannitol), loop diuretic (furosemide), IV steroids
- **Prophylaxis and treatment of complications**
  - ◼ Rebleeding
    - ○ **Bedrest**
    - ○ **Analgesia:** pain is associated with transient ↑BP, therefore increasing risk of rebleeding; treatment with codeine
    - ○ **Sedation:** short-acting benzodiazepine, eg midazolam
    - ○ **Stool softeners:** prevent straining
  - ◼ Vasospasm
    - ○ **Calcium–channel blockers:** nifedipine (prophylaxis)
    - ○ **IV fluids:** irrespective of ↑ICP; dehydration → vasospasm
    - ○ **If symptomatic vasospasm:** triple 'H' therapy
      - ☐ **H**ypertension
      - ☐ **H**ypervolaemia
      - ☐ **H**aemodilution
  - ◼ **Seizures:** phenytoin (antiepileptic)
- **Surgical therapy**
- **Urgent neurosurgical opinion:** if ↓conscious level, progressive focal neurological deficit, cerebellar haematoma
  - ◼ **Endovascular coil:** first-line treatment method in Europe, and is of proved benefit; or
  - ◼ **Clipping aneurysm:** first-line method in USA
- **Cerebellar haematoma:** urgent evacuation

Prognosis
- Almost all mortality is within first month; of those who survive, 90% live to 1 year
- Poorer prognosis with altered conscious level; almost 100% if comatose

6.3.3 Subdural haemorrhage
Bleeding beneath the dura mater (within the subdural space).

Pathophysiology
Three meninges (pia, arachnoid and dura maters); bleeding from bridging veins between the cortex and dura into the subdural space is most commonly due to decelerating injury (traumatic).

Epidemiology
- **Male:female ratio is 2:1**
- **Elderly** (↑risk of subdural haemorrhage due to more brain atrophy than younger patients, making bridging veins more vulnerable to decelerating injury)

Risk factors
- Patients at ↑risk of falls, eg elderly, epileptics, alcoholics
- Long-term anticoagulation therapy
- Bleeding disorders (coagulopathies, thrombocytopenia)
- Hypertension
- Diabetes mellitus

Causes
- **Traumatic:** head injury (commonest)
- **Atraumatic (spontaneous):** bleeding disorders, eg coagulopathies and anticoagulation therapy

Clinical features
- **Acute subdural haemorrhage**
  - ◼ Symptoms
    - ○ Altered conscious level (fluctuating)
  - ◼ Signs
    - ○ Ipsilateral pupil dilatation and failure to react to light (CN III palsy)
    - ○ Contralateral hemiparesis
    - ○ Others (less common), eg papilloedema and CN VI palsy (↑ICP)
- **Chronic subdural haemorrhage**
  - ◼ Symptoms
    - ○ Altered conscious level (fluctuating)
    - ○ Headache, **sleepiness**, unsteadiness, physical and intellectual **slowness** (cognitive dysfunction), ↓memory, personality change, motor deficit, eg hemiparesis, aphasia, seizures
  - ◼ Signs
    - ○ ↑ICP: drowsiness, confusion, nausea and vomiting, seizures, papilloedema; late features include ↑BP, ↓PR and irregular RR
    - ○ Localising neurological signs (late onset ~ 2 months)

Differential diagnosis
- Brain tumour
- Evolving stroke
- Dementia

Investigations
- **Bloods:** FBC, U&E, coagulation studies (INR, activated partial thromboplastin time, thrombin time), group and save
- **Radiology**
  - ◼ **CT** (always indicated): long, irregular, crescent-shaped haematoma ± midline shift
  - ◼ **MRI** (not preferred)

Management
- **Urgent neurosurgery**
  - **Acute subdural haemorrhage** [>5mm thickness (axial CT), mass effect on CT (midline shift), neurological signs (lethargy, focal neurological deficit, coma)]
  - **Chronic subdural haemorrhage** (symptomatic, or mass effect)
  - **If otherwise, interventional neurosurgery contraindicated:** serial imaging (CT)
- **Surgical therapy**
  - **Burr hole:** liquefied chronic subdural haemorrhage
  - **Craniotomy:** non-liquefied chronic subdural haemorrhage, or acute subdural haemorrhage
    - **Pre-op:** phenytoin (within 7 days of head injury; not effective after that date)
    - **Intra-op:** USS to locate any intraparenchymal clots that may require evacuation
    - **Peri-op:** antibiotics
    - **Post-op:** CT scan follow-up (24 hours; urgent if signs of ↑ICP), coagulation studies and platelet count, hydration and flat head on bed to aid brain re-expansion after chronic subdural haemorrhage
- **Medical therapy**
  - **Treatment of ↓prothrombin time (INR) and ↓platelet count:** fresh frozen plasma
  - **Treatment of ↑ICP:** intubation and hyperventilation at head-up tilt; others – osmotic agent (IVI mannitol), loop diuretic (furosemide), IV steroids

Prognosis
- Full recovery following evacuation of haematoma; 80% resume their pre-haematoma level of function
- No correlation has been found between pre-operative CT scan and post-operative outcome

6.3.4 Extradural haemorrhage
Bleeding outside the dura mater (within the epidural space).

Pathophysiology
Commonly head injury (2% of patients with head injuries) fractures of pterion, temporal, or parietal bones, resulting in laceration of and bleeding from the middle meningeal artery and vein, but can also be from the dural venous sinus.

Extradural haemorrhage may be acute (58%), subacute (31%), or chronic (11%).

Causes
- **Traumatic (commonest):** head injury
- **Atraumatic:** spontaneous extradural haemorrhage, eg bleeding disorders (coagulopathies)

Clinical features
- **Symptoms**
  - **Lucid interval** (interval post-head injury in which patient had no loss of consciousness, or loss of consciousness followed by recovery) **followed by deteriorating conscious level**
- **Signs**
  - **↑ICP:** drowsiness, confusion, nausea and vomiting, seizures, papilloedema; late features (Cushing's reflex) include ↑BP, ↓PR and irregular RR
  - **Tentorial herniation:** Hutchinson's sign (CN III compression results in ipsilateral pupil dilatation, unreactive to light) ± contralateral hemiparesis (decussating motor tracts compression), upper motor neurone lesion (upgoing plantars, brisk reflexes) and, finally, respiratory arrest

Investigations
- **Bloods:** FBC [packed cell volume (Hct), platelet count], U&E, coagulation screen (INR, activated partial thromboplastin time, thrombin time), blood glucose, group and save
- **Radiology**
  - **CT (always indicated):** lens-shaped (biconvex) haematoma
  - **Skull X-ray:** may show fracture
- **Practical:** lumbar puncture is contraindicated

Management
- **Urgent neurosurgical opinion** – not all cases of acute extradural haemorrhage require immediate surgical evacuation; some can be delayed. Urgent if large haematoma, midline shift and worsening neurological signs
  - **Burr hole:** surgical evacuation of haematoma is definitive treatment
- **Treatment:**
  - **↑ICP:** intubation and hyperventilation at head-up tilt ± osmotic diuretic (mannitol), loop diuretics (furosemide), IV steroids
  - **Coagulopathies:** vitamin K, protamine, fresh frozen plasma, platelet exchange
  - **Fever:** paracetamol
- **Prophylaxis**
  - **Seizures:** phenytoin
  - **Peptic ulcer disease:** antacids
  - **Venous thromboembolism:** TED stockings and consider aspirin, or low-molecular-weight heparin if immobile

Prognosis

- Good if patient treated early; poor if patient is comatose and has late signs of ↑ICP
- Mortality:
  - Mortality rate associated with epidural haematoma has been estimated to be 5%–50% (↑if bilateral or posterior fossa)
  - The level of consciousness prior to surgery has been correlated with mortality rate

6.3.5 Cerebral vein thrombosis

Cerebral venous sinus thrombosis ± cortical vein thrombosis.

Pathophysiology

Partial thrombosis, or external compression, eventually resulting in complete occlusion, which can lead to cortical vein infarction.

Causes

- **Idiopathic** (30%)
- **Virchow's triad**
  - **Hypercoagulability**
    - Hereditary
    - Drugs
    - Infectious: meningitis, cerebral abscess, septicaemia, otitis media
    - Hyperviscosity: polycythaemia, sickle cell disease, myeloma, vasculitis
    - Pregnancy/post-partum
  - **Stasis**
    - Dehydration
    - Diabetes mellitus
  - **Vessel wall damage**
    - Surgery

Clinical features

Non-specific, usually:

- **Isolated sagittal sinus thrombosis** (50%):
  - ↑ICP: headache, confusion, drowsiness/coma, vomiting, seizures, papilloedema, Cushing's reflex (↑BP, ↓PR and irregular RR)
  - Often accompanied by:
    - Lateral sinus thrombosis (35%): CN palsies (VI and VII), field defects, otalgia
    - Cavernous sinus thrombosis: central retinal vein thrombosis, grossly oedematous eyelids, chemosis
    - Sigmoid sinus thrombosis: cerebellar signs, lower CN palsies
    - Inferior petrosal sinus thrombosis: CN palsies (V and VI) – Gradenigo's syndrome

- **Cortical vein thrombosis:** 'thunderclap' headache, encephalopathy, seizures, cortical vein infarction (± focal neurological signs)

Differential diagnosis

- Stroke
- SAH
- Meningitis
- Migraine

Investigations

- **Bloods:** FBC, ESR, platelet count, U&E, liver function tests, D-dimer, sickle cell testing
- **Radiology**
  - MRI and magnetic resonance venography: gold standard
  - CT: initially normal → ~1 week delta sign
- **Practical procedure**
  - Lumbar puncture if CT negative (normal; or xanthochromia and RBCs)

Management

- Urgent neurosurgical opinion
- Anticoagulation therapy: heparin and warfarin (improves outcome)

6.4 SPINAL SURGERY

6.4.1 Spinal tumours

Aetiology
- **Primary**
  - **Extradural**
    - **Myeloma**
    - **Neurofibroma**
    - **Lymphoma**
  - **Intradural**
    - **Meningioma**
      - □ Genetic
      - □ Cranial irradiation
    - **Schwannoma**
  - **Intramedullary**
    - **Ependymoma**
    - **Gliomas**
      - □ **Astrocytoma**
- **Secondary (metastatic)**
  - Breast
  - Lung
  - Prostate
  - Renal

Clinical features

- Meningioma
  - Seizures
  - Compression: spastic paraparesis
- Schwannoma/neurofibroma
  - Cutaneous: *café au lait* spots, mostly asymptomatic
  - Neurological: slowly advancing spastic paraparesis with a unilateral band of pain and distorted sensation at the level of the lesion
- Ependymoma
  - Nausea and vomiting
  - Headache
  - Behavioural changes: irritability, anorexia, lethargy
  - Cerebellar symptoms: gait abnormalities
- Astrocytoma
  - Seizure and headache
- Metastatic
  - **Back pain and tenderness ± pathological fractures:** collapse of vertebrae
  - **Spinal cord compression:** progressive limb weakness, sensory loss and sphincter dysfunction
  - **Cauda equina syndrome:** sensory loss in saddle distribution and sphincter dysfunction
  - **Neoplastic features:** weight loss, anorexia, night sweats, fatigue

Investigations

- **Bloods:** Routine bloods
- **Radiology**
  - Plain radiograph
  - CT head
  - MRI
  - Myelography
- **Biopsy:** histology and cytology

Management

- Medical
  - Analgesia
- Surgical
  - Metastases: decompressive laminectomy
  - Intradural/intramedullary tumours: excision of the tumour ± decompressive surgery
- **Radiological:** local radiotherapy
- Palliative

6.4.2 Spinal trauma

Classification

- Fractures
  - **Stable:** spinal cord is rarely damaged and movement of the spine is safe

  - **Unstable:** spinal cord may well have sustained damage and, if not, may do so if the patient is moved
- Subluxation
- Dislocation

Risk of spinal injury

- Road traffic accidents (RTA)
- Falls
- Sports injuries
- Birth injuries
- Non-accidental injuries (NAI)

Mechanisms of spinal injury

Most injuries involve a combination of forces.

- Vertical (axial) compression
- Hinge injury
  - Forced flexion
    - Compression or crush fractures
    - Whiplash injury
    - Seatbelt fracture
  - Forced extension
    - 'Hangman' fracture
- Rotation or shearing
- **Avulsion:** tearing or forcible separation of part of a structure, eg tendon from bone

Assessment of a patient with a possible spinal injury in A&E

- Advanced Trauma Life Support (ATLS)
- Stabilise spine (immobilisation)
  - C-spine: hard collar
  - Thoracolumbar: spinal board
- **Clinical features:** pain, loss of function, swelling, deformity, erythema, bleeding, crepitus
- Examination
  - Inspect: open/closed fracture, bruising, erythema, swelling, deformity, bleeding
  - Palpate: Log-roll patient, palpate spinous processes for bony and soft tissue tenderness
  - Neurological examination
    - Sensory and motor deficit
    - Head injury
- **Grading spinal cord injury:** Frankel grading system A–E (Box 6.6)

Box 6.6: Frankel grading system

A	Complete lesion
B	Partial sensory lesion. No motor function
C	Variable sensory lesion. Useless motor function
D	Variable sensory lesion. Useful motor function
E	No lesion

Investigations
- **Bloods:** FBC, U&E, LFT, XM G+S, glucose
- **Radiology:**
  - ■ Spinal X-ray
    - ○ C-spine: lateral, AP and odontoid views
    - ○ Thoracolumbar: lateral and AP views
  - ■ CT: if spinal X-ray inadequate
  - ■ MRI: spinal cord injury

Management
- **General management**
  - ■ Immobilise patient's spine: spinal boards, Ked splints and hard cervical collars
  - ■ Splint all fractures
- **Specific management:** the general principles involved in the management of spinal fractures are as follows:
  - ■ **Stable fractures**
    - ○ Conservative: bedrest and support in a position that will not cause further strain
  - ■ **Subluxation and dislocations**
    - ○ Manipulation
    - ○ Traction
    - ○ Open reduction
  - ■ **Unstable fractures**
    - ○ Cervical spine: traction
    - ○ Lumbar spine: immobilisation in an appropriate position ± internal or external fixation
- **Continued care and rehabilitation:** physiotherapy

6.4.3 Spinal cord compression

Epidemiology
- **Prevalence:** 5%–10% of patients with cancer
- **Incidence:** 0.5–2.5 per 100 000 population
- **Commonest cause:** vertebral metastases
  - ■ 60% in the thoracic spine
  - ■ 30% in the lumbosacral spine
  - ■ 10% in the cervical spine

Pathophysiology
Spinal cord: extends from C1 to L2 (spinal cord level) and is located inside the vertebral canal, which is formed by the foramina of 7 cervical, 12 thoracic, 5 lumbar and 5 sacral vertebrae.

Cauda equina: formed by the lumbar and sacral nerve roots from L2 (spinal cord level), which occupy the spinal canal below L1 (vertebral body) and extend into the pelvis and thigh.

Spinal cord compression is characterised by **progressive history** of neurological deficit. On examination, a **sensory level is evident (hallmark)**, **lower motor neurone lesion signs** occur at the level of compression, and **upper motor neurone lesion signs occur below the level of compression**.

It is a **neurological emergency** because:

- Later stages results in **ischaemia (irreversible)**
- Patient may become **wheelchair-bound**, and **incontinent of urine**

Sensory (ascending) pathways (Figure 6.9)
- **Spinothalamic tract:** mediates pain and temperature. Lies anterolaterally (supplied by anterior spinal artery) in spinal cord, and decussates (crosses) in the spinal cord (hence spino-). Lesions give rise to **anterior cord syndrome**, which is typically due to anterior spinal artery infarction
  - ■ Above lesion level: normal
  - ■ At lesion level: ipsilateral loss of pain and temperature
  - ■ Below lesion level: contralateral loss of pain and temperature, with paralysis

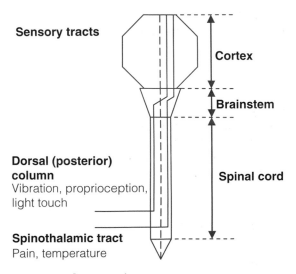

Figure 6.9: Sensory pathways

- **Posterior (dorsal) column:** mediates joint position sense (proprioception), vibration sense and light touch. Lies posteriorly (supplied by posterior spinal artery) in spinal cord and decussates at the medulla (brainstem)
  - Above level of lesion: normal
  - At level of lesion: contralateral loss of pain and temperature
  - Below level of lesion: ipsilateral loss of pain and temperature

Motor (descending) pathways

Descending motor pathways form two systems, the ventromedial and dorsolateral systems; their names correspond to their sites in the spinal cord:

- **Ventromedial system:** modulated by **medial cerebellar system**, and includes pontine reticulospinal, lateral vestibulospinal and tectospinal tracts. They do not decussate (exception is tectospinal tract), and descend ipsilaterally; therefore, effects are ipsilateral to spinal cord lesions
- **Dorsolateral system:** modulated by **lateral cerebellar system**, and includes corticospinal, rubrospinal and medullary-reticulo tracts. They decussate and descend contralaterally; therefore, effects are contralateral to cerebral lesions, and ipsilateral to spinal cord lesions

Ventromedial system

- **Pontine reticulospinal tract**
  - Origin: pontine reticular nucleus in pons
  - Lower motor neurone (LMN): postural muscles
  - Function: excites extensors and inhibits flexors
- **Lateral vestibulospinal tract**
  - Origin: vestibular nucleus in pons and medulla
  - LMN: anti-gravity muscles
  - Function: ↑anti-gravity (stance phase), inactive early swing, active late swing and extension, excites extensors

- **Tectospinal tract**
  - Origin: superior colliculus in midbrain; receives peripheral retinal input
  - LMN: proximal girdle and neck muscles
  - Function: orientation and flinching, ballistic reaching, navigation

Dorsolateral system

- **Corticospinal tract**
  - Origin: cerebral motor cortex
  - LMN: digits
  - Function: flexion of single digits, excites flexors, speed and agility
- **Rubrospinal tract**
  - Origin: red nucleus
  - LMN: pectoral girdle muscles
  - Function: flexion of shoulder girdle, excites flexors, active in swing phase
- **Medullary–reticulo tract**
  - Origin: medullary reticular formation
  - Function: inactive in simple gait, active in complex gait

Causes

Spinal cord compression

- **Commonest cause: vertebral body metastases** (breast, lung and prostate account for 15%–20% of cases of spinal cord compression)
- **Rare**
  - Infectious: epidural abscess
  - Iatrogenic: warfarin (haematoma)
  - Neoplastic: primary tumour (astrocytoma, ependymoma, haemangioblastoma)
- **Others (specific to cauda equina)**
  - Canal stenosis
  - Lumbosacral nerve lesions

	UMN lesions *Affect muscle groups, not individual muscles*	LMN lesions *Affect muscles supplied by involved cord segment*
Bulk	Normal	Wasting ± fasciculation
Tone	↑Spasticity; affects large muscle groups, eg flexors of arms (biceps) and extensors of legs (quadriceps) that can suddenly be overcome (clasp-knife feel)	↓Flaccidity (hypotonia)
Power	Weakness or paralysis	Weakness or paralysis
Reflexes	Hyperreflexia (brisk reflexes) ± clonus	↓ Or absent reflexes
Plantars	Upgoing (extensor; positive Babinski sign)	Downgoing (flexor; negative Babinski sign)

Table 6.8: Comparison of upper (UMNL) and lower (LMNL) motor neurone lesions

Paraplegia (weakness of both legs)

- Commonest cause: spinal cord compression
- Others
  - **Chronic spastic paraparesis:** multiple sclerosis, intrinsic cord tumours, syringomyelia, motor neurone disease, subacute combined degeneration of the cord (B_{12} deficiency), syphilis
  - **Chronic flaccid paraparesis:** tabes dorsalis, peripheral neuropathies, myopathies
  - **Unilateral foot drop:** common peroneal nerve palsy, diabetes mellitus, stroke, intervertebral disc prolapse
  - **No sensory loss:** motor neurone disease, parasagittal meningioma
  - **Absent knee jerk and extensor plantars:** 'MAST' – **m**otor neurone disease, Fredreich's **a**taxia, **s**ubacute combined degeneration of the cord, **t**aboparesis (syphilis)

Clinical features

Essential note

Upper motor neurones (UMNs) occur in the brain, brainstem and spinal cord, down to the ventral horn of the spinal cord. Lower motor neurones (LMNs) are the neurones extending from the ventral horn of the spinal cord along the length of the peripheral nerve. Strokes will result in UMN lesion signs. Spinal cord insults will result in a combination of UMN and particular LMN lesion signs, depending on the spinal level affected. A comparison of UMN and LMN lesion signs is summarised in Table 6.8.

Spinal cord compression

- **Presentation:** back pain is the commonest symptom (83%–95% of patients), usually described as sharp, shooting, deep, or burning; precipitated by coughing, bending, sneezing, or, in 20% of patients, simply lying flat
- Symptoms
  - Progressive **weakness** of limbs and **sensory loss** (may be preceded by spinal/root pain); if rapidly progressing then emergency
  - **Sphincter dysfunction** (bladder and rectal; late feature)
- Signs (depend on site of lesion)
  - Upper cervical cord lesion
    - **Motor and reflex level:** upper motor neurone lesion signs with tetraplegia
    - **Sensory level:** absent/decreased sensation below lesion, sensory ataxia (loss of proprioception leads to high steppage and unsteady gait; exacerbated by closing eyes, positive Romberg's sign)
      - Incontinence
  - Lower cervical cord lesion
    - Motor and reflex level
      - Above level of lesion: normal
      - At level of lesion: lower motor neurone signs of upper limb, eg C5 lesion results in absent biceps reflex
      - Below level of lesion: upper motor neurone lesion signs of lower limb with paraplegia
    - **Sensory level:** absent/decreased sensation below lesion, sensory ataxia
    - Incontinence
  - Thoracic cord lesion
    - **Motor and reflex level:** upper motor neurone lesion signs with paraplegia
    - **Sensory level:** absent/decreased sensation below lesion, sensory ataxia
    - Incontinence
  - Lumbar cord lesion
    - **Motor and reflex level:** lower motor neurone lesion signs of lower limb
    - **Sensory level:** absent/decreased sensation below lesion, sensory ataxia
    - Incontinence

Cauda equina (nerve roots) syndrome

- **Presentation: loss of sensation** in a **saddle distribution;** 60%–80% of these patients have **sphincter dysfunction** (in particular, decreased anal sphincter tone)
- Symptoms
  - Back pain, and radicular (nerve root) pain down the legs
  - Sensory loss (root distribution)
  - Sphincter dysfunction (bladder and rectal)
- Signs
  - Motor and reflex level
    - Above lesion: normal
    - Below lesion: asymmetrical lower motor neurone lesion signs of lower limb with **paraplegia**
  - **Sensory impairment:** depends on root distribution

Brown–Séquard syndrome (hemicordectomy or hemisection; rare)

- Signs
  - At level of lesion: ipsilateral loss of spinothalamic tract (pain and T°)
  - Below level of lesion:
    - Ipsilateral loss of dorsal column (proprioception, vibration sense and light touch)
    - Contralateral loss of spinothalamic tract (pain and T°; beginning perhaps two to three segments below)
    - Upper motor neurone lesion signs with hemi/monoplegia

Head, neck and neurosurgery

Anterior cord syndrome
- **Cause:** typically anterior spinal artery infarction
- **Signs:** below level of lesion – paralysis, and loss of pain and temperature sensation

Differential diagnosis
Transverse myelitis (acute inflammation of cord from viral infection, syphilis, or radiotherapy), multiple sclerosis, Guillain–Barré, carcinomatous meningitis, cord infarction [spinal artery thrombosis (rare), trauma, dissecting aneurysm, vasculitis, eg panarteritis nodosa].

Investigations
- Imaging
  - **MRI:** gold standard for diagnosing epidural disease, spinal cord compression and for treatment planning
  - **Spinal X-ray (cervical and thoracic):** can be helpful, but has false-negative rate of 10%–17%
  - **Chest X-ray:** tuberculosis, cancer, metastasis
- **EMG with post–myelography CT**
- **Haematology:** FBC, ESR, B_{12}, folate, syphilis serology
- **Biochemistry:** U&E, liver function tests, prostate-specific antigen

Management
- Malignancy:
  - **Steroid** (dexamethasone)
  - Radiotherapy/chemotherapy ± surgical decompression (laminectomy; poor results); depends on tumour type, quality of life and prognosis
- **Epidural abscess: surgical decompression** + antibiotics
- **Management of paraplegic complications**
  - Avoid pressure sores: turn regularly, pressure mattress
  - Avoid venous thromboembolism: aspirin, TED stockings, consider low-molecular-weight heparin for immobile patients
  - Bladder care: catheterisation, bladder drill
  - Manual evacuation or suppositories
  - Exercise

Prognosis
- Prognosis and survival related to severity of neurological deficit at presentation
- 75%–100% of patients who are ambulatory (able to walk pre-disease) remain ambulatory; 50% of those who survive a year after treatment are still ambulatory
- If paraplegia and sphincter involvement have occurred, then recovery is uncommon; however 15% of paraplegic patients regain 'useful' function after radiotherapy, whereas 80% of incontinent patients do not

6.4.4 Cervical spondylosis and myelopathy
Spondylosis (stiffening or fixation of the joint) affecting cervical vertebrae, intervertebral discs and surrounding soft tissues.

If cord compression ensues (50%), it is called 'myelopathy'.

Epidemiology
- Incidence
  - Accounts for **25% of patients** presenting with **non-traumatic myelopathic signs**
  - Commonest cause of non-traumatic progressive spastic paralysis (paraparesis, tetraparesis, or quadriparesis) and sensory loss below the neck
- **Prevalence:** increases with age
- **Gender:** affects males earlier than females
- **Age:** most commonly >40 years old

Pathophysiology
Progressive degeneration of cervical intervertebral discs ± bony spurs (osteophytes) results in narrowing of the spinal canal and intervertebral foramina. This leads to cord damage as the neck flexes and extends, because the cord is dragged over the protruding osteophytes and ossification of the ligamentum flavum posteriorly contributes to anterior cord compression, resulting in cervical spondylosis.

Cause
- Age-related changes in intervertebral discs

Risk factors
- Repeated trauma, familial, smoking

Clinical features
- Presentation
  - Neck: pain and stiffness
  - Arm: pain (brachialgia)
  - Leg: spasticity, weakness ± ataxia
- Symptoms
  - **Intermittent cervicalgia (neck and shoulder pain; most common):** radiates into shoulders or occiput, often accompanied by stiffness
    - Chronic or episodic, with long periods of remission
    - One-third present with headache
    - More than two-thirds present with unilateral or bilateral shoulder pain
  - **Chronic suboccipital headache**
  - **Radiculopathy:** most commonly C6 and C7 nerve roots are compressed affecting biceps and deltoid (C5, C6), triceps and finger extensors (C7)
    - Pain, paraesthesiae and lower motor neurone lesion weakness

- **Paraparesis, tetraparesis or quadriparesis**
  - Asymmetrical spastic leg weakness ± ataxia
  - Numbness (anaesthesia) and tingling (paraesthesia) of feet and hands
  - Bladder dysfunction (rare; hesitancy, urgency and frequency)
- Signs
  - **Painful neck movements and stiffness ± crepitus**
  - **Positive Lhermitte sign:** neck flexion may result in tingling down spine
  - **Positive Spurling sign:** neck compression test
  - Arms:
    - At level of lesion: lower motor neurone lesion weakness most commonly affects triceps ± hand intrinsic muscles, and wasting of intrinsic muscles of hand
    - Below level of lesion: upper motor neurone lesion and sensory loss (especially pain and temperature); positive Hoffman sign
  - **Legs:** upper motor neurone (± positive Babinski sign) and sensory loss (especially proprioception and vibration sense)

Differential diagnosis
- Multiple sclerosis
- Subacute combined degeneration of the cord

Investigations
- **MRI:** diagnostic imaging modality
- **Serum B$_{12}$:** exclude subacute combined degeneration of the cord
- Others
  - Haematology: Hb, mean cell volume, white cell count, platelet count, peripheral blood smear
  - EMG
  - Cervical myelography

Management
- Avoid heavy lifting
- Analgesia
  - Non-steroidal anti-inflammatory drugs: aspirin, paracetamol, ibuprofen, naproxen, diclofenac
  - Corticosteroids
  - COX-2 inhibitor: celecoxib (Celebrex)
- **Muscle relaxants:** diazepam, short course if muscle spasm
- **Neck immobilisation:** firm neck collar (<1/52; 50% improvement with use)
- Physiotherapy
- Surgical therapy
  - Carries significant risks

- Symptomatic resolution 75%–90% (post-cervical root decompression)
- Halts myelopathic progression, but not if chronic symptoms and signs
- Indications
  - Abnormal neurology
  - Persistent, progressive or intermittent (rarely warrants surgery) brachialgia ± abnormal neurology
- **Procedures:** usually combined with spinal fusion
  - **Removal of osteophytes**
  - **Laminectomy:** wide decompression, eg from C3 to C7
  - **Foraminectomy:** root decompression

6.5 NEUROPATHIES

6.5.1 Mononeuropathies
Defined as an individual nerve abnormality (peripheral and cranial).

When several individual nerves are affected, it is called 'mononeuritis multiplex'. (Table 6.9).

Carpal tunnel syndrome (median nerve entrapment) is the commonest mononeuropathy.

Causes
- **Common – trauma, idiopathic** (most cases of carpal tunnel syndrome)
- **Uncommon –** diabetes mellitus, leprosy
- **Pregnancy and rheumatoid arthritis** are most likely causes of carpal tunnel syndrome in young patients

Table 6.9: Causes of mononeuritis multiplex	
• Wegner's granulomatosis	• Polyarteritis nodosa (PAN)
• Amyloidosis	• Leprosy
• Rheumatoid arthritis	• Carcinomatosis
• Diabetes mellitus	
• Sarcoidosis	

Clinical features
See Table 6.10 for clinical features of common mononeuropathies.

Investigations
- **EMG:** site and severity of lesion
- **Imaging:** MRI, X-ray if indicated
- **Bloods:** FBC, blood glucose, ESR, biochemistry (U&E, thyroid function test), immunology (ANA)

Table 6.10: Clinical features of common mononeuropathies

Nerve	Sensory supply	Motor supply	Compression
Median	Lateral 3½ of fingers, palm and nails	Abductor pollicis brevis, (thenar eminence) Lateral two lumbricals, Opponens pollicis Flexor pollicis brevis	**Sensory signs:** *Paraesthesia* over lateral 3½ of fingers, palm and nails *Pain* may extend proximally, to shoulder region **Motor signs:** *Weakness* (↓tone, power and reflexes) *Wasting* (thenar eminence)
Ulnar (bicyclist's neuropathy)	Medial 1½ of fingers and palm	Flexors, interossei, medial two lumbricals, hypothenar eminence	**Sensory signs:** *Paraesthesia* over medial 1½ of fingers and palm **Motor signs:** *Claw hand* *Wasting* (hypothenar eminence)
Radial (Saturday night palsy)	Root of thumb on dorsum	Extensors	**Sensory signs:** *Paraesthesia* over dorsum of thumb root **Motor signs:** *Wrist drop*
Sciatic	Below knee laterally	Hamstring muscles and all muscles below knee	**Sensory signs:** *Paraesthesia* over lateral side of leg below knee **Motor signs:** *Foot drop, paralysis of leg*
Common peroneal	Dorsum of foot	Foot dorsiflexion and eversion	**Sensory signs:** *Paraesthesia* over dorsum of foot **Motor signs:** *Foot drop*

Carpal tunnel syndrome

Median nerve entrapment in the carpal tunnel.

Usually bilateral, although the dominant hand tends to be more severely affected; commoner in females (3F:1M); 60% of patients are between 40 and 60 years.

Associations
- Pregnancy, diabetes, hypothyroidism, rheumatoid arthritis, trauma, acromegaly, amyloid, sarcoid

Examinations
- **Phalen's test:** maximal flexion elicits symptoms
- **Tinel's test:** tapping wrist elicits symptoms

Diagnosis
- Increased pain and paraesthesiae at night combined with reduced nerve conduction across the wrist (EMG) are diagnostic of carpal tunnel syndrome

Management
- Wrist splint
- Analgesia (WHO analgesic ladder)
- Local steroid injection ± surgical decompression

6.6 NECK SURGERY

6.6.1 Neck lumps

Differential diagnosis
- Skin
- Soft tissue
- Bone
- Branchial apparatus
- Lymph node (LN)
- Salivary gland
- Vascular
- Thyroid gland

Clinical features
- **History**
  - Site: site of lump
  - Onset: slow-growing, or acute onset
  - Character: painful/non-painful
  - Radiation: development of new lumps
  - Associated features: fever, sore throat, catarrh, cough, dysphonia, anorexia, weight loss, night sweats
  - Timing: duration of lump
  - Exacerbating factors: palpation tenderness
  - Progress: enlarging/regressing
- **Examination**
  - **Inspect**
    - Site: in relation to a bony prominence
    - Size: rough estimate in mm/cm
    - Shape: regular or irregular
    - Edge
    - Colour: overlying skin erythema, skin colour
  - **Palpate**
    - Consistency: cystic or solid (firm)
    - Mobility: mobile or tethered (in relation to skin/ muscle)
    - Tenderness
    - Warmth
    - Reducibility
    - Tethering: skin or muscle
    - Pulsation
    - Regional lymph node examination
  - **Percuss:** enlarged thyroid gland – percuss for a retrosternal goitre
  - **Auscultate:** enlarged thyroid gland – listen for a **bruit**

Investigations
- **Fine needle aspiration (FNA)**
- **Biopsy**
  - Core biopsy
  - Open biopsy
- **Bloods:** FBC, U&E, thyroid function tests, liver function tests, C-reactive protein, ESR
- **Throat swabs**
- **Radiology:** USS of lesion, CT, MRI

Management
- **Conservative:** observe, 'wait and watch'
- **Surgical:** excision of lesion

Causes of lumps in the neck (based on tissue of origin; Figure 6.10)

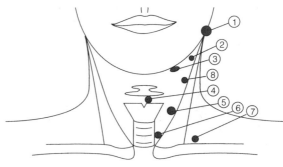

1 Parotid tumour	5 Branchial cyst
2 Tonsillar node	6 Thyroid nodule
3 Swollen submandibular gland	7 Virchow's node
4 Thyroglossal cyst	8 Cartoid body tumour

Figure 6.10: Differential diagnosis of neck lumps

Skin: epidermis and dermis
- Benign:
  - Epidermoid (sebaceous) cyst
- Malignant:
  - Malignant melanoma
  - Carcinoma (basal cell carcinoma and squamous cell carcinoma)

Soft tissue
- Subcutaneous fat: lipoma (most common)
- Muscles: leiomyosarcoma
- Nerves: neuroma
- Connective tissues
  - Infectious: abscess
  - Inflammatory: systemic lupus erythematosus, Sjögren's disease, scleroderma

Bone
- Cervical rib
- Malignant
  - Primary (rare)
  - Secondary (metastatic)

Head, neck and neurosurgery

Branchial apparatus
- Branchial cyst
- Pharyngeal pouch

Lymph node
- See Section 6.6.2

Salivary glands: submandibular and parotid glands
- **Infectious**
  - Viral: mumps
- **Inflammatory**
  - Sarcoidosis
  - Sjögren's disease
- **Neoplastic**
  - Benign: pleomorphic adenoma (commonest)
  - Malignant: adenoid cystic carcinoma, mucoepidermoid carcinoma and acinic cell tumour

Vascular
- Cystic hygroma (lymphangioma)
- Carotid body tumour (rare)
- Carotid artery aneurysm

Thyroid gland
- **Congenital**
  - Thyroglossal cyst
- **Inflammatory**
  - Acute thyroiditis
  - Subacute thyroiditis (De Quervain's disease)
  - Lymphocytic thyroiditis (Hashimoto's disease)
  - Riedel's thyroiditis (rare)
- **Hyperplastic**
  - Graves' disease
  - Endemic hyperplasia
  - Sporadic hyperplasia
- **Neoplastic**
  - Adenoma
  - Carcinoma
  - Lymphoma

Common conditions causing lumps in neck

Cervical rib
- **Aetiology:** congenital
- **Anatomy:** overdevelopment of the costal element of the seventh cervical vertebra
- **Clinical features:** firm immobile lump in the lower posterior triangle causing pressure-related symptoms secondary to compression of subclavian artery causing thoracic outlet syndrome, or the brachial plexus

- **Investigation**
  - Radiology: neck X-ray confirms diagnosis (although some are cartilaginous)
- **Management**
  - Conservative: physiotherapy
  - Medical: analgesia
  - Surgical: removal of rib or band division

Branchial cyst
- **Aetiology:** congenital lesion
- **Anatomy:** arises from the vestigial remnants of the second branchial cleft
- **Clinical features:** presents in young adults as a non-painful, non-tender cystic mass which protrudes from beneath the anterior border of the sternocleidomastoid muscle
- **Investigation**
  - Fine-needle aspiration: histology and cytology
- **Management**
  - Fine-needle aspiration
  - Surgical excision
- **Prognosis:** may recur after aspiration, indicating surgical excision

Pharyngeal pouch
- **Aetiology:** acquired lesion
- **Pathophysiology:** spasm or failure of relaxation of the cricopharyngeus muscle leads to increased cricopharyngeal pressure, resulting in formation of diverticulum if prolonged
- **Anatomy:** formed by a protrusion through the posterior pharyngeal wall
- **Clinical features:** presents in late adult life or the elderly as dysphagia and regurgitation ± swelling in the lateral neck (often left-sided)
- **Investigation**
  - Barium swallow
- **Management**
  - Conservative
    - Nil by mouth + IV fluids
    - Nasogastric tube feeding
  - Surgical: myotomy of the cricopharyngeus ± excision of the pharyngeal pouch

Cystic hygroma (lymphangioma)
- **Aetiology:** congenital
- **Clinical features:** presents during infancy or at birth as a slow-growing non-painful, non-tender, soft cystic lump, with no systemic features
- **Investigation**
  - Fine needle aspiration
  - Biopsy

- Radiology: USS, CT, MRI
- **Complications:** mass effect
- **Management**
  - Medical: interferon-α, absolute alcohol (sclerosing agent)
  - Surgical: excision

Carotid body tumour (rare)

- **Clinical features:** presents in middle age as a pulsating lump at the carotid bifurcation, which characteristically moves from side to side (not up or down)
- **Investigation**
  - Biopsy needs to be avoided due to risk of haemorrhage
  - Carotid angiogram (confirms diagnosis)
- **Management:** surgical excision

6.6.2 Cervical lymphadenopathy

Anatomy
See Figure 6.11.

Aetiology
- **Infectious**
  - **Viral:** pharyngitis, infectious mononucleosis (Epstein–Barr virus), cytomegalovirus
  - **Bacterial:** TB
  - **Fungal:** toxoplasmosis (classically presents as a single enlarged occipital lymph node in a young female)
- **Inflammatory**
  - Sarcoidosis
- **Neoplastic**
  - Primary
    - Lymphoma
      - □ Hodgkin's disease
      - □ Non-Hodgkin's lymphoma (NHL)
    - Leukaemia
  - Secondary (metastatic)

Clinical features
- **Infectious:** short history of feeling unwell, pharyngitis, palatine tonsillitis, pyrexia and a tender, firm, slightly mobile neck lump (often >1)
- **Inflammatory**
  - Systemic features, eg malaise, fever, generalised aches, night sweats
  - Respiratory features, eg cough
  - Cutaneous features, eg erythema nodosum
  - Ocular features, eg uveitis, keratoconjunctivitis sicca
- **Neoplastic**
  - **Lymphoma**
    - Hodgkin's disease
      - □ Asymptomatic ('A')

- □ Systemic ('B') symptoms: pyrexia of unknown origin or Pel-Ebstein fever (alternates with long periods of normo/hypothermia), weight loss, night sweats, cachexia
- □ Others: anorexia, fatigue, alcohol-induced pain in lymph nodes
  - NHL
    - □ Systemic symptoms: similar to Hodgkin's disease
    - □ Bone marrow suppression (pancytopenia)
  - **Leukaemia**
    - Bone marrow infiltration
      - □ Anaemia: pallor, fatigue, dyspnoea
      - □ Immunosuppression: infection
      - □ Bleeding: petechiae
      - □ Disseminated intravascular coagulation: bruising, bleeding, acute renal failure, gangrene
    - Leukaemic infiltration
      - □ Bone: pain
      - □ CNS: spinal cord compression, cranial nerve palsies
      - □ Liver/spleen: hepatosplenomegaly, massive splenomegaly (chronic myelogenous leukaemia)
      - □ Lymph nodes: lymphadenopathy
    - Neoplastic features: weight loss, weakness, malaise, fever

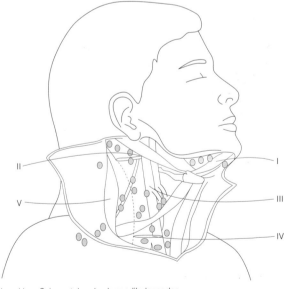

Level I	Submental and submandibular nodes
Level II	Upper jugular from the level of the hyoid to the skull base
Level III	Middle jugular nodes from the hyoid to the cricoid cartilage
Level IV	Lower jugular from the cricoid cartilage to the clavicle
Level V	Posterior triangle nodes subdivided into upper, middle and lower by the planes dividing levels II to IV
Level VI	Anterior compartment nodes from the hyoid bone to the suprasternal notch, bounded laterally by the medial border of the carotid sheath
Level VII	Nodes in the superior mediastinum

Figure 6.11 Levels of lymph nodes in the neck

Investigations
- **Bloods:** FBC, U&E, liver function tests, Ca^{2+}, angiotensin-converting enzyme, monospot test, rubella and toxoplasma serology
- **Urinalysis:** dipstick, MC+S, calcium
- Biopsy
  - Fine-needle aspiration
  - Core
    - Reed –Sternberg cells: Hodgkin's disease
- Radiology
  - Chest X-ray: bihilar lymphadenopathy (BHL)
  - High-resolution CT
  - Staging CT (chest/abdomen/pelvis)
- Others
  - Throat swab MC+S and virology
  - Respiratory
    - Sputum MC+S
    - Lung function tests
  - Bone marrow
    - Bone marrow aspiration
    - Trephine biopsy

Management
- **Infectious nodes**
  - Conservative: watchful waiting and treat symptoms
  - Medical: antipyretic, analgesic, antibiotic
  - Surgical: excision biopsy
- **Inflammatory nodes**
  - Medical: steroids
- **Neoplastic nodes**
  - Lymphoma
    - Hodgkin's disease
      - Surgical: excision of constantly enlarged lymph nodes
    - NHL
      - Chemotherapy
  - Leukaemia
    - Bone marrow transplant
    - Chemotherapy
    - Radiotherapy

Breast surgery

CONTENTS

Breast surgery

EDITOR'S NOTE

Breast surgery deals with virtually all disorders of breast tissue, both medical and surgical. It is an important topic for both students and doctors of any specialty. Although it is not commonly examined in the clinical setting for obvious reasons, the epidemiology and features of breast disorders are common written exam topics. Communication skills form a very important part in the practice of breast surgery and this may also be examined in OSCE stations.

Revision objectives

You should know:

- How to assess symptoms and signs of breast disease and arrive at a differential diagnosis
- How to investigate breast diseases further, including 'triple assessment'
- The clinical features and epidemiology of benign and malignant breast diseases
- The principles of managing breast disease, including surgical, oncological and endocrine therapy
- The features of screening test design and screening for breast cancer in the UK
- Briefly, the clinical features and causes of male breast disease

7.1 INTRODUCTION TO BREAST DISEASE

Breast disease is an important problem as cancer of the breast remains the commonest malignancy in women and the second commonest cause of cancer death in women in the UK. Breast problems account for about 15% of all referrals to a general surgery department, with over 90% of cases being benign. A basic understanding of breast disease in addition to an adequate clinical assessment and management plan is essential for doctors from every specialty.

7.1.1 Assessment of breast disease

Breast symptoms cause considerable morbidity and anxiety as women are often worried about breast cancer. Every breast lump should be regarded as a cancer until proved otherwise. A clear and rapid assessment should be performed in every patient and is always accomplished using the 'triple assessment'. This is usually offered in 'one-stop' breast clinics in most hospitals.

Triple assessment includes:

- Clinical assessment (history and examination)
- Radiological assessment (imaging)
- Pathological assessment (histology or cytology)

Clinical assessment

History

- Age and ethnic origin
- **Breast symptoms** (Box 7.1)
  - Breast lumps
  - Pain in the breast
  - Nipple abnormalities or discharge
  - Breast enlargement
- **Risk factor assessment**
  - Family history of breast cancer or disease
  - Previous history of breast cancer
  - Parity and history of breastfeeding
  - Age at menarche and menopause
  - Exposure to exogenous oestrogens [oral contraceptive pill (OCP) or hormone replacement therapy (HRT)]
  - Previous history of chest radiation
  - Smoking and alcohol consumption

Examination

Examination is performed at 45° inclination and with a chaperone.

- **Observation** at rest and with both hands raised above the head for
  - Asymmetry
  - Masses
  - Scars
  - Skin changes (redness, puckering, *peau d'orange*)
  - Nipple retraction
- **Palpation** with both hands behind the head
  - Both breasts, one at a time, starting with the asymptomatic one
  - Systemic palpation of all quadrants, including the axillary tail
  - Assessment of any specific mass or lump
  - Expression of discharge from the nipple (colour and nature)
  - Axillary and supraclavicular palpation for nodes (number, fixation)
- **General examination**
  - Chest for pleural effusion or consolidation
  - Abdomen for hepatomegaly and ascites
  - Spine for bony tenderness

Box 7.1: Presentation of breast disease

Breast lumps
- Benign skin lesions
  - Sebaceous cyst
  - Lipoma
- ANDI – aberrations of normal development and involution
  - Fibroadenoma
  - Fibroadenosis
  - Breast cyst
- Inflammatory
  - Breast abscess
  - Duct ectasia
  - Fat necrosis
- Neoplastic
  - Carcinoma and carcinoma-in-situ
  - Phyllodes tumour
  - Fibroadenoma
  - Duct papilloma
- Physiological
  - Galactocoele

Pain in the breast
- Cyclical mastalgia
- Non-cyclical mastalgia
  - Inflammatory – fat necrosis, mastitis, abscess
  - Duct ectasia
  - Carcinoma (<15% of cases)
- Non-breast causes
  - Costochondritis (Tietze's disease)

- Mondor's disease (superficial thrombophlebitis)
- Cardiopulmonary and oesophageal disorders

Nipple abnormalities or discharge
- Nipple discharge
  - Serous – early pregnancy or malignancy
  - Milky – lactation, late pregnancy, prolactinoma, post-lactational
  - Purulent – breast abscess
  - Yellowish, brown, or green – duct ectasia, benign nodularity (ANDI)
  - Thick creamy – duct ectasia (ANDI)
  - Blood-stained – intraduct papilloma, intraduct carcinoma, Paget's disease
- Nipple retraction
  - Congenital
  - Duct ectasia
  - Carcinoma
- Nipple inflammation
  - Eczema
  - Paget's disease

Breast enlargement
- Pregnancy
- Hyperplasia
- Cancer
- Lymphoedema
- Fibroadenoma
- Phyllodes tumour

Radiological assessment

First-line investigations include mammography and/or ultrasound examination.

- Age is an important factor in deciding investigation choice:
  - <35 years – ultrasound only
  - >35 years – mammography ± ultrasound.
- **Mammography** is the investigation of choice to start with in women over the age of 35. Below this age, ultrasound should be used as the breasts are too dense and the sensitivity of the investigation decreases.
- Mammography views should ideally be taken in at least two different planes.
- **Ultrasound** is best used in focal symptomatic breast disease to localise lesions. It can aid in the diagnosis of breast cancer in patients with a very dense background

pattern on mammography. It is also used in the biopsy of both palpable and impalpable lesions whilst on scanning in the breast as well as in tissue sampling of lymph nodes showing abnormal morphology.

Second-line investigations include magnetic resonance imaging (MRI) and magnetic resonance mammography (MRM), computed tomography (CT) and isotope scanning.

- MRI is the most sensitive technique for detecting breast cancer, in-situ carcinoma and for multifocal disease although it is not used widely due to the lack of scanner availability and cost.
- MRI is the best technique for imaging women with breast implants.
- There is a high false-positive rate and so needle sampling may also be required.

- MRI can also be used to detect recurrence and can reliably distinguish between scar tissue and recurrent tumour after at least 18 months post-surgery.
- CT scanning and breast scintigraphy are not used in primary imaging of the breast and their role is to detect metastatic disease in breast cancer patients.

Pathological assessment

It is important to have a tissue diagnosis in order to establish a diagnosis and management plan for further treatment. Ideally this should be obtained under image guidance such as ultrasound, however in clinically palpable and obvious lesions, an attempt can be made to obtain a sample directly. The methods of obtaining samples include:

- Fine-needle aspiration (FNA)
- Core biopsy – taken using a Trucut biopsy device (non-surgical)
- Surgical (open) excision biopsy

It is always better to obtain a tissue sample for histology than cells for cytology as the sensitivity of diagnosis increases with better cellular structure and sampling.

Reporting of assessment is provided using the scoring systems given in Table 7.1. This aids the clinician in deciding the accuracy of the confidence with which the reporting has been made and allows a decision to be made about further investigation or treatment.

Gradings are a combination of the mode of assessment plus the score (eg a definitely malignant mammogram is reported as M5):

Table 7.1: Scoring systems for pathological assessment of breast samples

U = Ultrasound	1 = Definitely benign
M = Mammography	2 = Probably benign
C = Cytology	3 = Equivocal
B = Biopsy (histology)	4 = Probably malignant
	5 = Definitely malignant

7.1.2 Screening

Cancer screening remains an important issue within the UK. It is provided to reduce morbidity and mortality from breast as well as other cancers. Approximately 25% of breast cancers are not clinically palpable. (See also Section 2.6.7.)

Breast cancer screening

Breast cancer screening was set up in 1987 following the Forrest report (Forrest, 1986) and has been modified through the years.

Current breast cancer screening guidelines within the UK:

- All women aged 50–70 are invited for 3-yearly screening mammography
- Double-view mammograms taken
- Single radiological reading
- Women with abnormal mammograms are recalled to specialist units for further assessment

Screening test design

Disease screening prerequisites (Wilson and Jungner, 1968)

Screening test should be:

- Sensitive and specific
- Safe and acceptable to the patient
- Inexpensive

The disease being screened should:

- Be an important disease with a known natural history
- Be treatable using local facilities
- Have a detectable latent or pre-clinical phase

Overall factors to consider in screening:

- Benefits of treatment should outweigh adverse effects of the test
- Must result in reduced mortality and morbidity
- Results must be audited and criteria for inclusion must be met

7.2 BENIGN BREAST DISORDERS

7.2.1 ANDI – aberrations of normal development and involution

Benign changes affect women from puberty to menopause while the physiology of the breast is under cyclical hormonal influence. Much proliferation and regression of the breast occurs during the frequent cyclical changes, and abnormalities arising from this process are referred to as 'aberrations of normal development and involution' (ANDI). This should not be regarded as a disease, rather a disorder affecting most women due to the nature of the breast cycle.

Clinical presentation

- ANDI disorders can present with any combination of breast symptoms and signs
- General presenting symptoms are those of a breast lump with or without pain or nipple discharge
- General examination finding are:
  - Diffuse lumpiness of the breasts, particularly in the upper outer quadrant

- A smooth spherical lump, either hard or fluctuant depending on the nature of the lump
- Bilateral signs or symptoms with a cyclical change

ANDI collectively encompasses the following individually known conditions:

- Breast cysts
- Sclerosing lesions, including sclerosing adenosis (fibroadenosis)
- Epithelial hyperplasia
- Cyclical mastalgia
- Fibroadenoma and duct papilloma

Breast cysts
- Present as discrete lumps and may be painful
- Cysts are often multiple and bilateral
- More common in perimenopausal women
- Palpation reveals a smooth, tense mass which may be fluctuant
- Needle aspiration reveals yellow–green or brown fluid which should disappear on aspiration
- Blood-staining and troublesome recurrence are indications for biopsy
- There is no increased risk of malignancy with cysts
- 1% of patients with cysts have carcinoma

Sclerotic lesions
- Include radial scars from previous surgery and sclerosing adenosis (fibroadenosis)
- Characterised pathologically by small-duct proliferation and fibrosis
- Sclerosing adenosis may present with a firm, mobile breast lump or mastalgia
- May be detected on screening and warrant further biopsy as they can calcify and mimic carcinoma
- There is an increased incidence of malignancy with sclerosing adenosis
- 30% of radial scars are associated with malignancy

Epithelial hyperplasia
- Due to an increase in the number of cells lining the terminal lobular unit
- Atypical hyperplasia has an increased risk of developing into breast carcinoma whereas simple hyperplasia does not
- Atypical ductal hyperplasia may represent the benign end of a spectrum leading to ductal carcinoma-in-situ (DCIS) and eventually ductal carcinoma
- Usually presentation is detected on mammographic screening although it may rarely present as a breast lump
- Cellular atypia requires annual examination and mammographic screening

Cyclical mastalgia
- Cyclical breast pain and heaviness experienced at a variable time before each period with symptoms often settling with the onset of menstruation
- Has an unknown aetiology but may be due to increased tissue sensitivity and hormonal imbalance
- Peak age of occurrence is in mid-30s; also seen in post-menopausal women on HRT
- Usually affects the upper outer quadrant of the breast as it is most glandular
- Clinical presentation may be with unilateral or bilateral breast tenderness and engorgement and marked nodularity
- Treatment involves reassurance, simple analgesics, supportive bra and advice to avoid caffeine
- Other measures that may help include evening primrose oil, danazol, bromocriptine, tamoxifen, and luteinising hormone-releasing hormone (LHRH) antagonists
- Symptoms settle after the menopause provided HRT is not taken

Fibroadenoma
- The commonest benign breast tumour in women; results from an aberration of lobular development
- Typically occurs after puberty and in young women
- Clinical presentation is that of a very mobile but smooth and firm breast lump often referred to as 'breast mouse' ranging from <1 cm to <5 cm in size
- Very large fibroadenomata arising in middle-aged or older women are referred to as 'phyllodes tumour' and may even ulcerate overlying skin due to pressure necrosis
- Phyllodes tumours may undergo malignant sarcomatous change and should be excised accordingly
- Normally treated with reassurance, but can be readily excised if it is large and uncomfortable, or if there is diagnostic uncertainty

Duct papilloma
- Arises from epithelial hyperplasia of the duct lining resulting in a polyp
- Affects women aged 35–50 years
- Often asymptomatic, but clinical presentation may also be with a blood-stained or serous nipple discharge, or a small palpable lump just under the nipple
- Requires the usual triple assessment in addition to nipple discharge cytology; ductography or ductoscopy may also be performed
- There is a slight increase in the risk of developing breast carcinoma
- Treatment is by duct excision (microdochectomy)

7.2.2 Inflammatory breast conditions

Common inflammatory conditions affecting the breast include:

- Acute bacterial mastitis (breast abscess)
- Duct ectasia
- Fat necrosis

Other less common causes of breast inflammation include mammary duct fistula, mastitis of the newborn, mumps mastitis, and chronic breast abscesses due to tuberculosis and other infections.

Acute bacterial mastitis

- The commonest and most important cause of acute inflammation of the breast
- Arises from infection ascending from a cracked nipple
- Usually caused by *Staphylococcus aureus* or streptococci
- Majority occur during lactation and affects about 3% of breastfeeding mothers, usually within the first 12 weeks of breastfeeding
- Fewer than 10% of these develop an abscess
- Non-lactating breast abscesses are seen more commonly in middle-aged smokers, diabetics, immunosuppressed women and those with duct ectasia
- Clinical presentation is with cellulitis of the breast, resulting in breast pain, swelling, erythema and tenderness. A fluctuant mass may also be palpable if an abscess has developed
- Treatment is given by a combination of antibiotics, analgesics and drainage of the abscess
- Drainage may be via aspiration under ultrasound guidance or via an incision made formally to drain the collection
- Breastfeeding should be encouraged from both breasts or if this is not possible due to discomfort, then the affected breast should still be expressed regularly

Duct ectasia

- Results from abnormal dilatation of periareolar lactiferous ducts which then fill with secretions to produce a thick creamy greenish stagnant collection
- Also known as plasma cell mastitis due to the chronic inflammation which may result from repeated infections of the stagnant collection
- Chronic inflammation may lead to recurrent breast abscesses, fibrosis resulting in nipple retraction or thick, green nipple discharge
- Treatment involves reassurance and surgical duct excision if symptoms persist

Fat necrosis

- Trauma to the fat cells in the breast results in an inflammatory reaction with subsequent fibrosis and possibly calcification
- Seen following blunt trauma, motor vehicle accidents and after breast surgery
- No history of trauma in 50% of cases
- Clinical features of fat necrosis mimic those of breast carcinoma with symptoms of a breast lump, signs of skin dimpling and nipple retraction, and mammographic appearances of calcification
- Fat necrosis must be thoroughly investigated as a cancer can be excluded only by histology
- Ideally these should be excised unless a firm diagnosis has been established to exclude carcinoma and the patient wishes to avoid surgery

7.3 BREAST TUMOURS

7.3.1 Epidemiology of breast carcinoma

- Breast cancer is the commonest malignancy in women and the commonest cause of cancer death in women, both worldwide and in the UK.
- There is an increasing incidence worldwide with over 1 million new cases diagnosed annually (35 000 in the UK).
- Approximately 1 in 9 women in the UK will develop breast cancer at some stage in their life.
- Male breast cancers account for only 1% of all breast cancers in Western countries and only 0.1% of male cancer deaths.

Box 7.2: Risk factors for breast cancer

- Increasing age
- Female gender
- White ethnicity
- Previous breast cancer or hyperplasia
- Family history or genetic predisposition to breast cancer
- Smoking and alcohol consumption
- Obesity
- Exposure to oestrogens (OCP, HRT)
- Early menarche and late menopause (oestrogen exposure)
- Nulliparity and lack of breastfeeding
- Late age of first pregnancy
- Previous exposure to ionising radiation

- Death rate from breast cancer is approximately 28 deaths per 100 000 women per annum worldwide and approximately 14 000 deaths in the UK annually.
- 5% of breast cancer is hereditary and associated with *BRCA* gene defects and the remaining 95% are sporadic, with unknown aetiology.
- Risk factors increase the chances of developing breast cancer (see Box 7.2).

7.3.2 Genetics of breast carcinoma

Familial breast cancer accounts for 5% of all breast cancers and incorporates the handful of hereditary syndromes and genetic mutations that predispose to breast cancer listed below:

- Familial breast cancer *BRCA1*
  - Mutation on long arm of chromosome 17
  - Associated with breast, ovarian, prostate and colon cancers
- Familial breast cancer *BRCA2*
  - Long-arm of chromosome 13
  - Associated with male and female breast cancer and ovarian cancer
- Li-Fraumeni syndrome
  - *TP53* gene mutation
  - Cancer syndrome associated with breast, brain, adrenal cancer as well as sarcomas and leukaemia
- HNPCC (hereditary non-polyposis coli cancer)
- Ataxic telangiectasia

BRCA1 and *BRCA2* genes account for 2% of all breast cancers and carriers have a lifetime risk of >80% of developing breast cancer. Relatives and offspring of identified gene carriers should be tested at a genetics centre and referred for genetic counselling accordingly.

7.3.3 Pathology of breast carcinoma

Cancer of the breast is due to a malignant proliferation of epithelial cells (carcinoma) arising from either ductal (90%) or lobular (10%) epithelium. All carcinomas commence from a pre-malignant stage called carcinoma-in-situ (CIS) where malignant cells are present but have not breached the basement membrane. CIS is often picked up on screening and should be assessed and treated with the same urgency as invasive breast carcinoma. As CIS is not invasive, it is not capable of producing metastases However, it should be noted that just because an area of CIS has been identified on biopsy, the surrounding area not contained in the biopsy specimen may contain invasive areas and this is the argument for axillary sampling and treatment of CIS in the same manner as invasive breast cancer. Like invasive cancer, CIS is either ductal or lobular.

Ductal carcinoma-in-situ (DCIS)

- 40% of DCIS progresses to become invasive
- Presentation is the same as breast cancer, but it is more commonly picked up on screening
- Micro-calcifications are seen on mammography
- May be further classed into low-, intermediate-, or high-grade

Lobular carcinoma-in-situ (LCIS)

- Should be regarded as a marker of increased risk rather than a pre-invasive cancer
- Develops in the acini of the lobules
- Often an incidental finding as it is impalpable and has no radiological features
- Can be multifocal and bilateral
- Most commonly found in pre-menopausal women
- 20% of patients develop invasive breast cancer on the same side with 15% developing one on the other

Invasive breast cancer

Most invasive breast cancers are invasive ductal carcinomas. The invasive lobular variety is less commonly encountered and pathologically tends to be very poorly circumscribed.

Macroscopic types

- Scirrhous (majority) – these cancers are often hard in consistency and contain areas of grey necrosis and calcification
- Inflammatory
  - Associated with timing of pregnancy (mastitis carcinomatosis)
  - Infiltration of dermal lymphatics leading to a *peau d'orange* appearance
- Atrophic scirrhous – scar-like tumour in the elderly breast
- Papillary – ductal or cystic papillary
- Paget's disease of the nipple

Box 7.3: TNM classification of breast cancer

Tis – Carcinoma-in-situ
T0 – No tumour located
T1 – Tumour < 2 cm
T2 – Tumour 2–5 cm
T3 – Tumour >5 cm
T4 – Tumour extension to chest wall
N0 – No nodes involved
N1 – Mobile ipsilateral nodes in axilla
N2 – Fixed ipsilateral nodes in axilla
N3 – Ipsilateral supraclavicular nodes
M0 – No metastases
M1 – Distant metastases

Microscopic types
- Invasive ductal carcinoma (75%)
- Invasive lobular carcinoma (10%)
- Medullary carcinoma (5%)
- Tubular carcinoma (3%)
- Mucoid carcinoma (3%)
- Papillary carcinoma (2%)
- Other minor variants (2%)

Spread
- Direct extension
  - Skin and chest wall
- Lymphatic
  - Dermal lymphatics, causing *peau d'orange*
  - Spread to axillary, internal mammary nodes initially
  - Later spread to supraclavicular and further lymph nodes
- Bloodstream
  - Lungs, liver and bone (spine, skull, chest wall)
  - Further spread to brain, ovaries, adrenals
- Transcoelomic
  - Can spread across pleural and peritoneal cavities resulting in pleural effusion and ascites

Grading (cell type and behaviour)
- Grade I – well differentiated
- Grade II – moderately differentiated
- Grade III – poorly differentiated

Staging systems (invasiveness and spread)
- TNM staging system (Box 7.3)
- Manchester staging (Box 7.4)
- International Union Against Cancer (UICC) – stages 1, 2A-B, 3A-B and 4, based on TNM combinations (eg stage 2A is T1/T2, N0/N1 and M0)

Paget's disease of the nipple
Breast cancer can present as Paget's disease of the nipple. It can be difficult to distinguish from eczema of the nipple (Table 7.2). The nipple–areola complex undergoes changes to a red,

---

> **Box 7.4:** Manchester staging
>
> **Stage I** – Lump <5 cm and not deeply fixed
>
> **Stage II** – As for stage I but with mobile ipsilateral axillary nodes
>
> **Stage III** – Lump >5 cm or showing fixation to skin or chest wall, fixed nodes, presence of supraclavicular node, lymphoedema of arm, or *peau d'orange*
>
> **Stage IV** – Distant metastases

destroyed. It has an underlying cancer of the breast which may or may not be palpable. The current theory suggests that the nipple becomes infiltrated by malignant cells from the duct in which the tumour originated. Treatment is by mastectomy.

7.3.4 Clinical presentation of breast cancer
Presentation of breast cancer can be variable as patients may often be referred from screening and not exhibit any signs or symptoms. On the other end of the spectrum, a few unaware patients will have advanced breast cancer and present with symptoms and signs of metastatic spread. An adequate triple assessment will diagnose most problems, with few patients being referred for further investigations.

Symptoms
- Asymptomatic (referred from screening)
- Breast lump (usually painless)
- Nipple discharge (occasionally blood-stained)
- Nipple retraction
- Skin dimpling
- Asymmetry and breast enlargement
- Presentation from secondaries (bone pain, dyspnoea)

Signs
- Usually a hard, irregular breast mass which may or may not show signs of fixation to the skin or chest wall

---

Table 7.2: Comparison of Paget's disease of the nipple and eczema

	Paget's disease	*Eczema*
Unilateral/bilateral	Unilateral	Bilateral
Pruritus	No	Yes
Site	Starts at nipple, spread outwards	Starts at areola and may spread to nipple
History of atopy	No	Yes
Underlying breast disease	DCIS or invasive breast cancer	No

bleeding, eczematous lesion which eventually becomes

- Skin tethering may occur if the cancer involves Cooper's ligaments
- Skin ulceration
- *Peau d'orange* (skin oedema from infiltration of the lymphatics)
- Axillary or supraclavicular lymphadenopathy
- Metastatic signs such as bony tenderness, effusion, jaundice

7.3.5 Management of breast cancer

Breast cancer management can be challenging as there are many factors involved in treating the patient. Investigation is standard with initial triple assessment in the breast clinic. Once a diagnosis is established, the patient is staged and treatment options are discussed. A multidisciplinary approach to managing breast cancer is essential and involves surgeons, oncologists, pathologists, radiologists, radiotherapists and breast-care nurses. In addition to the standard medical therapies for these patients, there is a major role for counselling and support, which are equally important in providing a complete treatment.

In the simplest of terms, medical treatment may be divided into:

- Surgical
- Radiotherapy
- Systemic chemotherapy
- Systemic endocrine therapy

Breast cancer surgery

Breast cancer surgery involves removal of the tumour and sampling or clearance of the axillary lymph nodes in the initial stages, followed by the option of breast reconstruction if the patient wishes at a later stage.

The breast

Wide local excision

The breast tumour may be removed by performing a wide local excision (breast-conserving) for smaller (usually <4 cm) tumours, with a 1-cm margin.

Mastectomy

For larger tumours, a mastectomy is performed in which the breast, including some overlying skin with the nipple–areola complex, is removed.

Needle-localised wide local excision

Occasionally, the breast surgeon is challenged with the presentation of an impalpable breast tumour which has been found on screening and has a proved malignant or pre-

malignant histology. In this case, a wide local excision is performed and the affected area is identified with a pre-inserted guide wire or skin marker with the help of radiologists.

The axilla

Management of the axilla remains a controversial issue as unnecessary clearance can result in considerable morbidity and lymphoedema of the affected arm. The surgery is performed to achieve two main goals: firstly, to stage the axilla and, secondly, to treat the axilla if necessary.

Axillary clearance

Axillary node clearance provides the best treatment of affected nodes although it is difficult to assess in advance which nodes are affected.

Sentinel node biopsy

A relatively new technique called sentinel lymph node biopsy aims to identify the first affected node of drainage from the cancer and to excise it for detailed histology, looking for micrometastases. The theory suggests that if this node has evidence of metastases, then one can proceed to an axillary clearance to provide a better prognosis. Alternatively, if the node is clear, theoretically the patient has been saved an unnecessary axillary clearance.

Other procedures

Modified radical mastectomy

Surgery of the breast and axilla can also be combined to perform a modified radical mastectomy in which a mastectomy is performed in combination with an axillary clearance through a single incision and operation.

Skin-sparing mastectomy

A skin-sparing mastectomy can also be performed in patients without evidence of occult breast cancer who require a prophylactic mastectomy. Such patients are usually *BRCA* gene carriers and request a mastectomy before the breast is affected with cancer.

Complications of breast surgery

- Seroma formation (very common)
- Bleeding and haematoma formation
- Wound infection
- Wound breakdown
- Skin necrosis
- Lymphoedema of the arm
- Shoulder stiffness
- Poor cosmesis

- Nerve damage during axillary dissection with resultant sequelae involving:
  - Intercostobrachial nerve
  - Long thoracic nerve
  - Thoracodorsal nerve
  - Medial and lateral pectoral nerves

Radiotherapy

Radiotherapy is given as adjuvant treatment to all invasive breast cancer patients who have undergone breast-conserving surgery to minimise the incidence of local recurrence. It is also used to treat and prevent local chest wall and axillary recurrence in those patients with a high risk. For patients with stage III or IV lesions, radiotherapy can play a palliative role.

Systemic chemotherapy

Indications

Combination adjuvant chemotherapy is given to selected patients to reduce the risk of recurrence and mortality following surgery. It can also be given before surgery as neoadjuvant chemotherapy to assess the tumour's response to chemotherapy as well as to downstage and shrink the tumour prior to excision. Smaller tumours may be amenable to breast-conserving surgery whereas without it a mastectomy may have been required.

Drugs

Treatment is tailored to the individual. However, standard treatment involves six cycles of chemotherapy administered every 3 weeks. 5-Fluorouracil (5-FU) and cyclophosphamide are combined with either epirubicin (FEC) or methotrexate (CMF) to provide combination therapy. Alternatively, trastuzumab (Herceptin®, monoclonal antibody targeting the human epidermal growth factor receptor HER-2) should be given to HER-2-positive patients, as the presence of this receptor is found in 15%–25% of all breast cancers and is associated with worse overall and disease-free survival.

Systemic endocrine therapy

Pathologically, specimens taken from breast cancers may contain oestrogen receptors (ER+) or progesterone receptors (PR+) that are responsive to their respective hormones. Hormonal blockade therapy is given to such patients to decrease the risk of local, regional and distant recurrence, as well as contralateral breast cancer. The major classes are listed below.

Tamoxifen

- Tamoxifen is a selective oestrogen receptor blocker
- It is the first-line treatment for ER+/PR+ patients with invasive breast cancer

- It reduces the annual recurrence rate by 25% and mortality by 17%
- Side-effects result in a chemical menopause (vaginal dryness, hot flushes, weight gain)
- Contraindicated in thromboembolic disease
- Small but increased risk of endometrial carcinoma and thrombosis

Aromatase inhibitors

- Newer class of drugs that block the peripheral conversion of androgens to oestrogen as well as the synthesis of oestrogen in the tumour
- Can only be used in post-menopausal women as all oestrogen in that age group is produced in body fat by aromatase
- Examples include anastrozole (Arimidex®), exemestane, and letrozole
- Also suitable for primary treatment of elderly patients who are ER+ but unfit for surgery
- Better than tamoxifen at reducing recurrence and better side-effect profile, but there is an increased risk of musculoskeletal disorders and fractures

LHRH agonists

- Can be given to pre-menopausal women to induce a chemical menopause (reversible)
- Can be prescribed in combination with aromatase inhibitor
- Example includes goserelin (Zoladex®)

Ovarian ablation

- Can be accomplished using surgery, radiotherapy, or drugs
- Used in pre-menopausal women to decrease recurrence and mortality in ER+ patients

7.3.6 Prognosis of breast cancer

Prognosis of breast cancer depends on the presence of disease spread (staging) and aggressiveness of the tumour (grading). Prognosis can be calculated using the Nottingham Prognostic Index (NPI) (Box 7.5) or the traditional 5-year survival based on Manchester staging system (Table 7.3).

Table 7.3: Prognosis according to the Manchester staging system	
Stage	5-year survival
I	80%
II	50%
III	15%
IV	5%

Box 7.5: Nottingham Prognostic Index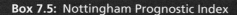

NPI = [tumour size (cm) × 0.2] +
(lymph node stage 1, 2, 3) + (histological grade 1, 2, 3)

Score	Category	10-year survival
0–2.4	Excellent prognosis (EPG)	96%
2.5–3.4	Good prognosis (GPG)	93%
3.5–4.4	Moderate prognosis I (MPGI)	82%
4.5–5.4	Moderate prognosis II (MPGII)	75%
5.5–6.4	Poor prognosis (PPG)	53%
6.5+	Very poor prognosis (VPG)	39%

7.4 CONDITIONS OF THE MALE BREAST

7.4.1 Gynaecomastia

Gynaecomastia is a benign hyperplasia of the ductal and connective tissue of the male breast. Males present with a unilateral or bilateral enlargement of the breast. All patients should undergo triple assessment to exclude male breast carcinoma.

Causes of gynaecomastia

- Physiological (birth, puberty)
- Alcohol excess
- Liver failure
- Renal failure
- Drugs (steroids, digoxin, cimetidine, spironolactone, cannabis, anti-androgens and others)
- Hyperthyroidism
- Klinefelter's syndrome
- Orchitis or cryptorchidism

Associations

- Testicular tumour
- Adrenal tumour
- Pituitary tumour

Treatment

- Reassurance
- Treat the cause
- Observe as it may regress in neonates and adolescents
- Subcutaneous mastectomy

7.4.2 Male breast cancer

- Male breast cancer is uncommon and represents <1% of all breast cancers
- About 200 cases per year in the UK
- Usually affects those over the age of 50
- Clinical presentation is similar to that in women and triple assessment should be the same
- Treatment is with mastectomy and axillary clearance
- Adjuvant treatment depends upon tumour's characteristics
- Prognosis is similar to women stage for stage

References

Forrest P. 1986. Breast Cancer Screening. Report to the Health Ministers of England, Wales, Scotland & Northern Ireland. London: HMSO.

Wilson J M G, Jungner G. 1968. Principles and practice of screening for disease. *WHO Chronicle*, **22(11)**, 473.

Endocrine surgery

CONTENTS

Endocrine surgery

Endocrine surgery was once a part of a general surgeon's routine workload. Although there are a few general surgeons still performing endocrine and general surgery, this has now become a specialised field in its own right. Endocrine disease may be jointly dealt with by endocrinologists and endocrine surgeons with a large degree of overlap. This chapter aims to complement the endocrine chapter from *Essential Revision Notes in Medicine for Students* (Kalra, 2006) and to provide a surgical viewpoint on the features, diagnosis and management of common endocrine disorders found in an endocrine surgeon's practice. Many of the topics from the endocrinology chapter in Kalra (2006) have been intentionally repeated in this book. This should indicate to students that it is an important topic to know as a practising doctor in any specialty as well as a common topic for the examinations.

Revision objectives

You should:

- Be aware of the anatomy and embryology of the endocrine glands and how disruption of this process can result in clinical disorders of these glands
- Know briefly the physiology of the endocrine glands and control of hormonal secretion
- Know the clinical features of benign and malignant endocrine diseases and how to assess further with investigations
- Know the basic surgical management of endocrine disease
- Know how to examine a thyroid gland and formulate a working diagnosis
- Know the indications and complications of thyroid surgery

8.1 PRINCIPLES OF ENDOCRINE SURGERY

Endocrine surgery has been in practice for over a century but in the past 30 years has become a specific specialty in its own right. The specialty mainly deals with disorders of the thyroid, parathyroid, adrenal glands and the endocrine pancreas. The pituitary gland is dealt with by neurosurgeons.

8.2 THYROID SURGERY

8.2.1 Embryology

An understanding of certain disease processes requires an appreciation of the developmental anatomy of the thyroid gland (Figure 8.1).

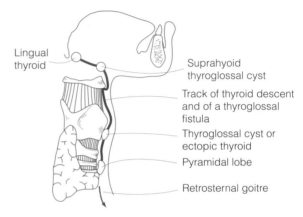

Lingual thyroid

Suprahyoid thyroglossal cyst

Track of thyroid descent and of a thyroglossal fistula

Thyroglossal cyst or ectopic thyroid

Pyramidal lobe

Retrosternal goitre

Figure 8.1: The descent of the thyroid, showing possible sites of ectopic thyroid tissue or thyroglossal cysts, and the course of a thyroglossal fistula. The arrow shows the further descent of the thyroid which may take place retrosternally into the superior mediastinum

The thyroid gland is derived from the floor of the pharynx, which later translates to a small pit after thyroid descent. This small pit is called the foramen caecum and is located at the junction of the anterior two-thirds and posterior third of the tongue in the midline. The gland then migrates inferiorly to lie anterior to the trachea. Following this migration there may be persistence of a thin tract – the thyroglossal duct – which normally closes. If the thyroglossal duct remains present it may lead to formation of a thyroglossal cyst or fistula.

Thyroglossal cyst

This presents as a small, painless, fluctuant lump in or close to the midline. The lump usually lies attached to or just above the hyoid bone. It is clearly recognised by specific features:

- It moves upwards on swallowing as it is attached to the pretracheal fascia.
- It moves up on protrusion of the tongue.
- It lies in the line of descent of the thyroid gland.

Thyroglossal cysts are removed via the 'Sistrunk' procedure, which involves surgical excision along with the remainder of the thyroglossal tract and the body of the hyoid bone.

Lingual thyroid

This occurs when thyroid tissue lies at the foramen caecum at the base of the tongue. It can interfere with speech or swallowing or can be symptomless. Treatment is by hormonal therapy to suppress thyroid-stimulating hormone (TSH) or by surgical excision, especially in the presence of obstructive symptoms.

8.2.2 Thyroid physiology

The thyroid gland produces the hormones thyroxine (T_4), triiodothyronine (T_3) and calcitonin (Figure 8.2). The gland itself is composed of follicular cells, which contain thyroid hormone-secreting colloid. Synthesis of thyroid hormones starts with the uptake of iodine from the diet and incorporation of this onto tyrosine residues on thyroglobulin (a glycoprotein that forms the basis of the thyroid hormones).

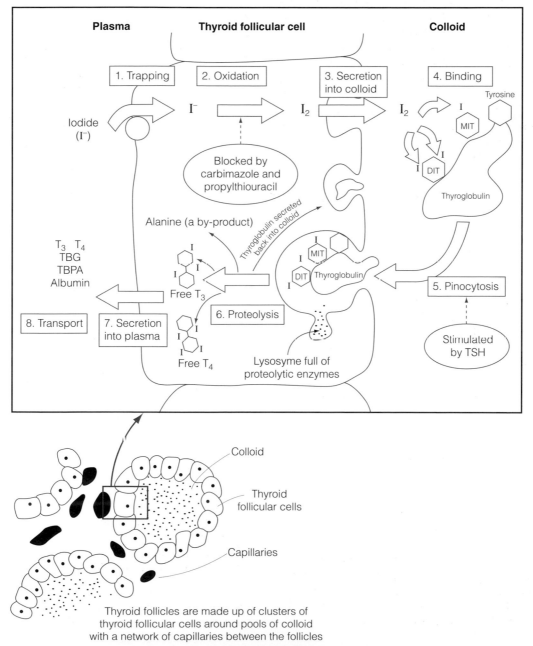

Figure 8.2: Synthesis of thyroid hormones. DIT = diidotyrosine; MIT = monoiodotyrosine; TBG = thyroxine-binding globulin; TBPA = thyroxine-binding pre-albumin; TSH = thyroid-stimulating hormone

221

Iodine from the diet is absorbed into the circulation as iodide and this is selectively absorbed by the thyroid gland. Iodide is taken up by the follicular cells and converted back into iodine by the enzyme thyroid peroxidase. Iodine is then bound to tyrosine residues on thyroglobulin by thyroid peroxidase to produce the iodine-containing residues – monoiodotyrosine (MIT) and diiodotyrosine (DIT). These residues are then coupled to produce T_3 or T_4. T_3 and T_4 are then bound to thyroxine-binding globulin and albumin in the circulation. In the main circulation, approximately 99% of T_3 and T_4 is bound to protein and the remaining 1% is biologically active. T_3 is believed to be the biologically active hormone and also results from the de-iodination of T_4 in the peripheries. Thyroid hormones circulate around the body and act by entering cells and attaching to nuclear receptors. These receptors bind DNA and lead to increased production of mRNA and the expression of certain genes.

The thyroid gland also secretes calcitonin from the parafollicular (medullary) C-cells. Calcitonin influences calcium homeostasis and drives to decrease the blood concentration of calcium by inhibiting calcium uptake from bone and gut.

T_3 and T_4 are controlled by a negative feedback mechanism axis called the hypothalamic–pituitary–thyroid axis. Thyrotropin-releasing hormone (TRH) is secreted from the hypothalamus and stimulates the release of TSH from the anterior part of the pituitary gland. TSH stimulates receptors on thyroid follicular cells and causes the release of T_3 and T_4. A rise in circulating levels of T_3 and T_4 causes a reduction in the release of TRH and TSH.

The control of thyroid hormone secretion

Carbimazole and thiouracils affect the uptake and concentration of iodine within the thyroid gland but do not affect the uptake of iodide. They also reduce the formation of DIT and thyroxine. They may be useful as short-term agents but prolonged use is associated with increased vascularity and growth of the thyroid gland as well as potent side-effects, which include agranulocytosis and hepatic impairment.

8.2.3 Clinical features of thyroid disease

Common modes in which a patient may present with thyroid disease are:

- Thyroid functional disturbance (ie hyper- or hypothyroidism)
- Goitre (an enlargement of the thyroid gland) or a lump in the neck
- Local symptoms of thyroid enlargement

Thyroid functional disturbances

Hyperthyroidism

Hyperthyroidism is otherwise known as thyrotoxicosis and may be caused by an excess of thyroid hormone from an overfunctioning gland or other source (Table 8.1).

Table 8.1: Causes of hyperthyroidism
• Graves' disease
• Solitary toxic nodule
• Toxic multinodular goitre
• Acute phase of thyroiditis
• Thyroxine overdose
• Thyroid carcinoma
• Iodine therapy
• Ovarian teratoma and choriocarcinoma
• Pituitary/hypothalamic tumours
• Drugs, eg amiodarone

Symptoms of hyperthyroidism
- Anxiety, irritability, nervousness
- Weight loss but with good or increased appetite
- Tremor
- Preference of cold temperature/heat intolerance
- Diarrhoea
- Palpitations
- Amenorrhoea or oligomenorrhoea
- Eye symptoms – see 'Signs of hyperthyroidism'

Signs of hyperthyroidism
- **General**
  - Anxiety and agitation
  - Weight loss
  - Pretibial myxoedema (thickening of the subcutaneous tissue of the shins)
  - Proximal myopathy
  - Tachycardia
- **Hands**
  - Fine tremor, thyroid acropachy (similar appearances to digital clubbing), sweating
- **Eyes** (seen only in Graves' disease)
  - Ophthalmoplegia – secondary to infiltration of the eye muscles
  - Exophthalmos – oedema and infiltration of orbital musculature and orbital fat
  - Chemosis – conjunctival oedema
  - Lid retraction – retraction of the upper eyelid due to overstimulation of levator palpebrae superioris
  - Lid lag – as the patient looks downwards the sclera is visible above the cornea

Management of hyperthyroidism
- Medical therapy (eg carbimazole)
- Radioactive iodine
- Surgery (thyroidectomy)

Hypothyroidism
Hypothyroidism is a clinical state of lack of thyroid hormone from an absent, suppressed, or underactive thyroid gland (Table 8.2).

Table 8.2: Causes of hypothyroidism
- Autoimmune thyroiditis (Hashimoto's, atrophic)
- Iodine deficiency
- Genetic defects of thyroid synthesis enzymes (eg Pendred's syndrome)
- Post-radiation
- Tumour infiltration
- Antithyroid medications
- Hypopituitarism
- Drugs (eg lithium)

Symptoms of hypothyroidism
- Tiredness, lethargy
- Weight gain with poor appetite
- Puffy eyes and dry skin
- Hair loss or thinning hair
- Constipation
- Menorrhagia or oligomenorrhoea
- Depression

Signs of hypothyroidism
- Hoarse voice
- Bradycardia
- Dry cool skin
- Dry, thinning hair
- 'Peaches and cream' complexion
- Periorbital oedema
- Peripheral oedema
- Slow-relaxing reflexes

Management of hypothyroidism
- Thyroxine replacement therapy

8.2.4 Examination of the thyroid gland
The thyroid examination should initially be carried out from the front of the patient to inspect the area. The thyroid should be inspected and the trachea palpated to confirm it is in the midline. The thyroid is then palpated with the fingertips of both hands whilst standing behind the seated patient. This is ideal with the neck muscles relaxed and can be achieved by tilting the neck slightly forwards. Palpation should confirm the presence of an enlarged or normal thyroid gland. Enlarged glands should be classified into smooth diffuse enlargement, multiple nodules that are palpable, or a palpable single nodule.

Allow the patient to have a glass of water to facilitate movement of the gland upwards with each swallow. Complete the neck examination by palpating the cervical lymph nodes for a thyroglossal cyst. Thyroglossal cysts can be confirmed by asking the patient to stick their tongue out and seeing if the lump moves upwards as the tongue protrudes. Return to standing in front of the patient to assess whether the thyroid gland extends retrosternally. It may be worthwhile having a look inside the patient's mouth to assess for the presence of a lingual thyroid. The upper sternum can also be percussed for examination purposes and the thyroid gland auscultated in Graves' disease to assess for the presence of a bruit.

The remainder of the systemic examination may now be completed if not done initially and this should confirm an over- or underactive thyroid state. This involves an assessment of the hands, pulse, hair, skin, eyes, tongue and weight for the features listed above under signs of hyperthyroidism and of hypothyroidism.

Essential note

The two most important parts of a clinical assessment of the thyroid gland are:

- The patient's clinical thyroid status (hyperthyroid, euthyroid, or hypothyroid)
- Classification of the type of goitre present (single nodule, multinodular, diffuse enlargement)

Goitre
A goitre is an enlargement of the thyroid gland.

The main classification of thyroid enlargement (which should be determined on palpation) are as follows:

- **Diffusely, smoothly enlarged** – toxic – seen in Graves' disease
- **Diffusely, smoothly enlarged** – euthyroid – endemic goitres, physiological enlargement (in puberty or pregnancy)
- **Diffusely, smoothly enlarged** – hypothyroid – in Hashimoto's thyroiditis

- **Multinodular enlargement** – seen in toxic or euthyroid patients (commonest presentation)
- **Solitary thyroid nodule** – usually non-functioning. May be dominant nodule of a multinodular goitre, a cyst, adenoma, primary carcinoma or metastatic carcinoma. May be a single nodule and the remainder of the gland may be normal. Need to exclude malignancy

Local symptoms of thyroid enlargement/compression of adjacent structures
- Dysphagia
- Dyspnoea
- Change in voice/hoarse voice
- Lymphadenopathy

8.2.5 Investigations

Thyroid function tests
Measurement of TSH (initially) and free T_3 and T_4 (second-line). Measurement of thyroid autoantibodies to thyroglobulin, microsomal antigens and thyroid peroxidise may be helpful for identifying Graves' disease or Hashimoto's thyroiditis.

Imaging investigations
Ultrasound of the thyroid may identify the nature of thyroid enlargement and the presence of solid or cystic nodules.

Thyroid scintigraphy involves ^{123}I, which is injected intravenously, and a gamma probe detects whether nodules are 'hot', ie functioning, or 'cold'.

CT scans can be useful in determining whether a goitre extends retrosternally.

Cytology/biopsy
Cytological diagnosis can be performed mainly via fine-needle aspiration (FNA) and histology by core biopsy. This may be performed either clinically or under ultrasound guidance.

Essential note

Think of thyroid investigations as similar in manner to the breast 'triple assessment' with a slight difference:

- Clinical
- Thyroid function test (bloods)
- Imaging

Biopsy or FNA can be performed as part of the clinical exam or under imaging guidance

8.2.6 Benign thyroid disease

Simple hyperplastic goitre

Causes
- Iodine deficiency
- Physiological – pregnancy or puberty

Clinically the patient is usually euthyroid with a smooth, diffusely enlarged thyroid gland.

Toxic goitre

Causes
- Diffuse enlargement (Graves' disease)
- Solitary toxic adenoma
- Toxic multinodular goitre

Clinically the patient is hyperthyroid with a low TSH and high free T_3 and T_4.

Graves' disease is an autoimmune disorder that is classically seen in women aged 20–40 years. It is characterised by autoantibodies that stimulate the TSH receptor, resulting in clinical hyperthyroidism. The effect of lymphocytic infiltration in the retrobulbar area and thyroxine on the orbital muscles in patients with Graves' disease results in ocular signs in 75% of patients.

Multinodular goitre
Multinodular goitre is an enlarged and irregular gland due to multiple nodules. It is the commonest cause of goitre in the UK. There are no known causes; they arise spontaneously. Symptoms and signs may be due to compression, cosmesis, or toxicosis if nodules are hyperfunctioning.

Hashimoto's disease
Hashimoto's is an autoimmune disease with diffuse lymphocytic infiltration of the thyroid and is the commonest cause of hypothyroidism in adults. A diffuse non-tender goitre is present with eventual clinical hypothyroidism. Blood tests show a raised TSH, low T_3 and T_4 and possibly raised antimicrosomal and antithyroglobulin antibody titres.

De Quervain's (subacute thyroiditis)
A self-limiting inflammatory condition of the thyroid gland associated with hyperthyroidism initially. May be associated with a recent viral upper respiratory tract infection.

Clinically presents with malaise, myalgia, a tender swollen thyroid gland, sore throat and elevated ESR. Acute symptoms can last up to 2 weeks.

Riedel's thyroiditis

Riedel's thyroiditis is an inflammatory condition resulting in a 'woody-hard' goitre that can infiltrate adjacent strap muscles and the carotid sheath. It can resemble anaplastic carcinoma or lymphoma and a biopsy or thyroidectomy may be necessary. It is associated with sclerosing cholangitis, retroperitoneal fibrosis and fibrotic diseases. Clinically it may present with hypothyroidism or compression symptoms on the trachea or oesophagus.

8.2.7 Management of thyroid disturbances
See Figure 8.3.

Simple hyperplastic goitre

Iodine supplements may help in cases of iodine deficiency. Thyroidectomy would be indicated for symptoms of compression or cosmesis.

Solitary thyroid nodule

A solitary thyroid nodule may be a dominant nodule in a multinodular goitre or a true solitary nodule. If adenoma detected on FNA cytology is impossible to distinguish from carcinoma, then excision is advised via ipsilateral thyroid lobectomy.

Multinodular goitre

If a multinodular goitre is long-standing with no features of compression or increasing size, it may be managed conservatively. If any other indications for surgery are present then options include thyroid lobectomy (hemithyroidectomy) or total thyroidectomy. Subtotal thyroidectomy is no longer widely advocated in thyroid surgery.

Non-operative options for toxic multinodular goitre or Graves' disease

Antithyroid drugs such as carbimazole or propylthiouracil are associated with a significant rate of relapse and have significant side-effects such as agranulocytosis, which is potentially very harmful but luckily occurs in only a small proportion of patients. Patients on antithyroid drugs require regular monitoring of blood counts.

Beta-adrenergic antagonists may give symptomatic relief from thyrotoxicosis.

Radioactive iodine is a useful mode of treating hyperthyroidism. However, there is a risk of malignancy and it is not advocated for use in female patients of childbearing age and must be avoided in pregnancy or breastfeeding.

Hashimoto's disease

First treatment is thyroxine replacement. Thyroid surgery may be necessary for compression symptoms.

De Quervain's (subacute thyroiditis)

Symptomatic relief is with steroids and aspirin. Rarely, a total thyroidectomy is needed for persistent inflammation.

Riedel's thyroiditis

Initial treatment of symptoms can be with steroids and thyroxine. Tamoxifen treatment has also resulted in shrinking of the goitre. Surgery is often required to confirm the diagnosis and rule out cancer. Compressive symptoms may also be treated with surgery.

8.2.8 Indications for surgery
- Rapid increase in size
- Hyperthyroidism refractory to medical therapy
- Compressive symptoms (oesophageal/tracheal), eg dysphagia/dyspnoea
- Vocal change
- Retrosternal extension
- Solitary nodule/follicular lesion
- Suspicion of malignancy/diagnosis confirmation
- Multiple endocrine neoplasia (MEN) syndrome/genetic predisposition
- Cosmesis

8.2.9 Complications of thyroid surgery

Bleeding and airway compromise

Haemostasis is critical in thyroid surgery, as bleeding within the confined space of the neck may compress the trachea and result in airway compromise. Clips and suture removers should be close by the patient post-operatively, as they may be required in an emergency to relieve tracheal pressure from an expanding haematoma.

Recurrent laryngeal nerve injury

This nerve supplies the muscles to the vocal cord except cricopharyngeus. If injured on one side there will be weakness and hoarseness of the voice. If injured bilaterally the patient will be virtually unable to speak and there may be airway compromise post-extubation. Emergency intubation and subsequent permanent tracheostomy will be required in cases of permanent bilateral nerve injury.

Superior (external) laryngeal nerve injury

The superior (exterior) laryngeal nerve can be injured at the superior pole of the thyroid. It supplies the cricopharyngeus and injury to this nerve results in an inability to reach high notes and mild weakness of the voice.

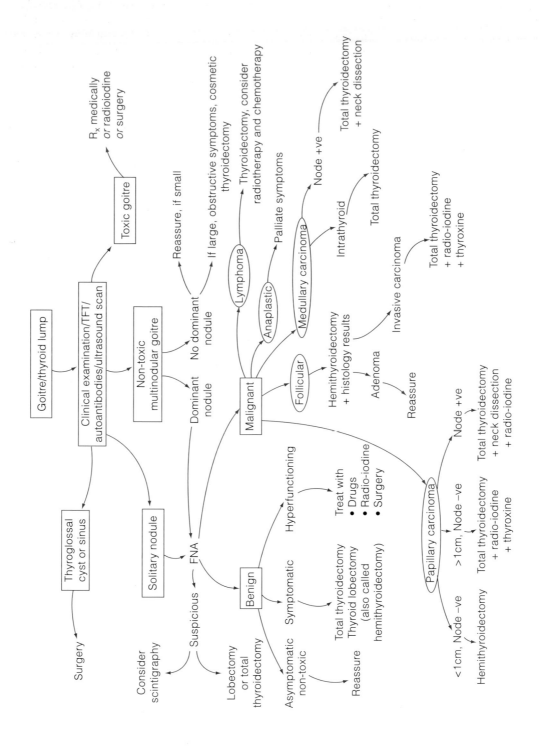

Figure 8.3: The management of thyroid nodules

Hypocalcaemia

Hypocalcaemia occurs secondary to removal, ischaemia, or injury of adjacent parathyroid glands. Clinical manifestations can include tetany, circumoral paraesthesia, Chvostek's sign and carpopedal spasms in severe hypocalcaemia. Treat with 10% calcium gluconate and oral calcium.

Hypothyroidism/need for thyroxine replacement

If thyroid tissue remaining after treatment is inadequate for the body's requirements, hypothyroidism may occur. This is treated with thyroxine replacement.

Thyrotoxic storm

Post-operative release of T_4 from the thyroid gland results in hyperpyrexia, sweating, confusion, agitation and arrhythmias (tachycardia). This is not seen commonly due to careful pre-operative preparation. Treat with steroids, β-blockers, and potassium iodide.

Laryngeal oedema

Laryngeal oedema results in respiratory distress, necessitating intubation. Settles spontaneously.

General complications

Infection and scarring (including keloid and hypertrophic scarring).

8.2.10 Thyroid cancer

Thyroid cancers are rare, with an incidence of approximately 2 per 100 000 people in the UK. They are twice as common in females as in males and cause 0.5% of cancer deaths.

There are five main classifications of thyroid carcinoma:

- Papillary
- Follicular
- Medullary
- Anaplastic
- Lymphoma

Papillary carcinoma

This is the most frequently encountered thyroid carcinoma, with a frequency of approximately 60%–70% of all thyroid malignancies. It is commonest in people aged between 30 and 50 years. The tumour is slow-growing, can be TSH-dependent and tends to spread via the lymphatics. Papillary thyroid carcinoma can present with cervical lymphadenopathy. These tumours are often found incidentally or at autopsy. The cure rate in small tumours is very high (approaching 100%).

Follicular carcinoma

This is the second most common thyroid carcinoma and has a mean age range of onset of between 40 and 60 years. It accounts for approximately 15% of all thyroid malignancies. It most commonly spreads haematogenously to lung and bone and rarely via lymphatics. It is usually unifocal in nature and commonly found in areas of low iodine.

Management of papillary and follicular thyroid carcinoma

The mainstay of treatment involves surgical excision of the affected thyroid lobe and block dissection of surrounding lymph nodes. If there is lymph node involvement then total thyroidectomy is generally advocated. Following surgery thyroxine replacement is instituted to suppress TSH production. Radio-iodine treatment with ^{131}I may be used to ablate remaining thyroid tissue or to treat recurrences. Lifelong thyroxine-suppressing TSH can also be administered. Serum thyroglobulin may be used as a tumour marker for recurrence. Bony metastases may best be treated with radiotherapy.

Medullary carcinoma

Medullary carcinoma accounts for approximately 5% of all thyroid cancers and originates from the parafollicular C-cells of the thyroid. C-cells produce calcitonin and this allows detection by blood assay. Seventy-five per cent occur sporadically, but there is an autosomal-dominant pattern of inheritance (25%) and it may also be associated with MEN type 2 syndrome (multiple endocrine neoplasia), when it presents with co-existing phaeochromocytoma and parathyroid hyperplasia. It can be multifocal in nature and may spread via the lymphatics.

Management of medullary thyroid carcinoma

If there is a family history or genetic basis of inheritance then family members should undergo screening for the *RET* proto-oncogene. Those with screen-detected medullary thyroid carcinomas should undergo prophylactic thyroidectomy, which can be performed in childhood. Total thyroidectomy and block dissection of surrounding lymph nodes is the mainstay of treatment, accompanied by thyroxine replacement. Recurrence can be monitored using plasma calcitonin.

Anaplastic carcinoma

Anaplastic carcinoma (<5%) generally occurs in the elderly and often presents with expansion of, or pressure symptoms from, a pre-existing goitre. This spreads rapidly, locally and via haematogenous and lymphatic spread. Patients with anaplastic carcinoma have a poor prognosis and few patients survive longer than 1 year.

Management of anaplastic carcinoma
Surgery may be used to excise or debulk the tumour, followed by radiotherapy. Palliative care is usually required.

Lymphoma

Thyroid lymphoma is very rare and represents a small proportion of thyroid malignancies.

It is part of the disease process of non-Hodgkin's lymphoma. There is an increased incidence in patients with Hashimoto's disease. Staging is performed with a staging CT scan as for all lymphomas.

8.3 PARATHYROID DISEASE

8.3.1 Anatomy and embryology

The parathyroids are four small ovoid glands which lie in pairs either side of the thyroid gland. Each gland is approximately the size and shape of a grain of rice and each gland normally weighs approximately 30 mg.

It is important to understand the developmental anatomy of the parathyroids. The superior parathyroids arise from the fourth branchial pouch and the inferior parathyroids arise from the third branchial pouch. Because of their complex developmental anatomy the parathyroid glands may vary in anatomical location. The superior glands are usually more reliable in their location and lie close to where the inferior thyroid artery passes the recurrent laryngeal nerve. The inferior glands are more variable and may occasionally lie within thymic tissue or even the superior mediastinum.

8.3.2 Parathyroid physiology and control of calcium

The role of the parathyroid glands is to secrete parathyroid hormone (PTH), which acts in a homeostatic mechanism with vitamin D and calcitonin to control calcium to normal levels.

Parathyroid hormone acts via the following mechanisms:

- Increasing reabsorption of calcium from the renal tubules by inhibiting the reuptake of phosphate; the net effect is to increase serum calcium and decrease serum phosphate concentrations.
- It stimulates the activity of osteocytes (initially) and osteoclasts (long-term) in bone, leading to mobilisation of calcium stores into the circulation.
- It stimulates the rate at which vitamin D is converted to 1,25-dihydoxycholecalciferol in the kidney.

8.3.3 Hyperparathyroidism

This condition is characterised by overactivity of the parathyroid glands, resulting in excessive secretion of PTH. It is classed as primary, secondary or tertiary depending on the pathology; only primary and tertiary hyperparathyroidism are surgically treated. Hyperparathyroidism may also rarely be caused by an ectopic secreting source, such as a squamous cell carcinoma of the lung.

Primary hyperparathyroidism

This condition has a mean incidence at age 30–50 years although any age can be affected; females are affected most commonly. In 85% of cases the cause is a solitary parathyroid adenoma with the remainder of normal glandular tissue being suppressed; in approximately 2%–5% there may be adenomata of multiple glands. In 10%–15%, primary hyperparathyroidism may be secondary to hyperplasia and in very few cases the raised calcium may be secondary to parathyroid carcinoma, although this is extremely rare. Blood tests reveal raised PTH and calcium levels and lowered phosphate levels. There is also increased urinary excretion of calcium. Surgical parathyroidectomy is the treatment of choice.

Secondary hyperparathyroidism

This is a feature of chronic renal failure or malabsorption, which leads to hyperplasia of all four glands secondary to a chronically decreased plasma calcium. The chronic hypocalcaemia leads to hyperplasia of the parathyroids due to long-term stimulation. Blood tests reveal a normal or lowered calcium, high phosphate levels, and raised creatinine levels, as expected in renal failure. PTH levels are very high. The hyperplasia tends to resolve with correction of the hypocalcaemia. Treat the cause.

Tertiary hyperparathyroidism

If secondary hyperparathyroidism persists, then parathyroid hyperplasia may become autonomous, even when hypocalcaemia is corrected. This generally results in hypercalcaemia and is best treated by parathyroidectomy.

Clinical features of primary hyperparathyroidism

These features are secondary to excessive secretion of PTH leading to hypercalcaemia. Classically referred to as 'bones, stones, abdominal groans and psychiatric moans', the features consist of:

- Bone demineralisation, which can lead to bone pain or pathological fractures
- Renal calculi

- Abdominal pain, which may be secondary to duodenal and gastric ulceration or pancreatitis, which are associated with hyperparathyroidism
- Mental disturbances and depression

Most cases of hyperparathyroidism are incidental findings on blood tests done for other reasons. It is important to consider other causes of hypercalcaemia, which include malignancy, myeloma, sarcoidosis, thyrotoxicosis and ectopic PTH secretion from tumours such as squamous cell lung carcinoma (see Box 8.1).

There are usually no findings on physical examination.

Box 8.1: Causes of hypercalcaemia

- Hyperparathyroidism[a]
- Malignancy, including multiple myeloma[a]
- Excess vitamin D intake
- Sarcoidosis
- Addison's disease
- Paget's disease
- Tuberculosis
- Long-term immobility
- Drugs, esp. thiazide diuretics and lithium
- Milk-alkali syndrome
- Familial hypocalciuric hypercalcaemia
- Thyrotoxicosis
- Phaeochromocytoma

[a]These make up more than 80% of the causes of hypercalcaemia

---

Investigations

To make a diagnosis
- Serum calcium will be raised usually to more than 2.70 mmol/l and is normally corrected for serum albumin
- PTH concentration is elevated (usually greater than 10 ngl/l)
- Raised 24-hour urinary calcium
- Bone mineral density scan (DEXA scan) will identify evidence of bone demineralisation

Parathyroid localisation studies
Ultrasound scan of the neck may be helpful in identifying the adenoma in 60%–70% of cases.

CT or MRI can be useful for identifying ectopic or difficult-to-find adenomas.

Radionuclide isotope scanning using sestamibi can identify the adenomatous gland more accurately. In selected cases or redo surgery, parathyroid venous sampling may enable accurate

localisation of adenomatous tissue by taking serial measurements from different locations within the venous system and finding the region with the highest PTH levels.

Treatment
Treatment is by surgical excision of the affected gland via a cervical exploration. Frozen section may be employed to identify adenomatous change and the affected gland is removed. If hyperplasia is present then three of four glands may be removed and in cases of persistent hypercalcaemia the surgeon may choose to remove all parathyroid tissue and replace calcium with supplements and vitamin D. Postoperatively one must monitor the patient for hypocalcaemia and supplement calcium if required.

8.4 ADRENAL DISORDERS

The adrenal (or suprarenal) glands are situated on the upper pole of each kidney. The glands are triangular in shape and are approximately 8 cm long and 2.5 cm high. Each consists of a cortex (the outer portion), which is derived from mesodermal tissue, and an adrenal medulla (the central portion), which is derived from neural crest ectodermal tissue.

8.4.1 The adrenal cortex
There are three zones of tissue within the adrenal cortex:

- **The zona glomerulosa** – secretes mineralocorticoids – dysfunction leads to primary hyperaldosteronism (Conn's syndrome)
- **The zona fasciculata** – secretes adrenal glucocorticoids – dysfunction leads to primary hypercortisolism (Cushing's syndrome)
- **The zona reticularis** – secretes androgenic steroids – dysfunction leads to virilism or the adrenogenital syndromes such as congenital adrenal hyperplasia

Insufficiency of the adrenal cortex results in Addison's disease, with deficiency of mineralocorticoids and glucocorticoids. Treatment of this condition is by hormone replacement therapy.

8.4.2 Cushing's syndrome
Cushing's syndrome is an excess and chronic hypersecretion of glucocorticoids. There are a number of causes. When secondary to a pituitary cause (excess stimulation from the hypothalamic–pituitary axis), which occurs in approximately 70%–80% of cases, this is called Cushing's disease. If it is due to an adrenal tumour (in about 20% of cases) or any other cause, this is called Cushing's syndrome.

Endocrine surgery

Causes

ACTH–dependent
- Pituitary tumour causing adrenal hyperplasia via hypersecretion of ACTH (Cushing's disease)
- Ectopic ACTH production – typically from small-cell/oat cell tumours of the lung
- Iatrogenic – from ACTH administration

ACTH–independent
- Adrenal tumour – adenoma or carcinoma
- Iatrogenic – treatment with steroids

Clinical features
- Weight gain, especially central distribution
- Proximal myopathy and muscle wasting
- 'Buffalo hump' of fat distribution across the upper back
- 'Moon face'
- Thin skin and easy bruising
- Acne
- Oedema
- Hirsutism
- Depression
- Psychosis
- Menstrual irregularities
- Hypertension
- Glucose intolerance
- Peptic ulcers
- Pancreatitis
- Hyperpigmentation
- Cataracts
- Skin striae
- Osteoporosis
- Avascular necrosis of bone

Blood tests
- Hypokalaemia
- Hypernatraemia
- Hyperglycaemia
- Loss of diurnal variation in plasma cortisol
- Raised free urinary cortisone
- ACTH levels variable depending on cause

Investigation and diagnosis

Screening tests
- Serum cortisol – raised and loss of diurnal variation
- 24-hour urinary cortisol – raised
- Urea and electrolytes
- Fasting serum glucose levels

Further tests
- A **dexamethasone suppression test** may demonstrate a failure to suppress cortisol production following dexamethasone administration. There are two types of suppression tests: low-dose and high-dose. The normal response to dexamethasone administration should be suppression of cortisol levels. The low-dose test shows no suppression of cortisol levels following dexamethasone administration and is used to confirm Cushing's, regardless of cause. The high-dose test will help to distinguish between a pituitary cause (Cushing's disease) and ectopic ACTH or a non-ACTH cause. In the high-dose test, negative feedback from the high dexamethasone intake suppresses the pituitary secretion of ACTH and therefore a normal suppression of cortisol is seen in Cushing's disease. High-dose dexamethasone has no effect on ectopic suppression of ACTH or on autonomously secreting adrenal lesions and no suppression of cortisol is seen.
- Plasma ACTH may assist in localisation of the problem as this will be undetectable in adrenal disease but may be elevated in pituitary or ectopic production.
- A chest radiograph (CXR) may detect an underlying lung carcinoma.
- CT/MRI brain may detect a pituitary lesion and abdominal CT will identify an adrenal lesion.

Treatment
If iatrogenic – remove the cause.

Surgical management
Adrenalectomy may be undertaken for adrenal adenoma or carcinoma, which may be undertaken via an open or laparoscopic approach. Steroid replacement must be given peri-operatively to prevent an adrenal crisis. For bilateral hyperplasia, a bilateral adrenalectomy can be carried out with permanent oral steroid replacement.

Ectopic ACTH production (eg from small-cell lung carcinoma) may be amenable to surgery but these tumours usually have a poor prognosis. Chest radiotherapy may be an option in some selected cases.

Pituitary tumours can be resected via a trans-sphenoidal or transfrontal approach if amenable.

For patients unsuitable for surgery or occasionally patients waiting for surgery, metyrapone, a cortisol production inhibitor, may be administered.

8.4.3 Conn's syndrome (primary hyperaldosteronism)

This syndrome refers to a single adrenal cortical adenoma secreting excessive amounts of aldosterone; however, it may rarely be due to carcinoma or bilateral adrenal hyperplasia.

This condition may be asymptomatic or present with resistant hypertension. Fatigue, muscle weakness, polyuria and polydipsia are other clinical features that may be present.

Conn's syndrome should be distinguished from secondary hyperaldosteronism which may be due to renal artery stenosis or organ failure (cardiac, nephrotic syndrome, liver cirrhosis). The two types of hyperaldosteronism are managed differently, hence the reason for early identification.

Investigations
- Urea and electrolytes will show a similar picture to that of Cushing's disease, with hypokalaemia and hypernatraemia.
- Plasma aldosterone levels are elevated.
- Plasma renin levels are decreased – if this is raised consider secondary hyperaldosteronism.
- CT scan may reveal an adrenal adenoma or carcinoma.

Treatment
Some control of blood pressure and symptoms may be achieved with aldosterone antagonists (eg spironolactone) but the mainstay of treatment is adrenalectomy if an adrenal lesion is identified.

> **Essential note**
>
> Think of Conn's syndrome in any patient presenting with hypertension and hypokalaemia

> **Essential note**
>
> Blood results in hyperfunctioning adrenal cortical disorders such as Cushing's and Conn's syndrome are all similar, with hypernatraemia and hypokalaemia. The reverse is seen in Addison's disease, with hyponatraemia and hyperkalaemia. It is also convenient to remember that glucose follows the sodium concentrations in Cushing's, with a hyperglycaemia. Hypertension follows adrenal hyperfunction; hypotension follows hypofunction

8.4.4 The adrenal medulla
Tumours may arise from the adrenal medulla which can require surgical excision. The main tumours are phaeochromocytomas, which are derived from chromaffin cells within the adrenal medulla, and neuroblastomas, which are derived from the neural crest.

Phaeochromocytomas
Phaeochromocytomas are rare tumours secreting catecholamines such as adrenaline and noradrenaline. They are known as '10% tumours' for the following reasons:

- 10% are malignant
- 10% are bilateral
- 10% are extra-adrenal (in sympathetic nervous tissue)
- 10% are found in children
- 10% are familial or are associated with MEN syndrome (MEN type 2)

Clinical features
These are essentially the effects of adrenergic stimulation from the sudden release of catecholamines. They are **paroxysmal** symptoms, consisting of:

- Hypertension
- Sweating
- Headache
- Palpitations
- Chest pain
- Dyspnoea
- Pallor
- Blurred vision
- Feelings of anxiety/impending doom
- There may be features of a multiple endocrine neoplasia (MEN) syndrome

> **Essential note**
>
> Always consider endocrine disorders such as phaeochromocytoma, thyrotoxicosis, carcinoid syndrome and MEN in patients presenting with anxiety

Investigations
- Serum catecholamines and glucose
- 24-hour urinary collection for catecholamines, metanephrines and vanillylmandelic acid (VMA)
- Ultrasound
- CT scan
- MRI scan
- MIBG scan (metaiodobenzylguanidine) involves injection of a radionuclide isotope that is a precursor for adrenaline and enables localisation of the tumour

Management
Management is by surgical excision, but with careful pre-operative preparation to prevent uncontrolled release of

catecholamines. Pre-operative blockade, first with phenoxybenzamine and then β-blockade (with propranolol) is normally employed with bedrest and under controlled conditions. Insulin may be required to control blood sugar because of the gluconeogenic effect of excess catecholamines. Surgical excision may be open or laparoscopic and via a trans-abdominal or retroperitoneal approach.

Indications for surgery

- Tumour secreting catecholamines
- Tumours greater than 4 cm in size (increasing suspicion of malignancy)
- Tumours causing pressure symptoms, eg flank pain
- Extra-adrenal tumours (carry an increased chance of malignancy)

8.5 MEN SYNDROME (MULTIPLE ENDOCRINE NEOPLASIA)

MEN types 1 and 2 are inherited in an autosomal dominant manner.

8.5.1 MEN 1 syndrome (Werner syndrome)

MEN 1 syndrome is characterised by development of:

- Parathyroid hyperplasia (hyperparathyroidism)
- Pancreatic islet cell adenomas (insulinomas, gastrinomas)
- Pituitary adenomas (prolactinomas)

8.5.2 MEN 2 syndrome

MEN 2 syndrome is characterised by medullary thyroid cancer. There are two variants:

MEN 2A (Sipple syndrome)

- Medullary thyroid cancer
- Phaeochromocytoma
- Parathyroid hyperplasia

MEN 2B

- As per MEN 2A but with phenotypic marfanoid features and mucosal neurofibromas

Screening for MEN 1 is biochemical, with the following studies:

- Serum calcium, PTH, prolactin
- Fasting blood glucose
- Serum pancreatic polypeptide and gastrin and plasma chromogranin A

Screening for MEN 2 is genetic and involves searching for the *RET* mutation. If this mutation is found, a thyroidectomy

should be performed to prevent medullary carcinoma development.

8.6 CARCINOID SYNDROME

This condition is characterised by hypersecretion of 5-hydroxytryptamine (5-HT) secondary to a tumour of argentaffin cells. These tumours occur commonly in the appendix, rectum, lung and ovary or testis. Tumours are often benign but those of larger size may behave in a malignant fashion and may metastasise. Ten per cent of cases have an association with MEN type 1.

Tumours tend to present late but may cause symptoms of an abdominal mass, present as intussusception or appendicitis. Carcinoid syndrome usually occurs with tumours of larger size or with metastases. This consists of symptoms of flushing, diarrhoea, abdominal pain and bronchospasm. Most cases arising from abdominal organs are asymptomatic, as 5-HT released from the carcinoid lesion will be metabolised by the liver first. Only when the capacity of the liver to metabolise is exceeded or the tumour metastasises to the liver can the carcinoid result in a syndrome. This is because 5-HT is now being secreted into the general circulation and can exert its effects.

8.6.1 Investigation of carcinoid syndrome

Urinary 5-HIAA (5-hydroxyindoleacetic acid) may be elevated and the tumour may be localised with CXR or CT imaging of the abdomen.

8.6.2 Treatment of carcinoid syndrome

If the tumour is small then surgical resection should be undertaken; if metastatic (or carcinoid syndrome is present) then surgical debulking may help symptoms. Octreotide (a somatostatin analogue) may help relieve symptoms.

8.7 PANCREATIC ISLET-CELL ENDOCRINE TUMOURS

Tumours of the pancreatic islet cells are derived from APUD (amine precursor uptake and decarboxylation) cells. Pancreatic islet cells consist of alpha (α) cells which secrete glucagon, beta (β) cells producing insulin, and other cells which produce a combination of somatostatin and serotonin. Tumours may produce other active hormones such as vasoactive polypeptide (VIPomas) and gastrin (gastrinomas.) Some islet cell tumours are part of MEN syndromes, usually associated with pituitary and parathyroid gland tumours or hyperplasia.

The main islet-cell tumours are described below.

8.7.1 Insulinomas

Insulinomas are mainly benign and extremely rare (1 per million of the population). They can present with hypoglycaemic episodes, disturbed consciousness and odd behaviour. Diagnosis is usually made by finding elevated insulin levels accompanying low blood glucose. C-peptide is raised with insulinoma and may allow one to exclude exogenous insulin administration as a cause. CT and MRI can locate the lesion and treatment is by surgical excision due to the risk of malignant transformation.

8.7.2 Gastrinomas (Zollinger–Ellison syndrome)

Gastrinomas (Zollinger–Ellison syndrome) result in elevated serum gastrin levels, which leads to excessive gastric acid secretion and subsequent peptic ulceration. The ulceration is usually severe and refractory to standard treatment. The syndrome is associated with MEN type 1 in 30% of cases but may occur in sporadic form. Sixty per cent of gastrinomas are malignant at diagnosis and they can have multiple metastases. The severe peptic ulceration may often result in perforation or bleeding and can cause significant morbidity. Investigations consist of serum gastrin estimation and acid secretion tests which reveal hypersecretion. Treatment involves surgical excision when the pancreatic tumour can be located, but, if this is not possible, control may be achieved with proton-pump inhibitors and acid suppression. Vagotomy and pyloroplasty, or total gastrectomy may be options in poorly localised or metastatic tumours.

8.7.3 Glucagonomas

Glucagonomas are tumours of the pancreatic α cells and are extremely rare. They present with diabetes and a bullous rash. Treatment is similar to that of insulinomas.

8.7.4 VIPomas

VIPomas are tumours that secrete vasoactive intestinal peptide (VIP). They are very rare and present with watery diarrhoea, hypokalaemia and achlorhydria. Raised VIP levels are characteristic and treatment by surgical excision is curative.

Reference

Kalra P. 2006. *Essential Revision Notes in Medicine for Students*. Knutsford: PasTest.

Plastic surgery

CONTENTS

Plastic surgery

Revision objectives

You should:

- Know the factors affecting wound healing and the different methods available for wound reconstruction, including grafts and flaps
- Know the different types of benign and malignant skin lesions and how to distinguish between them
- Know the classification of the different types of burns injuries and their clinical features
- Know the management and complications of burns injuries
- Know the clinical features of cleft lip and palate
- Know the clinical features of hand infections and how to assess and manage hand conditions, including tendon injuries and acute infections of the hand
- Know briefly about the different cosmetic surgical techniques

9.1 INTRODUCTION TO PLASTIC SURGERY

Plastic surgery is a highly specialised branch of surgery, and is not linked to particular parts of the body in the way that, for example, cardiac and urological surgery are. It should not be confused with cosmetic or aesthetic surgery, which makes only a small part of the workload of plastic surgeons in the UK. This chapter will focus on the common conditions and problems faced by plastic surgeons, including wound closure, craniofacial defects, hand diseases, burns, skin cancers and cosmetic surgery.

9.2 WOUNDS

9.2.1 Wound closure and delayed healing

Referral to plastic surgeons from other specialist teams is often for wound closure. When closing wounds, there are multiple factors that need to be taken into consideration. These include:

1 The ability for the wound to heal
2 Functional outcome
3 Cosmetic outcome

The ability of the wound to heal is dependent on a number of factors. Wound healing is dealt with in Chapter 2 in much more detail, but it is important to recap as follows. Factors that may impair healing can be classed as local or general and include:

Local causes
- Infection
- Ischaemia
- Foreign body
- Malignancy

General causes
- Poor nutrition
- Diabetes mellitus
- Immunosuppressive agents
- Age

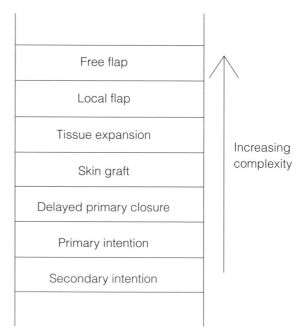

Figure 9.1: The reconstructive ladder

The reconstructive ladder

When deciding how to close wounds, it is best to choose the simplest method and decide if that will suffice. Often the more complex or extensive the defect, the more radical the closure option will be. The reconstructive ladder is a general scheme for thinking about closure, where each rung on the ladder constitutes a more complex closure method than on the rung below. It is outlined in Figure 9.1 and starts from the bottom working upwards.

Secondary intention

This describes a method of healing where the edges of the wound are not brought back together, but the wound ultimately heals either exposed to the air or with a covered dressing.

Primary intention

This is the most common method of wound closure surgically, and is where the edges of a wound are brought together and held in that position with, for example, stitches, glue or staples.

Delayed primary intention

This is otherwise known as tertiary intention. This method of closure is used for dirty wounds, where closing the wound primarily would result in an increased risk of infection. In tertiary intention, the wound is first washed and cleaned, and then closed at a later date if it remains clean.

9.2.2 Grafts

Skin can be taken from one area of the body (donor site) and attached onto another area (recipient site). This skin that is taken is known as a graft. Two types of graft exist: split-skin and full-thickness grafts. The blood supply is detached, in contrast to a flap, and thus requires the recipient site to be well vascularised in order to 'take'. The factors that lead to graft failure include:

- Haematoma formation (commonest cause)
- Poorly vascularised tissue
- Infection
- Seroma formation
- Movement of the graft
- Tension on the graft
- Poor tissue handling

Split-skin graft (SSG)

- Consists of epidermis and upper papillary dermis only
- Commonly taken from the arms, thighs, abdomen or back
- Used to cover large defects where cosmesis is less important

- Advantages:
  - Donor site heals quicker than a full-thickness graft
- Disadvantages:
  - Cosmetic mismatch – hair, meshed appearance
  - Graft contracture
  - Poor tissue strength

An SSG is harvested with either a knife or a power dermatome. It can then be 'meshed', either freehand or by passing it through a mesher. The principle of this is that making holes in the graft allows it to be stretched out, which offers two advantages:

- Allows a greater surface area to be covered, eg in burns patients
- Reduces the chance of blood or serous fluid becoming trapped between the graft and recipient site, which may otherwise prevent the graft from being accepted

Full-thickness graft

- Consists of epidermis and dermis, ie also contains skin elements, including hair follicles and sweat glands
- Commonly taken from supraclavicular, post-auricular, nasolabial areas
- Used to cover small defects where cosmesis and low risk of contracture are important, eg face, hands, over joints
- Donor site closed either by primary intention or with an SSG
- Advantages:
  - More resistance to trauma than ssg
  - Better cosmetic appearance
  - Lower risk of contracture
- Disadvantages:
  - Higher risk of graft failure
  - Donor site takes longer to heal

Management of graft sites

Donor site

Split-skin graft donor sites heal by re-epithelialisation. They are covered with a dressing material such as paraffin gauze (eg Jelonet®), alginate dressing (eg Kaltostat®) or synthetic semi-permeable membranes. The presence of a dressing allows the tissues to heal and, depending on which is used, may in fact promote healing. Clinically, the dressings on donor sites can start to smell or ooze exudate. This is normal. If this happens, these dressings should be left alone for several days to allow the newly epithelialised tissue to form. Removing dressings prematurely removes the healing layer with the dressing and prevents recovery of the tissue.

Full-thickness graft donor sites are either closed by primary intention, or are covered with an SSG.

Recipient site

The recipient site needs to be cleaned with saline. The graft is then sutured at a few points, and then can be secured all around the edges of the wound. Care is taken to handle the graft carefully, and to keep it moist. Petroleum gauze is placed on top of the graft to prevent haematoma formation, and further dressings are applied. The wound is then left untouched for 5 days to allow it to take. The dressings are then changed every 48 hours.

Tissue expansion

- Involves stretching skin to provide wound coverage.
- Most commonly, a saline-filled silicone implant is placed under the skin or muscle and filled with more saline twice weekly.
- The overlying tissue is subsequently stretched and when there is sufficient extra tissue, the implant is removed and the tissue harvested as a flap.
- The tissue expander may be placed for 4 weeks to 6 months, the length of time being determined by the size of coverage required.

9.2.3 Flaps

- Flaps are defined as units of tissue transferred from one site to another while maintaining their own blood supply.
- Indications for a flap include:
  - Skin coverage over poorly vascularised sites, eg directly over tendon, bone or cartilage
  - Areas where padding is required, eg pressure areas such as the sacrum
  - Facial reconstructive surgery.

Classification of flaps

There are three ways to classify a flap. One is based on blood supply, one on the type of tissue and the final way is by the location of the donor site.

Method 1: random vs axial flap

A **random flap** is where the blood supply is not derived from a recognised artery but rather comes from many little unnamed vessels. Most cutaneous flaps are random flaps. **Axial flaps** are where the blood supply comes from a recognised artery or group of arteries. Most muscle flaps are axial flaps.

Method 2: type of tissue transferred

The contents of the flap can include skin, fascia, muscle, bone or viscera or be a mix of all or some of these. Examples include latissimus dorsi myocutaneous flaps consisting of muscle and skin used in breast reconstruction, or a fibula osseocutaneous flap consisting of bone and skin used in mandibular reconstruction.

Method 3: local vs distant flap

Tissue transferred from an area adjacent to the defect is known as a **local flap**. Tissue transferred to a remote site is known as a **distant flap**. Distant flaps themselves can be classified as either a pedicle or a free flap. A **pedicle flap** is where tissue is left attached to the donor site and simply transposed to a new location keeping the 'pedicle' intact as a conduit to supply the tissue with blood. A **free flap** is where the tissue, along with its blood supply, is detached from the original location ('donor site') and then transferred. With a free flap, the blood supply is reconstituted using microsurgery. The term 'free flap' can be misleading as it can also be regarded as a graft; however, the unique blood vessels carried with the tissue allow it to be classed as a flap.

9.3 BENIGN SKIN LESIONS

Skin lesions can be either benign or malignant. History taking will involve asking about the duration of symptoms, if there are any precipitating or predisposing factors, and whether there are sinister features. Examination will determine the physical characteristics and planning for surgical removal if appropriate. Benign skin lesions will be discussed first, detailing which lesions are found in which layer of skin, and skin cancers will be discussed later. Note that not all skin lesions require or warrant surgical removal.

9.3.1 Lesions derived from the epidermis

Papilloma

- Pedunculated overgrowth of skin
- Also known as a skin tag
- Occur anywhere on the body
- Soft and flesh-coloured

Wart

- Has a rough surface
- Caused by human papillomavirus
- Commonly found on hands, feet and face

Seborrhoeic keratosis

- Also known as a senile wart
- Mostly found in elderly people
- Slightly raised, well-defined plaque
- Surface is velvety or warty
- Have a stuck-on appearance
- Can be picked off

Pigmented naevus

- Also known as a mole

- Can be flat or raised, rough or smooth and may or may not contain hair
- Should be differentiated from malignant melanoma

9.3.2 Lesions derived from the dermis

Dermatofibroma
- Benign neoplasm of dermal fibroblasts
- Small pink or brown lesion ranging from a hemispherical lump to a flattened disc
- Firm 'woody' feel
- Fully mobile from deeper tissues as they are in the skin
- Commonest on lower limbs

Pyogenic granuloma
- Bright red or blood-encrusted hemispherical nodule
- Soft, fleshy consistency
- Classically associated with a preceding penetrating injury

9.3.3 Lesions derived from skin appendages

Sebaceous cyst
- Very common
- Smooth hemispherical swelling of a blocked sebaceous gland
- Central punctum (pathognomic) is present in 50%
- Attaches to skin and therefore moves with it
- Can become infected, ulcerated, calcified and, very rarely, undergo malignant transformation

Keratoacanthoma (adenoma sebaceum)
- Overgrowth and subsequent regression of hair follicle cells
- Resembles a volcano, with a lump of normal skin colour with a central keratin crater
- Appears over 6 weeks, stays at a constant size for 6 weeks, and usually regresses spontaneously over a few months
- A variant is a keratin horn, which forms a dry, hard spike and does not regress spontaneously

Furuncle
- Also known as a boil
- Represents an infection of a hair follicle
- Usually caused by *Staphylococcus aureus*
- Superficial and occurs in isolation

Carbuncle
- Extensive collection of hair follicle infections
- Adjacent infected follicles are linked by tracts, and form draining sinuses
- May appear necrotic

Hidradenitis suppurativa
- Chronic, recurrent infection of sweat glands
- Most commonly affects the groins and armpits
- May require radical excision followed by full-thickness skin grafts

9.3.4 Lesions derived from vascular structures

Campbell de Morgan's spots
- Small, red capillary naevus
- No clinical significance

Telangiectasia
- Dilatation of normal capillaries
- Can be part of Osler–Weber–Rendu syndrome, also known as hereditary haemorrhagic telangiectasia or can be secondary to skin irradiation

Spider naevus
- Variant of telangiectasia
- Associated with liver disease and pregnancy
- Central arteriole with branches that blanch on applied pressure

Port-wine stain
- Present from birth and does not regress
- Occurs as a result of vascular malformation

Cavernous haemangioma
- Also known as a strawberry naevus
- Resembles a bright-red strawberry
- Present from birth
- Over half regress spontaneously by the age of 3 years

9.3.5 Lesions not derived from skin layers
Lumps and bumps referred to plastic surgeons may not derive from the skin. Below are three conditions which are important to know and may be included in a differential diagnosis.

Lipoma
- Very common
- Benign tumour of adipocytes
- Distinct lesion of varying size, with a lobulated surface
- Skin is not adherent, in contrast to a sebaceous cyst (for which it is most commonly mistaken)

Dermoid cyst
- Smooth, soft, spherical swelling
- Skin-lined cyst deep to the skin

Plastic surgery

- Congenital cysts occur along lines of fusion of skin dermatomes (midline)
- Acquired cysts occur following forced implantation of skin into subcutaneous tissues following injury

Ganglion
- Smooth, hemispherical, fluctuant swelling
- Cystic myxomatous degeneration of fibrous tissue
- Results in a swelling arising out of a joint or tendon sheath

9.4 SKIN CANCERS

Over 75 000 cases of skin cancer are reported each year in the UK alone. There are three main types of skin cancer:

- Malignant melanoma
- Squamous cell carcinoma
- Basal cell carcinoma

Risk factors for skin cancer include:

- Sunlight (UV radiation)
- Age
- Ionising radiation
- Chemicals

9.4.1 Malignant melanoma
Presents with a pigmented skin lesion. Features suggestive of malignancy include:

- Increasing size
- Irregular margin
- Bleeding or itching
- Variation in skin colour within the lesion
- Presence of a halo
- Presence of satellite lesions
- Ulceration or change in surface appearance

Five types of melanoma exist (in order of frequency):

- Superficial spreading (most common)
- Nodular
- Lentigo maligna
- Acral lentiginous
- Amelanotic

Staging is based on the depth of invasion, and also gives prognostic information whereby increasing depth correlates with a lower survival rate. The two staging systems used are **Breslow's depth**, which measures the thickness of the tumour, and **Clark's levels**, which state which layer the tumour extends down to. It is worth noting that Breslow's depth has superseded

Clark's levels as the main staging tool due to its ease in accurately determining the stage of disease.

Treatment
- Surgical excision of the lesion plus removal of affected lymph nodes
- Malignant melanoma is neither radio- nor chemo-sensitive

9.4.2 Squamous cell carcinoma
- Usually arises in sun-exposed areas
- Edge is raised and everted
- Red–brown in colour due to vascularity
- Treated with surgical excision. Radiotherapy or block dissection can be performed for lymph node involvement

9.4.3 Basal cell carcinoma
- Most common skin cancer
- Usually arises in sun-exposed areas such as the face
- Different types include nodular (most common type, with a raised, rolled edge), pigmented, cystic, superficial, micronodular and morpheaform
- Can present as an ulcer with a raised, rolled, 'pearly' edge appearance
- Treatment options include surgical excision, Mohs micrographic surgery, curettage, radiotherapy and cryotherapy

9.5 BURNS

A burn is a coagulative destruction of the surface layers of the body. Causes of burns include:

- Heat (most common)
- Electricity
- Chemicals
- Friction
- Radiation
- UV light

9.5.1 Classification of burns
Burns can be classified according to the depth to which they penetrate.

Superficial burns
- Formerly called first-degree burns
- Example is sunburn
- Involves epidermis only
- Germinal matrix not involved
- Clinically painful with erythema but no blistering
- Normally heals within 5–7 days
- Usually heals on its own without scarring

Partial-thickness burns

- Formerly called second-degree burns
- Involves epidermis and varying degrees of dermis
- Clinically painful with marked blistering
- Germinal matrix intact
- Can be split into superficial partial-thickness and deep partial-thickness burns
- Superficial partial-thickness burns heal on their own in 1–3 weeks
- Deep partial-thickness burns appears paler, with drier skin and decreased skin sensation
- May require skin grafts to heal

Full-thickness burns

- Formerly called third-degree burns
- Involves all layer of the skin, including subcutaneous tissue
- Germinal matrix destroyed
- Clinically painless (due to destruction of nerve endings) with minimal blistering. Appear white, grey or leathery
- Require skin grafts to heal

9.5.2 Extent of burns

Two methods exist for estimating the total body surface area (BSA) of a burn. The first is to use to use **the rule of palm**. This states that the patient's palm (not including fingers or wrist) is 1% of the BSA. Another method is the **rule of nines**. This rule is only applicable to adults and states that the body can be divided into 12 regions, 11 regions each making up 9% of the BSA, with the perineum region constituting the final 1% (see Figure 9.2).

Burns in babies and children cannot be estimated with the rule of nines. This is because the trunk is smaller relative to the rest of the body. The surfaces in babies are as follows:

- Head and neck – 21%
- Each arm – 10%
- Back – 13%
- Abdomen and chest – 13%
- Each leg – 13.5%
- Buttocks – 5%
- Genital area – 1%

9.5.3 Management of burns

First aid

- Remove the insult and expose the burnt area
- If evidence of smoke inhalation, ensure there is a clear airway
- Run cold water over a thermal burn, or neutralisation solution over a chemical burn
- Decide if the patient needs to come to hospital

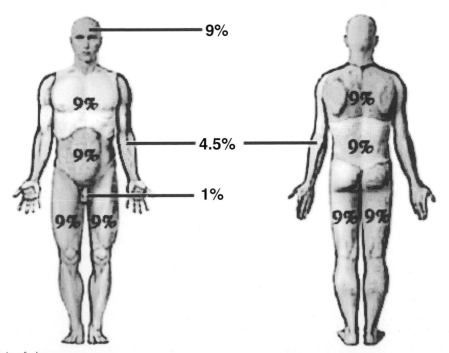

Figure 9.2: Rule of nines

Hospital phase

- Assess resuscitation requirements
  - Clear airway
  - Ensure breathing is adequate
  - Ascertain if circulation is compromised and correct if required
  - Administer analgesics as appropriate
- Take a history, noting the nature of the cause of the burn, duration of contact and any associated inhalation injuries
- Estimate the depth and extent of burn
- Decide on need for referral to a specialist unit
- If referral is not required, clean and dress the burn
- If referral is required, commence IV fluids, dress the burn, and transfer the patient so that specific injuries may be addressed and complications watched for

Fluid resuscitation

One of the complications of burns is hypovolaemia. This needs to be corrected with IV fluids. The **Parkland formula** (see below) is commonly used to calculate the fluid required to resuscitate the patient, but be aware that maintenance fluids are required in addition.

$$\text{Fluid in the first 24 hours (ml)} = 4 \times m \,(\text{kg}) \times$$
$$\% \text{ BSA of second-/third-degree burns}$$

where m is mass (in kg) and BSA is body surface area; 50% of this fluid is then given in the first 8 hours, and the remaining 50% over the next 16 hours.

Criteria for referral to a specialist burns unit

- Associated airway injury or facial burns with a suspicion of inhalation injury
- Partial-thickness burns >5% of total BSA in a child
- Partial-thickness burns >10% of total BSA in an adult
- >1% full-thickness burn
- Partial- or full-thickness burns to face, perineum, external genitalia, feet and hands, and over joints
- Circumferential injury
- Chemical and electrical burns
- Extremes of age
- Non-accidental injury
- Co-morbidity
- Non-healed burn 3 weeks after injury

9.5.4 Complications of burns

Local complications

- **Tissue loss** – the severity of the burn may devitalise tissue, requiring skin grafts at a later stage.
- **Contracture** – circumferential full-thickness burns around the chest or limbs can contract and cause breathing difficulties or limb ischaemia. Escharotomy needs to be performed to relieve this.
- **Infection** – infections can develop (usually *Streptococcus pyogenes* or *Pseudomonas aeruginosa*).

General complications

- **Inhalation injury** – suggested by the presence of burnt skin and soot around the mouth and nostrils, as well as elevated carboxyhaemoglobin levels on arterial blood gas samples. Burns can cause oedema of the airways, necessitating oxygen to correct hypoxia, and potentially intubation to facilitate ventilation.
- **Anaemia** – arises from destruction of red cells within the affected skin capillaries, and also toxic depression of bone marrow if the burn site becomes infected.
- **Shock** – arises from plasma loss where the loss of skin allows seepage of plasma out of the capillaries.
- **Renal failure** – occurs secondary to plasma loss and exacerbated by rhabdomyolysis, which occurs in full-thickness burns.
- **Acute respiratory distress syndrome** (ARDS) – the mechanism by which ARDS develops in burns patients is unclear.
- **Acute peptic ulcer** – also known as a Curling's ulcer. Precipitated by the stress response.

9.6 CLEFT LIP AND PALATE

Craniofacial disorders are operated on by plastic, ENT, neuro- or maxillofacial surgeons, depending on the disorder itself. Often the surgeons will be one part of a multidisciplinary team. The most common craniofacial disorder is cleft lip (Figure 9.3) and/or palate (Figure 9.4) with an incidence of 1 in 700. Cleft lip with or without cleft palate is more common than cleft palate alone.

- A cleft lip denotes a vertical fissure (otherwise known as a cleft) in the upper lip.
- It can be either unilateral or bilateral.
- It can be incomplete where the nose is not involved, or complete where it does.
- Surgery is indicated for cosmesis, though suckling difficulties may occasionally arise.

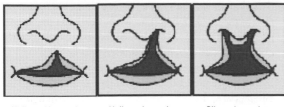

Unilateral incomplete cleft lip   Unilateral complete cleft lip   Bilateral complete cleft lip

Figure 9.3: Cleft lip

- A cleft palate denotes a failure of the palatal shelves to come together on either side of the mouth and join in the midline.
- It may involve the soft palate or both the hard and soft palate.
- Bilateral cleft palates usually involve both hard and soft palates.
- Surgery is indicated to prevent difficulties in breathing and feeding, to prevent malalignment of the mouth later in life, and to reduce the risk of respiratory tract and ear infections.

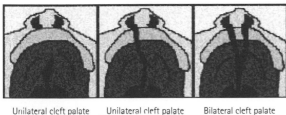

Unilateral cleft palate cleft lip   Unilateral cleft palate and lip   Bilateral cleft palate and lip

Figure 9.4: Cleft palate

- Surgery is performed in one of the ten specialist centres in the UK.
- Surgery for cleft lip is classically performed on the basis of the rule of tens – the baby is 10 weeks old, weighs 10 pounds, and the Hb is 10 g/dl.
- Outcome for cleft lip surgery is good, usually with no functional sequelae.
- Surgery for cleft palate is classically performed at 12–18 months. The principles of surgery are to:
  - Separate the oral and nasal cavities
  - Separate the oropharynx and nasopharynx.
- Any feeding difficulties occurring before surgery are overcome with the use of special bottles and teats, and occasionally a feeding tube.
- Cleft palate surgery is associated with satisfactory speech in 80% of patients. Further operations may be required to correct residual speech abnormality or jaw malalignment.

Hand surgery is a specialist branch of either plastic or orthopaedic surgery, with the two most common presentations being hand infections and tendon rupture.

9.7.1 Tendon injuries

- The hand and wrist contain a number of tendons.
- The extensors are found on the dorsal aspect, and flexors on the volar aspect.
- The hands can be split into anatomical zones:
- Rupture of the tendons is usually post-traumatic, eg following a laceration.
- Tendons will not heal unless the edges are brought back together. This requires surgery due to the pull of the originating muscle separating one part of the tendon from that attached to its insertion.
- The blood supply of tendons is poor. Careful handling and minimal iatrogenic trauma are required to promote healing of the tendon and to prevent re-rupture.

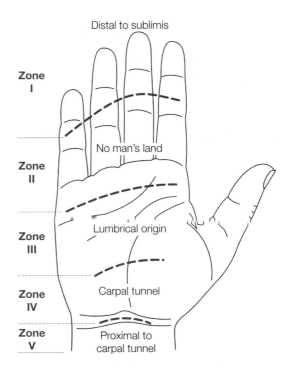

Figure 9.5: Zones of the hand on the volar surface

Management involves:

- History
- Examination of the function of the movements of the wrist and fingers. This should identify which tendon or tendons are damaged; associated neurovascular deficits should be identified
- X-rays to identify associated fractures
- Antibiotic and tetanus cover
- Irrigation of the wound
- Repair of the tendon
- Immobilisation of the tendon to allow healing
- Physiotherapy

Classically, extensor tendons are repaired either in the Emergency department or by the general orthopaedic/plastics team as a day-case procedure under local anaesthetic. Flexor tendons, however, are repaired by specialist hand surgeons or general plastic surgeons in theatre under general or regional anaesthetic.

9.7.2 Hand infections

Although rarer since the introduction of antibiotics, infections involving the hand are potentially disastrous if not appropriately recognised and managed. History should explore:

- Dominance, ie left- or right-handed
- Occupation
- Resulting function and disability
- Underlying hand conditions, eg arthritis, Raynaud's disease
- Predisposing susceptibility, eg presence of trauma, immunocompromised state
- Treatment involves antibiotics for all acute infections plus possible surgical treatment

9.7.3 Paronychia

- Denotes a nail-bed infection.
- Also known as a whitlow.
- Pus is found in the cuticle and may track underneath the nail.
- If acute presentation, think of *Staphylococcus aureus* as the main cause.
- If chronic presentation, think of fungal agents (eg *Candida*) as the main cause.
- Initial treatment is antibiotics or antifungal agents.
- Further treatment may involve drainage of pus and possible removal of the nail.

9.7.4 Pulp space infection

- Also known as a felon.
- *Staphylococcus*, *Streptococcus* and anaerobes are the commonest causative organisms.

- Usually arises following a minor penetrating injury in the pulp of the finger. This is followed by accumulation of pus, which may either collect or spontaneously discharge.
- Fibrous septa arise from the dermis to the terminal phalanx. If the infection collects between the septa, the condition mimics compartment syndrome and can lead to terminal ischaemia.
- Infection may also track down to the bone, causing osteomyelitis.
- Treatment involves drainage of the pus, taking care to break down the septa.

9.7.5 Infectious flexor tenosynovitis

- Also known as a flexor tendon sheath infection.
- This is a **hand emergency** and should not be missed.
- Pus accumulates within the tight sheath giving rise to Kanavel's four cardinal signs:
  - Intense pain on extension of the affected digit (the first and most reliable sign)
  - Flexion of the affected digit (this position allows more space within the sheath-making it more comfortable)
  - Uniform swelling along the digit
  - Percussion tenderness of the flexor tendon.
- Main complication is destruction and rupture of the flexor tendon.
- If recognised within the first 24–48 hours, intravenous antibiotics and elevation of the limb may suffice.
- Most cases require opening of the sheath and irrigation of the sheath to wash out any pus, followed by intravenous antibiotics.
- Commonest causative organism is *Staphylococcus aureus*.
- *Neisseria gonorrhoeae* is a common cause in the absence of trauma.

9.7.6 Midpalmar and thenar space infection

- Infection can convert a potential space into a true space after accumulation of pus.
- There are two potential spaces deep to the flexor tendons, but superficial to the interossei. These are the:
  - Midpalmar space – occurs between the middle, ring and little finger flexor tendons and volar interosseous muscles. Extends from the hypothenar muscles to the midpalmar septum
  - Thenar space – separated from the midpalmar space by the midpalmar septum, and occurs volar to the adductor pollicis muscle over the second and third metacarpal.
- Infection in these two spaces is rare, but may arise following trauma or infectious flexor tenosynovitis. Pain and swelling of the affected region on the palm of the

hand are the first manifestations of infection. This swelling rapidly accumulates in the palm and worsens, causing flexion of the affected digits, which is painful on extension.

- Non-surgical treatment alone is rarely advocated since the penetration of antibiotics into this space is poor. Incision and drainage of the space, followed by intravenous antibiotics is the treatment of choice. Simple measures such as elevation of the hand in a Bradford sling will also help reduce swelling and encourage lymphatic drainage.

9.7.7 Bites

- Can cause cellulitis or an abscess.
- Human bites are more infectious than animal bites.
- Oral commensal bacteria are the infective agents, commonly anaerobes.
- Animal bites, especially dog bites, are associated with other traumatic injuries, eg tendon rupture, fractures. This is due to the more violent nature of the attack.
- Management of bites begins with antibiotic prophylaxis and tetanus cover. The bite should be washed out and explored for the presence of foreign bodies. Devitalised skin edges should be debrided. Care should be taken to manage associated injuries. For animal bites, the wound can be closed primarily if it is clean and healthy. For human bites, delayed closure of the wound is employed due to the risk of infection.

9.8 COSMETIC SURGERY

Cosmetic or aesthetic surgery is a specialised branch of plastic surgery, where a different patient demographic exists. It is important to ascertain patient expectations before an operation, and to make sure that they are psychologically and physically prepared for the planned procedure. This section will briefly discuss different cosmetic operations.

9.8.1 Breast surgery

Augmentation mammoplasty

- Otherwise known as a 'breast enhancement'
- Indicated for unilateral or bilateral small breasts
- Prostheses can be filled with silicone or saline
- Implant either superficial or deep to pectoralis major
- Approaches include inframammary, periareolar, transaxillary or transumbilical
- Complications include:
  - Capsular thickening around the implant, resulting in deformed appearance and discomfort
  - Leakage of implant material

Reduction mammoplasty

- Otherwise known as a 'breast reduction'
- Indicated for symptomatic large breasts causing
  - Back, shoulder or neck ache
  - Kyphosis
  - Cosmetic abnormality
  - Skin irritation or ulceration in the submammary region or under bra straps
  - Gynaecomastia
- Involves removal of breast tissue, with superior transposition of the nipple in women
- Complications include:
  - Disruption of the blood supply, resulting in nipple or flap necrosis

Reconstruction following mastectomy

- Performed either at time of mastectomy or months later
- Implants used if adequate soft tissue is present and pectoralis major preserved
- Flap used following more extensive surgery and can be combined with an implant
- Two most common are:
  - Latissimus dorsi myocutaneous flap
  - Transverse rectus abdominis myocutaneous (TRAM) flap

9.8.2 Rhinoplasty

- Otherwise known as a 'nose job'
- Indications are cosmesis or function (breathing abnormalities)
- Re-formed using controlled nasal and facial fracture with excision of varying amounts of bone, cartilage and skin

9.8.3 Pinnaplasty

- Otherwise known as 'ear pinning'
- Indicated for bat ears, ie where the ears do not lie flat against the head
- Performed by reshaping the cartilage within the ear and, if necessary, pinning the ear closer to the head

9.8.4 Blepharoplasty

- Otherwise known as an 'eye job'
- Performed on either upper or lower eyelids
- Indicated in upper lids where the skin is excessively droopy, causing cosmetic dysfunction or problems from overhang, eg visual impairment, headache
- Indicated in lower lids for puffy skin

9.8.5 Rhytidectomy

- Otherwise known as a 'facelift'
- Indicated to help restore a younger look
- Method:
  - Make incisions above the hairline, in the pre- and post-auricular areas
  - Separate the skin from the fat and muscle below
  - Remove excess fat
  - Tighten underlying muscle
  - Pull the skin back and trim the excess

9.8.6 Abdominoplasty

- Otherwise known as a 'tummy tuck'
- Indicated for removal excess skin or fat on the abdomen, or repair of divarication of the recti
- Different types of abdominoplasty exist depending on whether just skin and fat need removal, whether the umbilicus needs repositioning and whether the divarication of the recti requires repair

9.8.7 Liposuction

- Indicated to contour specific areas of fat accumulation for cosmesis
- Not indicated for weight loss in generalised obesity
- Performed by:
  - Introducing suction cannulae into the subcutaneous deep fat layer
  - Removing fat using a high-suction vacuum attached to the cannulae
- Complications include:
  - Poor cosmetic outcome with contour irregularities following uneven fat removal

9.8.8 Dermal fillers

- Indicated to treat wrinkles
- Performed by injecting filler substance along the line of the wrinkle
- Either biocompatible
  - For example, collagen
  - Limited duration of 6 months
- Or synthetic
  - For example, polyacrylamide gel
  - Permanent effects
  - Higher risk of rejection, migration, granuloma formation, inability to change to the ageing face

9.8.9 Botulinum toxin type A

- Indicated cosmetically to reduce frown lines
- Non-cosmetic indications include axillary hyperhidrosis, cervical dystonia, strabismus
- Acts as a neuromuscular blocking agent

Cardiac surgery

CONTENTS

Cardiac surgery

10.1 INTRODUCTION TO CARDIAC SURGERY

10.1.1 Pre-operative assessment of the cardiac surgical patient

Cardiac surgery, including coronary artery bypass grafting (CABG) and surgery for valvular disease, represents one of the most common classes of surgical procedure performed worldwide. Due to recent developments in catheter-guided techniques, an increasing number of older and sicker patients are being referred for cardiac surgery. In addition, far more patients with depressed left ventricular function, multiple co-morbidities, failed interventional procedures and prior revascularisation operations are now being referred for cardiac surgery. The pre-operative evaluation and risk assessment of patients undergoing cardiac surgery has therefore become even more critical to ensure the safety of cardiac surgical procedures and the achievement of low complication and low mortality rates.

Physical examination

The pre-operative physical examination is an essential aspect of a patient's evaluation for cardiac because since the findings can greatly influence peri-operative management.

Aspects that require special attention include:

- **The patient's risk of endocarditis**
  - Examination of the head, eyes, ears, throat and teeth for infection is helpful in the assessment of an individual's risk of endocarditis in valvular surgery.
  - Inspection of the patient's skin is helpful in detecting and preventing infection (eg the presence of tinea pedis on the lower extremities increases the risk of lower extremity cellulitis).
- **The presence of aortic insufficiency**
  - Regurgitation can worsen during cardiopulmonary bypass and acute left ventricular distension can develop.
- **The presence of vascular disease**
  - Assess the patency of the venous system in the lower extremities, as extensive varicosities may necessitate the use of arm veins or arteries such as bilateral internal mammary arteries or radial artery as conduits.
  - Identify potential contraindications to the use of an intra-aortic balloon pump.
- **The neurological status**
  - Pre-operative identification of any baseline neurological deficits provides an important reference in the event of neurofunctional deterioration post-operatively.

Laboratory investigations

Basic laboratory testing prior to cardiac surgery should include a full blood count, coagulation screen, serum chemistry profile, faecal occult blood, evaluation of ventricular function and assessment of coronary anatomy via cardiac catheterisation (Box 10.1). Any abnormalities detected should be corrected before surgery.

Pre-operative risk estimation

Pre-operative risk assessment has important implications for patient well-being, and is needed to identify peri-operative issues in need of improvement. The major risk factors for adverse outcome during cardiac surgery include advanced age, emergency surgery, history of prior cardiac surgery, dialysis dependency, and creatinine levels of 2 mg/dl or higher.

Contraindications for cardiac surgery

In the presence of irreparable myocardial damage or irreversible end-organ failure (lung, liver, kidneys), correction of cardiac defects may be contraindicated.

Box 10.1: Pre-operative laboratory investigations in cardiac surgical patients

- Full blood count to exclude anaemia and infection
- Coagulation screen to exclude prolonged bleeding time, an elevated prothrombin time (PT) or activated partial thromboplastin time (aPTT) and exclude thrombocytopenia
- Serum biochemistry to exclude renal impairment, abnormal liver function, electrolyte disturbances and nutritional deficiencies
- Faecal occult blood to exclude active bleeding
- Pulmonary function tests and chest X-ray (CXR) to guide post-operative respiratory management
- Echocardiography and electrocardiography (ECG) to assess ventricular function, valvular structure and function and congenital defects
- Coronary angiography (cardiac catheterisation) to assess coronary anatomy, perform haemodynamic measurements and assess status of existing grafts
- Magnetic resonance imaging (MRI), radionuclide scanning and Doppler investigations to assess further cardiac function as needed

---

10.1.2 Cardiopulmonary bypass

Cardiopulmonary bypass (CPB) is a technique that temporarily takes over the function of the heart and lungs during surgery on the heart and/or great vessels. The CPB pump itself is often referred to as a 'heart-lung machine'. CBP pumps are operated by allied health professionals known as perfusionists, in association with surgeons who connect the CPB pump to the patient's body. CPB is a form of extracorporeal circulation.

Uses of cardiopulmonary bypass

CPB is commonly used in heart surgery (Box 10.2) because of the difficulty of operating on the beating heart. Operations requiring opening of the heart's chambers require the use of CPB to support the circulation during that period.

CPB can be used for the induction of total body hypothermia, a state in which the body can be maintained for an hour or more without perfusion (blood flow). If blood flow is stopped at normal body temperature, permanent brain damage normally occurs in 3–4 minutes – death may follow shortly afterwards.

Components of cardiopulmonary bypass

CPB consists of two main functional units: the pump and the oxygenator, which remove oxygen-deprived blood from a patient's body and replace it with oxygen-rich blood through a series of hoses. A CPB circuit consists of a systemic circuit for oxygenating blood and re-infusing blood into a patient's body, and a separate circuit for infusing cardioplegic solution to stop the heart and provide myocardial protection.

Cardioplegia is the intentional and temporary cessation of cardiac activity, primarily for use in cardiac operations. The most common procedure for accomplishing asystole is called cold crystalloid cardioplegia. This process is considered the most successful because it protects the myocardium from damage. In most cases, the patient is first exposed to hypothermia. Then an ice-cold solution of 4°C dextrose with a high concentration of potassium chloride and other ingredients is introduced into the coronary circulation via specialised cannulae.

Box 10.2: Surgeries in which cardiopulmonary bypass is used

- Coronary artery bypass surgery
- Cardiac valve repair and/or replacement (aortic valve, mitral valve, tricuspid valve, pulmonary valve)
- Repair of large septal defects (atrial septal defect, ventricular septal defect, atrioventricular septal defect)
- Repair and/or palliation of congenital heart defects (tetralogy of Fallot, transposition of the great vessels)
- Transplantation (heart transplantation, lung transplantation, heart-lung transplantation)
- Repair of some large aneurysms
- Pulmonary thromboendarterectomy

Complications of cardiopulmonary bypass

CPB is a complex circuit and there are a number of associated problems (Box 10.3).

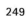

Box 10.3: Adverse effects associated with cardiopulmonary bypass

- Complement and neutrophil activation
- Vasoconstriction, with an increase in capillary permeability, leading to fluid shift into the interstitial compartment; increased risk of microemboli
- Platelet damage and release of vasoactive substances, resulting in increased capillary permeability, leading to further fluid shift into the interstitial compartment; impaired haemostasis
- Haemolysis of red blood cells (RBCs) resulting in jaundice
- Haemodilution, leading to lowered intravascular colloidal oncotic pressure (including pulmonary oedema and interstitial oedema)
- Alteration in fluid balance, urine output and an increase in interstitial renal perfusion volume, an increase or decrease in urine output, and an increase or decrease in intravascular volume
- Coagulopathies caused by inadequate heparin, haemolysis and bleeding reversal, heparin rebound, consumption of clotting factors and platelets, and platelet dysfunction
- Increase in catecholamine release leading to hypertension (which can lead to stress on suture sites and subsequent bleeding)
- Increase in levels of renin, angiotensin, aldosterone and antidiuretic hormone, leading to sodium and water retention
- Serum dilution; intracellular–extracellular fluid shifts, acid–base equilibrium processes; disturbances in electrolytes and cellular transport mechanisms (eg hypokalaemia, hypernatraemia, hyperchloraemia)
- Metabolic disturbances, including alteration in carbohydrate metabolism, suppression of hyperglycaemia, insulin release with concomitant stimulation of glycogenolysis by increase in adrenaline secretion
- Hypothermia due to an increase in systemic vascular resistance because of vasoconstriction; decrease in myocardial contractility and heart rate, resulting in decreased cardiac output and perfusion pressure (including renal perfusion, with subsequent decrease in urine output); hyperglycaemia due to impairment of insulin release by pancreatic islet cells and altered glucose transport across the cell membrane

- Alteration in cardiac function, including decreased cardiac output, cardiac arrhythmias (prolonged cardioplegic arrest of >60 minutes can result in prolonged ischaemic periods with tissue hypoxia, acidosis, subendocardial necrosis, release of myocardial enzymes and compromised cardiac performance)
- Alteration in central nervous system function, including cerebral dysfunction due to embolic (gas, atheromatous debris from aorta, fat) or ischaemic events
- Alteration in pulmonary function, including: pulmonary oedema; adult respiratory distress syndrome (ARDS); atelectasis (alveolar collapse) and retention of secretions; predisposition to microthrombi, which can increase pulmonary shunting, interstitial pulmonary oedema and anoxia
- Alteration in gastrointestinal function due to splanchnic vasoconstriction leading to bowel ischemia; bleeding

10.1.3 Myocardial protection

The term 'myocardial protection' refers to strategies and methodologies used to either attenuate or prevent post-ischaemic myocardial dysfunction, which occurs during and after heart surgery.

Post-ischaemic myocardial dysfunction is partly attributable to a phenomenon known as ischaemia/reperfusion-induced injury.

Clinically, it is manifest by low cardiac output and hypotension, and may be subdivided into two groups: reversible injury and irreversible injury. The two are typically differentiated by the presence of ECG abnormalities, elevations in the levels of specific plasma enzymes or proteins such as creatine kinase and troponin I or T, and/or the presence of regional or global echocardiographic wall motion abnormalities.

Strategies for myocardial protection

The strategies adopted for myocardial protection during cardiac surgery can be broadly classified as:

- **Cardioplegic techniques**
  - These are the commonly used techniques, which enable the cardiac surgeon to operate on a still heart in a bloodless field.
  - Cardioplegic solutions contain a variety of chemical agents that are designed to arrest the heart rapidly in diastole, create a quiescent operating field and provide reliable protection against ischaemia/reperfusion injury.

- **Non–cardioplegic techniques**
  - Intermittent cross-clamping with fibrillation is one of the earliest forms of cardioprotection and is still used in some centres today. This technique allows the surgeon to operate in a relatively quiet field (during ventricular fibrillation) and to avoid the consequences of the profound metabolic changes that occur with more prolonged periods of ischaemia.
  - Systemic hypothermia and elective fibrillatory arrest is an infrequently used technique. With this method, systemic hypothermia (28°C), elective fibrillatory arrest and maintenance of systemic perfusion pressure between 80 mmHg and 100 mmHg are the key elements.

10.1.4 Post-operative complications of cardiac surgery

- Respiratory failure from atelectasis or pulmonary oedema
- Acute tubular necrosis from renal underperfusion
- Jaundice as a result of haemolysis from CPB or multiple transfusions
- CPB-associated complications (Box 10.3)

10.2 ADULT CARDIAC SURGICAL DISORDERS

10.2.1 Ischaemic heart disease

Ischaemic heart disease or coronary artery disease (CAD) involves impairment of blood flow through the coronary arteries, most commonly due to atheroma. The atheromas are deposited below the intima in large and medium-sized coronary arteries. Less often, CAD is due to coronary spasm. Rare causes include coronary artery embolism, dissection, aneurysm (eg in Kawasaki disease), and vasculitis (eg in systemic lupus erythematosus, syphilis). Acute coronary syndromes (ACS) usually occur when an acute thrombus forms in an atherosclerotic coronary artery. CAD is the leading cause of death in developed countries. The incidence is rising in Central Europe and in Eastern Europe, but it is low in Japan. Epidemiological studies of differences between countries and regions have revealed dietary and environmental factors that contribute to disease (eg saturated fat, cholesterol, abdominal obesity, smoking, exposure to second-hand smoke) and also factors that protect against it (eg fish oils, vitamin C and other antioxidants, red wine or grape juice, anti-inflammatory agents).

Clinical presentation

Clinical presentations include silent ischaemia, angina pectoris, acute coronary syndromes [unstable angina, myocardial infarction (MI)] and sudden cardiac death.

- Classical presentation is with angina, which may be a vague, barely troublesome ache or may rapidly become a severe, intense precordial crushing sensation. It is rarely described as pain.
- Discomfort is most commonly felt beneath the sternum, although location varies. Discomfort may radiate to the left shoulder and down the inside of the left arm, even to the fingers; straight through to the back; into the throat, jaws and teeth; and, occasionally, down the inside of the right arm. It may also be felt in the upper abdomen.
- Some patients have atypical angina (eg bloating, gas, abdominal distress), often ascribing symptoms to indigestion; belching may even seem to relieve the symptoms.
- Between and even during attacks of angina, physical findings may be normal.
- During the attack, heart rate may increase modestly; blood pressure is often elevated; heart sounds become more distant; and the apical impulse is more diffuse.
- Palpation of the precordium may reveal localised systolic bulging or paradoxical movement, reflecting segmental myocardial ischaemia and regional dyskinesia.
- The second heart sound can become paradoxical because left ventricular ejection is more prolonged during an ischaemic attack.
- A fourth heart sound is common.
- A mid- or late systolic apical murmur – shrill but not especially loud – may occur if ischaemia causes localised papillary muscle dysfunction, producing mitral regurgitation.

Diagnosis

The diagnosis is suspected if chest discomfort is typical and is precipitated by exertion and relieved by rest. Patients whose chest discomfort lasts >20 minutes or occurs during rest or who have syncope or heart failure are evaluated for an acute coronary syndrome. Several other clinical conditions can cause chest discomfort and must be considered in the differential diagnosis (Box 10.4).

- If typical exertional symptoms are present, **ECG** is indicated. Because angina resolves quickly with rest, an ECG can rarely be done during an attack except during stress testing. If done during an attack, an ECG is likely to show reversible ischaemic changes: ST-segment depression (typically), ST-segment elevation, decreased R-wave height, intraventricular or bundle branch conduction disturbances and arrhythmia (usually ventricular extrasystoles).
- If a patient has a normal resting ECG and can exercise, **exercise stress testing with ECG** is done.
- **Coronary angiography** is the gold standard for diagnosing CAD but is not always necessary to confirm the diagnosis.

It is indicated primarily to locate and assess the severity of coronary artery lesions when revascularisation [percutaneous coronary intervention (PCI) or CABG surgery] is being considered. Angiography may also be indicated when knowledge of coronary anatomy is necessary to advise about work or lifestyle needs (eg discontinuing job or sports activities). Obstruction is assumed to be physiologically significant when the luminal diameter is reduced >70%.

Box 10.4: Differential diagnosis of ischaemic heart disease

- Anxiety
- Aortic dissection
- Aortic stenosis
- Arteritis
- Cardiomyopathy
- Congestive heart failure
- Constrictive pericarditis
- Costochondritis
- Gastro-oesophageal reflux
- Gastric ulcer
- Mitral valve prolapse
- Oesophageal spasm
- Oesophageal tear

Treatment

The treatment for CAD involves modification of risk factors, drugs and PCI and CABG surgery.

Modification of risk factors
- Reversible risk factors are modified as much as possible.
- Smokers should stop smoking; ≥2 years after stopping smoking, the risk of MI is reduced to that of people who never smoked.
- Hypertension is treated diligently because even mild hypertension increases cardiac workload.
- Weight loss alone often reduces the severity of angina.
- Sometimes, treatment of mild left ventricular failure markedly lessens angina.
- Aggressive reduction of total and low-density lipoprotein (LDL) cholesterol (via diet plus drugs as necessary) slows the progression of CAD, may cause some lesions to regress and improves endothelial function and thus arterial response to stress.
- An exercise programme emphasising walking often improves the sense of well-being, reduces CAD risk and improves exercise tolerance.

Drugs
The main aims of drug therapy in CAD are to relieve acute symptoms and prevent or reduce ischaemia. For an acute attack, sublingual glyceryl trinitrate is the most effective drug. To prevent ischaemia, all patients diagnosed with CAD or at high risk of developing CAD should take an antiplatelet drug daily. Beta-blockers, unless contraindicated or not tolerated, are given to most patients. For some patients, prevention requires calcium-channel blockers or long-acting nitrates.

Percutaneous coronary intervention
- PCI (eg angioplasty, stenting) should be considered if angina persists despite drug therapy and worsens quality of life, or if anatomical lesions (noted during angiography) put a patient at high risk of mortality.
- The choice between PCI and CABG surgery depends on the extent and location of the anatomical lesions, the experience of the surgeon and medical centre, and, to some extent, patient preference.
- PCI is usually preferred for one- or two-vessel disease with suitable anatomical lesions.
- Lesions that are long or near bifurcation points are often not amenable to PCI.
- Most PCI these days is done with stenting rather than balloon angioplasty alone, and as stent technology improves, PCI is being used for more complicated cases.
- The risk of PCI is comparable to that of CABG.
- Mortality rate is 1%–3%; MI rate is 3%–5%.
- In <3%, intimal dissection causes obstruction requiring emergency CABG.
- After stenting, aspirin is supplemented with clopidogrel for at least 1 month, but preferably 6–12 months, and a statin is added if not already being used.
- About 5%–15% of stents re-occlude in a few days or weeks, requiring placement of a new stent inside the original, or CABG. Occasionally, occluded stents are asymptomatic.
- Recently, drug-eluting stents have been used to treat CAD. These stents release antimitotic agents slowly and are thought to prevent stent restenosis.
- Angiography 1 year later shows an apparently normal lumen in about 30% of affected vessels.
- Patients may quickly return to work and usual activities, but strenuous activities should be avoided for 6 weeks.

Coronary artery bypass graft surgery
- CABG surgery (heart bypass or bypass surgery) is a surgical procedure performed to relieve angina and reduce the risk of death from CAD (Box 10.5).
- CABG uses sections of autologous veins (eg saphenous) or, preferably, arteries to bypass diseased segments. Most

patients will have at least the internal mammary artery as the arterial graft to the left anterior descending artery.

- At 1 year, about 85% of venous bypass grafts are patent, but after 10 years, as many as 97% of internal mammary artery grafts are patent. Arteries also hypertrophy to accommodate increased flow.
- CABG is preferred for patients with left main artery disease, three-vessel disease, diffuse CAD, poor left ventricular function, or diabetes mellitus.
- The terms **single bypass, double bypass, triple bypass, quadruple bypass** and **quintuple bypass** refer to the number of coronary arteries bypassed in the procedure. In other words, a double bypass means two coronary arteries are bypassed (eg the left anterior descending coronary artery and right coronary artery).
- CABG is typically performed using cardiopulmonary bypass with the heart stopped.
- For patients with a normal-sized heart, no history of MI, good ventricular function, and no additional risk factors, the risk is <5% for peri-operative MI, 2%–3% for stroke, and ≤1% for mortality.
- Risk increases with age and the presence of underlying disease. The operative mortality rate is 3–5 times higher for a second bypass than for the first; thus, the timing of the first bypass should be optimal.
- Alternative methods of minimally invasive coronary artery bypass surgery have been developed recently. Off-pump coronary artery bypass surgery (OPCAB) is a technique for performing bypass surgery without the use of cardiopulmonary bypass.
- Further refinements to OPCAB have resulted in minimally invasive direct coronary artery bypass (MIDCAB) surgery, which is a technique of performing bypass surgery through a 5–10-cm incision.

Prognosis

- The prognosis worsens with increasing age, increasingly severe anginal symptoms, presence of anatomical lesions and poor ventricular function.
- Lesions in the left main coronary artery or proximal LAD indicate particularly high risk.
- Although the prognosis correlates with the severity and number of coronary arteries affected, prognosis is surprisingly good for patients with stable angina, even those with three-vessel disease, if ventricular function is normal.

Box 10.5: CABG procedure

- The patient is brought to the operating room and moved onto the operating table
- An anaesthetist places a variety of intravenous lines and injects an induction agent (usually propofol) to render the person unconscious
- A double-lumen endotracheal tube is inserted and secured by the anaesthetist and mechanical ventilation is started
- The chest is opened via a median sternotomy and the heart is examined by the surgeon
- The grafts are harvested – common conduits are the internal mammary artery or bilateral arteries, radial arteries and segments of long saphenous vein
- The surgeon stops the heart and initiates cardiopulmonary bypass; or, in the case of 'off-pump' surgery, places devices to stabilise the heart
- One end of each graft is sewn onto the coronary arteries beyond the blockages and the other end is attached to the aorta
- The heart is restarted; or, in 'off-pump' surgery, the stabilising devices are removed
- The sternum is wired together and the incisions are sutured
- The person is moved to the intensive therapy unit (ITU) to recover
- After awakening and stabilising in the ITU (approximately 1 day), the person is transferred to the cardiac surgery ward until they are ready to go home (approximately 5–7 days)

10.2.2 Valvular heart disease

Any heart valve can become stenotic or insufficient causing haemodynamic changes long before symptoms. Most often, valvular stenosis or insufficiency occurs in isolation in individual valves, but multiple valvular disorders may co-exist.

Aortic stenosis

- Aortic stenosis (AS) is narrowing of the aortic valve, obstructing blood flow from the left ventricle to the ascending aorta during systole
- Causes include
  - Congenital bicuspid valve
  - Idiopathic degenerative sclerosis with calcification
  - Rheumatic fever
- Progressive untreated AS ultimately results in one or more of the classic triad of syncope, angina and exertional dyspnoea; heart failure and arrhythmias may develop

- A carotid pulse with small amplitude and delayed upstroke and a crescendo–decrescendo ejection murmur are characteristic (slow-rising)
- Diagnosis is by physical examination and echocardiography. Asymptomatic AS often requires no treatment
- For progressive severe or symptomatic AS in children, balloon valvotomy is used; adults require valve replacement

Aortic regurgitation

- Aortic regurgitation is incompetency of the aortic valve causing flow from the aorta into the left ventricle during diastole
- Causes include
  - Idiopathic valvular degeneration
  - Rheumatic fever, endocarditis
  - Myxomatous degeneration
  - Congenital bicuspid aortic valve
  - Aortic root dilatation or dissection
  - Connective tissue or rheumatological disorders (Marfan's syndrome)
- Symptoms include exertional dyspnoea, orthopnoea, paroxysmal nocturnal dyspnoea, palpitations and chest pain
- Signs include widened pulse pressure (water-hammer pulse) and an early diastolic murmur
- Diagnosis is by physical examination and echocardiography
- Surgical treatment is aortic valve replacement

Mitral stenosis

- Mitral stenosis is narrowing of the mitral orifice, impeding blood flow from the left atrium to the left ventricle
- The (almost) invariable cause is rheumatic fever
- Common complications are pulmonary hypertension, atrial fibrillation and thromboembolism
- Symptoms are those of heart failure; signs include an opening snap and a mid-diastolic murmur
- A presystolic crescendo murmur may also be present in patients without atrial fibrillation
- Diagnosis is by physical examination and echocardiography
- Prognosis is good
- Medical treatment includes diuretics, β-blockers or rate-limiting calcium-channel blockers and anticoagulants
- Effective treatment for more severe disease consists of balloon valvotomy, surgical commissurotomy, or valve replacement

Mitral regurgitation

- Mitral regurgitation (MR) is incompetency of the mitral valve, causing flow from the left ventricle (LV) into the left atrium during systole
- Common causes include
  - Mitral valve prolapse
  - Ischaemic papillary muscle dysfunction
  - Rheumatic fever
  - Annular dilatation secondary to LV systolic dysfunction and dilatation
- Complications include progressive heart failure, arrhythmias and endocarditis
- Symptoms and signs include palpitations, dyspnoea and a holosystolic apical murmur
- Diagnosis is by physical examination and echocardiography
- Prognosis depends on LV function and severity and duration of MR
- Patients with mild, asymptomatic MR may be monitored, but progressive or symptomatic MR requires mitral valve repair or replacement

Pulmonary stenosis

- Pulmonary stenosis is narrowing of the pulmonary outflow tract causing obstruction of blood flow from the right ventricle to the pulmonary artery during systole
- Most cases are congenital; many remain asymptomatic until adulthood
- Signs include a systolic crescendo–decrescendo ejection murmur
- Diagnosis is by echocardiography
- Symptomatic patients and those with large gradients require balloon valvuloplasty

Pulmonary regurgitation

- Pulmonary regurgitation (PR) is incompetency of the pulmonary valve causing blood flow from the pulmonary artery into the right ventricle during diastole
- The most common cause is pulmonary hypertension
- PR is usually asymptomatic
- Signs include a decrescendo diastolic murmur
- Diagnosis is by echocardiography
- Usually, no specific treatment is necessary except for management of conditions causing pulmonary hypertension

Tricuspid stenosis

- Tricuspid stenosis (TS) is narrowing of the tricuspid orifice that obstructs blood flow from the right atrium to the right ventricle
- Almost all cases result from rheumatic fever

- Symptoms include a fluttering discomfort in the neck, fatigue, cold skin and right upper quadrant abdominal discomfort
- Jugular pulsations are prominent, and a presystolic murmur is often heard at the left sternal edge in the fourth intercostal space and is increased during inspiration
- Diagnosis is by echocardiography
- TS is usually benign, requiring no specific treatment, but symptomatic patients may benefit from surgery

Tricuspid regurgitation

- Tricuspid regurgitation (TR) is insufficiency of the tricuspid valve causing blood flow from the right ventricle to the right atrium during systole
- The most common cause is dilatation of the right ventricle
- Symptoms and signs are usually absent, but severe TR can cause neck pulsations, a holosystolic murmur, and right ventricular-induced heart failure or atrial fibrillation. A pulsatile liver may also be palpable
- Diagnosis is by physical examination and echocardiography
- TR is usually benign and does not require treatment, but some patients require annuloplasty or valve repair or replacement

Essential note

Holo- or pansystolic murmurs may be caused by mitral regurgitation, tricuspid regurgitation, or by a ventricular septal defect (VSD). The key features to distinguish one from another is whether the murmur radiates to the axilla (MR), whether there are jugular venous pressure (JVP) signs with a pulsatile liver (TR), or neither, which may indicate a VSD

Essential note

Right-sided heart problems always result in JVP signs; left-sided heart problems usually do not

Choice of prosthetic valve for valve replacement

- Traditionally, a mechanical valve has been used in patients <65 years and in older patients with a long life expectancy, because bioprosthetic valves deteriorate over 10–12 years.
- Patients with a mechanical valve require lifelong anticoagulation to an INR of 2.5–3.5 (to prevent thromboembolism) and antibiotics before some medical or dental procedures (to prevent endocarditis).

- A bioprosthetic valve, which does not require anticoagulation beyond the immediate post-operative period, has been used in patients >65 years, in younger patients with a life expectancy <10 years, and in those with some right-sided lesions.
- However, newer bioprosthetic valves may be more durable than first-generation valves; thus, patient preference regarding valve type can now be considered.
- Women of childbearing age who require valve replacement and plan to become pregnant must balance the increased risk of teratogenicity from warfarin use required with mechanical valves against that of accelerated valve deterioration with bioprosthetic valves.
- These risks can be reduced by using heparin instead of warfarin in the first 12 weeks and last 2 weeks of the pregnancy, but management is difficult and careful discussion is required before surgery.
- Endocarditis prophylaxis is also indicated for nearly all patients with valvular heart disorders who have had valve replacement.

10.2.3 Aortic vascular disease

The aorta originates at the left ventricle above the aortic valve (aortic root), travels upwards (ascending thoracic aorta) to the first large-vessel branch of the aorta (brachiocephalic or innominate artery), arches up and behind the heart (aortic arch), and then turns downwards distal to the left subclavian artery (descending aorta) through the thorax (thoracic aorta) and abdomen (abdominal aorta). The abdominal aorta ends by dividing into the two common iliac arteries. Important conditions of the (thoracic) aorta of relevance to cardiothoracic surgeons include:

- Aortic dissection
- Aortic aneurysm

Aortic dissection

Aortic dissection is the most common catastrophe of the aorta, 2–3 times more common than rupture of the abdominal aorta. When left untreated, about 33% of patients die within the first 24 hours, and 50% die within 48 hours. The 2-week mortality rate approaches 75% in patients with undiagnosed ascending aortic dissection.

Aetiology

Aortic dissection is more common in patients with hypertension, connective tissue disorders, congenital aortic stenosis or bicuspid aortic valve, and in those with first-degree relatives with a history of thoracic dissections. These diseases affect the media of the aorta and predispose it to dissection.

Cardiac surgery

Classification

- Dissections of the thoracic aorta have been classified anatomically by two different methods
- The more commonly used system is the Stanford classification, which is based on involvement of the ascending aorta
- The **Stanford classification** divides dissections into two types, type A and type B. Type A involves the ascending aorta; type B does not. This system also helps delineate treatment. Usually, type A dissections require surgery, while type B dissections may be managed medically under most conditions

Clinical presentation

- Chest pain is the most common presenting symptom (Box 10.6) in patients with an aortic dissection
- Consider thoracic aortic dissection in the differential diagnosis of all patients presenting with chest pain
- The pain usually is described as ripping or tearing and often occurs between the shoulder blades
- Blood pressure may increase or decrease
- Hypertension may result from a catecholamine surge or underlying essential hypertension
- Hypotension is an ominous finding and may be the result of excessive vagal tone, cardiac tamponade, or hypovolaemia from rupture of the dissection
- A blood pressure differential of more than 20 mmHg in both arms is an independent predictor of aortic dissection and should increase the suspicion of aortic dissection
- Significant inter-arm blood pressure differentials are found in 20% of people without aortic dissection
- Neurological deficits are a presenting sign in up to 20% of cases. The most common neurological findings are syncope and altered mental status
- Syncope is part of the early course of aortic dissection in about 5% of patients and may be the result of increased vagal tone, hypovolaemia, or dysrhythmia
- Other causes of syncope or altered mental status include strokes from compromised blood flow to the brain or spinal cord and ischaemia from interruption of blood flow to the spinal arteries
- Peripheral nerve ischaemia can manifest with numbness and tingling in the extremities
- Hoarseness from recurrent laryngeal nerve compression also has been described
- Horner's syndrome is caused by interruption in the cervical sympathetic ganglia and presents with ptosis, miosis and anhidrosis
- Superior vena cava syndrome, caused by compression of the superior vena cava from a large distorted aorta, may occur

- Dyspnoea may be caused by congestive heart failure or tracheal or bronchial compression
- Dysphagia from compression of the oesophagus may be present
- Findings suggestive of cardiac tamponade, such as muffled heart sounds, hypotension, pulsus paradoxus, jugular venous distension, and Kussmaul sign, must be recognised quickly
- Other diagnostic clues include a new diastolic murmur, asymmetrical pulses and asymmetrical blood pressure measurements
- Pay careful attention to carotid, brachial and femoral pulses on initial examination and look for progression of bruits or development of bruits on re-examination
- Physical findings of a haemothorax may be found if the dissection ruptures into the pleura

Essential note

Consider any patient presenting with severe (10/10) and sudden-onset chest pain radiating between the shoulder blades to have an aortic dissection until proved otherwise

Diagnosis

- Aortic dissection must be considered in any patient with chest pain, thoracic back pain, unexplained syncope or abdominal pain, stroke, or acute-onset heart failure, especially when pulses or blood pressure in the limbs are unequal
- Such patients require a chest X-ray; in 60%–90%, the mediastinal shadow is widened, usually with a localised bulge signifying the site of origin. Left pleural effusion is common
- If chest X-ray suggests dissection, transoesophageal echocardiography (TOE), CT angiography (CTA), or magnetic resonance angiography (MRA) is done immediately after the patient is stabilised. Findings of an intimal flap and double lumina confirm dissection
- If TOE is unavailable, CTA is recommended; it has a positive predictive value of 100%
- MRA has nearly 100% sensitivity and specificity for aortic dissection, but it is time-consuming and ill-suited for emergencies. It is probably best used for stable patients with subacute or chronic chest pain when dissection is suspected
- Contrast aortography is an option if surgery is being considered. In addition to identifying the origin and extent of dissection, the severity of aortic regurgitation, and the

extent of involvement of the aorta's major branches, aortography helps determine whether simultaneous CABG surgery is needed

- Echocardiography should also be done to check for aortic regurgitation and so determine whether the aortic valve should be repaired or replaced concomitantly

Treatment

- Patients who do not immediately die of aortic dissection should be admitted to an ITU with intra-arterial BP monitoring; an indwelling urethral catheter is used to monitor urine output
- Blood should be typed and cross-matched for 4–6 units of packed RBCs when surgery is likely
- Haemodynamically unstable patients should be intubated
- Aggressive management of heart rate and blood pressure should be initiated
- Beta-blockers should be given initially to reduce the rate of change of blood pressure and the shear forces on the aortic wall
- The target heart rate should be 60–80 beats per minute
- The target systolic blood pressure should be 100–120 mmHg
- A trial of drug therapy alone is appropriate for uncomplicated, stable dissection confined to the descending aorta (type B) and for stable, isolated dissection of the aortic arch
- Urgent surgical intervention is required in type A dissections (Box 10.7)
- The area of the aorta with the intimal tear is usually resected and replaced with a Dacron graft. The operative mortality rate is usually less than 10%, and serious complications are rare with ascending aortic dissections
- All patients, including those treated surgically, are given long-term antihypertensive drug therapy, usually including β-blockers, calcium-channel blockers and angiotensin-converting enzyme (ACE) inhibitors
- Stent grafts that seal entry to the false lumen and improve patency of the true lumen, balloon fenestration (in which an opening is made in the dissection flap that separates the true and false lumina), or both may be non-invasive alternatives

Box 10.6: Symptoms in aortic dissection

- Anterior chest pain – ascending aortic dissection
- Neck or jaw pain – aortic arch dissection
- Interscapular tearing or ripping pain – descending aortic dissection
- Chest pain
- Myocardial infarction
- Neurological symptoms
- Syncope
- Stroke symptoms
- Altered mental status
- Limb paraesthesiae, pain, or weakness
- Hemiparesis or hemiplegia
- Horner's syndrome
- Dyspnoea
- Dysphagia
- Orthopnoea
- Anxiety and premonitions of death
- Flank pain if renal artery is involved
- Dyspnoea and haemoptysis if dissection ruptures into the pleura

Box 10.7: Indications for surgery in aortic dissection

- Involvement of proximal aorta
- Limb or visceral ischaemia
- Uncontrolled hypertension
- Continued aortic enlargement
- Extension of the dissection
- Evidence of aortic rupture (regardless of dissection type)
- Acute distal dissections in patients with Marfan's syndrome

Essential note

Blood pressure control with resuscitation and close monitoring are key to managing aortic dissections before surgery

Aortic aneurysm

Thoracic aortic aneurysms (TAAs) account for a quarter of aortic aneurysms. Men and women are affected equally. About 40% of TAAs occur in the ascending thoracic aorta (between the aortic valve and brachiocephalic, or innominate, artery); 10% occur in the aortic arch (including the brachiocephalic, carotid and subclavian arteries); 35% occur in the descending thoracic aorta (distal to the left subclavian artery); and 15% occur in the upper abdomen (as thoracoabdominal aneurysms).

Aetiology

- Most TAAs result from atherosclerosis
- Risk factors for both include prolonged hypertension, dyslipidaemia and smoking
- Additional risk factors for TAAs include the presence of aneurysms elsewhere and older age (peak incidence at age 65–70)

Clinical features

- Most TAAs are asymptomatic until complications (eg aortic regurgitation, dissection) develop
- Compression of adjacent structures can cause chest or back pain, cough, wheezing, dysphagia, hoarseness (due to left recurrent laryngeal or vagus nerve compression), chest pain (due to coronary artery compression) and superior vena cava syndrome
- Erosion of aneurysms into the lungs causes haemoptysis or pneumonitis
- Thromboembolism may cause stroke, abdominal pain (due to mesenteric embolism), or extremity pain
- Patients who do not immediately die of a ruptured TAA present with severe chest or back pain, hypotension, or shock; exsanguination most commonly occurs into the pleural or pericardial space
- When erosion into the oesophagus (aorto-oesophageal fistula) precedes rupture, patients may present with massive haematemesis
- Additional signs include Horner's syndrome due to compression of sympathetic ganglia, palpable downward pull of the trachea with each cardiac contraction (tracheal tug) and tracheal deviation
- Visible or palpable chest wall pulsations, occasionally more prominent than the left ventricular apical impulse, are unusual but can occur
- Syphilitic aneurysms of the aortic root classically lead to aortic regurgitation and inflammatory stenosis of the coronary artery ostia, which may manifest as chest pain due to myocardial ischaemia. Syphilitic aneurysms do not dissect

Diagnosis

- TAAs are usually first suspected when a chest X-ray incidentally shows a widened mediastinum or enlargement of the aortic knob
- CTA can delineate aneurysm size and proximal or distant extent, detect leakage and identify coincident pathology; MRA may provide similar detail
- TOE can delineate the size and extent and detect leakage of aneurysms of the ascending but not the descending aorta. TOE is especially useful for detecting aortic dissection

- Contrast angiography provides the best image of the arterial lumen but no information on extraluminal structures; it is invasive and has a significant risk of renal and extremity atheroembolism and contrast nephropathy
- Choice of imaging test is based on availability and local experience. However, if rupture is suspected, TOE or CTA, depending on availability, is done immediately
- Aortic root dilatation or unexplained ascending aorta aneurysms warrant serological testing for syphilis
- If a mycotic aneurysm is suspected, bacterial and fungal blood cultures are obtained

Treatment

- Survival rate of patients with untreated large TAAs is 65% at 1 year and 20% at 5 years
- Treatment is surgical repair and control of hypertension if present
- Recently, stent grafts have also been used for management of aneurysms in high-risk surgical candidates

10.3 CONGENITAL CARDIAC SURGICAL DISORDERS

Congenital heart disease (CHD) is malformation of the heart or the large blood vessels near the heart. CHD is the most frequent form of major birth defect in newborns, affecting close to 1% of newborn babies (8 per 1000). This figure is an underestimate because it does not include some common problems, namely:

- Patent ductus arteriosus in preterm babies (a temporary condition)
- Bicuspid (two cusps) aortic valve (the aortic valve usually has three cusps)
- Mitral valve prolapse
- Peripheral pulmonary stenosis (narrowing of the lung vessels well away from the heart)

10.3.1 Classification of congenital cardiac disorders

Congenital cardiac disorders are most easily classified into cyanotic and non-cyanotic forms. They can also be more broadly classified on the basis of morphology of defect as follows.

Detour defects within the heart

Defects may cause blood to take an abnormal route through the heart, passing directly between the right and left sides of the heart. This occurs when there is a defect in the septum that normally separates the right and left sides of the heart. The two most common types of septal defect are:

- Atrial septal defect (ASD)
- Ventricular septal defect (VSD)

Less common types of CHD with altered routes of blood flow include:

- Eisenmenger's complex
- Atrioventricular canal defect (also called an endocardial cushion defect)

Detour defect outside the heart

Patent ductus arteriosus (PDA) is a special type of a blood routing problem located outside the heart. The ductus arteriosus is a prenatal shunt between the pulmonary artery and the aorta that remains open (patent) after birth, letting blood that should flow through the aorta to the body return to the lungs.

Obstructive defects

A number of types of CHD obstruct blood flow within the heart or the great vessels near it. They do so via a narrowing that partly or completely blocks the flow of blood. The narrowing (a stenosis) can occur in heart valves, arteries or veins. The three most common forms of CHD with obstructed blood flow are:

- Pulmonary (valvular) stenosis
- Aortic stenosis
- Coarctation of the aorta

Less common forms of CHD with obstructed blood flow include:

- Bicuspid aortic valve
- Subaortic stenosis
- Ebstein's anomaly

Cyanotic defects

Some types of CHD cause cyanosis. The blood pumped to the body has less than normal amounts of oxygen. This results in cyanosis, a bluish discoloration of the skin. Typical cyanotic forms of CHD include:

- Tetralogy of Fallot
- Transposition of the great arteries
- Tricuspid atresia
- Truncus arteriosus
- Total anomalous pulmonary venous return
- Pulmonary atresia

Hypoplastic heart defects

Part of the heart may be selectively underdeveloped or hypoplastic, as in:

- Right heart hypoplasia
- Left heart hypoplasia

Other developmental heart defects

A number of other defects in heart development can occur, such as:

- Single ventricle
- Double outlet right ventricle (both the aorta and pulmonary artery emanate from the right ventricle)

10.3.2 Aetiology of congenital cardiac disorders

- The cause of most congenital heart defects is unknown.
- Where a cause is known, it may be of a multifactorial origin and/or a result of genetic predisposition and environmental factors.
- Known genetic causes of heart disease include chromosomal abnormalities such as trisomies 21, 13 and 18, as well as a range of newly recognised genetic point mutations, point deletions and other genetic abnormalities as seen in syndromes such as CATCH 22 (cardiac defects, abnormal facial features, thymic hypoplasia, cleft palate, hypocalcaemia), familial ASD with heart block, Alagille syndrome, Noonan syndrome and many more.
- Known antenatal environmental factors include maternal infections (rubella), drugs (alcohol, warfarin, phenytoin, lithium and thalidomide) and maternal illness (diabetes mellitus, phenylketonuria and systemic lupus erythematosus).

10.3.3 Diagnosis of congenital cardiac disorders

Congenital cardiac disorders may be diagnosed before birth, after birth or in adulthood.

Antenatal diagnosis

- Before birth, an obstetric ultrasound scan may be used to screen pregnant women for signs of CHD in their unborn babies.
- This screening scan is often performed around 20 weeks of pregnancy when the fast moving structures of the fetal heart are large enough to be more easily imaged.
- If CHD is suspected, a mother will be referred for a fetal echocardiograph, which is a more detailed, diagnostic ultrasound scan by a specialist cardiologist.
- It is increasingly possible for specialists to screen for CHD as early as 14 weeks, if CHD is suspected from other factors such as a family history.

Post-natal diagnosis

- After delivery, if CHD is present but has not been detected, then a newborn baby may appear blue or breathless.

- Signs of CHD are sometimes mistaken for an infection or illness, so it is important to rule this out.
- Blueness and/or breathlessness may take some time to present, depending on the type of CHD and whether there is a duct-dependent lesion (ie one relying on an open ductus arteriosus for blood flow).
- This duct usually closes within the first 3 days of life in babies born at term (ie at 9 months' gestation).

Diagnosis in adulthood
- Although the majority of CHD diagnoses are made in childhood, there are significant congenital heart defects which may go undetected until adulthood.
- These typically include defects that do not cause cyanosis in childhood but may cause problems over time, such as certain kinds of valve problems, transposition disorders, septal defects and abnormalities of the heart's major veins and arteries.
- Congenital heart defects are most commonly diagnosed through an echocardiogram – an ultrasound of the heart which shows the heart's structure.
- A chest X-ray may also be used to look at the anatomical position of the heart and lungs.
- Cardiac MRI is used to confirm CHD when signs or symptoms occur in the physical examination and the defect is a complex one in which the anatomy is hard to determine with echocardiography.
- A CT scan can also be used to visualise CHD.

10.3.4 Clinical features of congenital cardiac disorders
Clinical features are related to the type and severity of the heart defects. Some children have no signs while others may exhibit shortness of breath, cyanosis, chest pain, syncope, sweating, heart murmur, respiratory infections, underdevelopment of limbs and muscles, poor feeding, or poor growth. Most defects cause a murmur, as blood moves through the heart causing some of these symptoms.

10.3.5 Treatment of congenital cardiac disorders
Sometimes congenital cardiac disorders improve, with no treatment necessary. At other times the defect is so small that it does not require any treatment. Most of the time CHD is serious and requires surgery and/or medications. Medications include diuretics and digoxin, which improve features of cardiac failure by removing excess fluid and improving cardiac contractility respectively. Digoxin also has antiarrhythmic properties. Some defects require surgical procedures to repair as much as possible in order to restore circulation back to

normal. In some cases, multiple operations are needed to help balance the circulation. Interventional cardiology now offers patients minimally invasive alternatives to surgery. Septal defects can now be closed with devices with a standard transcatheter procedure using a closure device mounted on a balloon catheter.

10.3.6 Common congenital cardiac surgical disorders
Eight defects (listed below) are more common than all others and make up 80% of all CHDs, whereas the remaining 20% consist of many independently infrequent conditions or combinations of several defects. Ventricular septal defect (VSD) is generally considered to be the most common type of malformation, accounting for about one-third of all congenital heart defects.

- Atrial septal defect
- Ventricular septal defect
- Patent ductus arteriosus
- Coarctation of the aorta
- Tetralogy of Fallot
- Transposition of the great arteries
- Atrioventricular septal defect
- Hypoplastic left heart syndrome

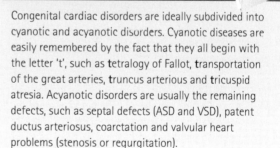

Essential note
Congenital cardiac disorders are ideally subdivided into cyanotic and acyanotic disorders. Cyanotic diseases are easily remembered by the fact that they all begin with the letter 't', such as **t**etralogy of Fallot, **t**ransportation of the great arteries, **t**runcus arterious and **t**ricuspid atresia. Acyanotic disorders are usually the remaining defects, such as septal defects (ASD and VSD), patent ductus arteriosus, coarctation and valvular heart problems (stenosis or regurgitation).

Atrial septal defect
- Atrial septal defects (ASDs) account for about 6%–10% of all cases of CHD. ASDs can be classified by location: **ostium secundum** (defect in the fossa ovalis – in the centre or middle part of the atrial septum), **sinus venosus** (defect in the posterior aspect of the septum, near the superior vena cava or inferior vena cava), or **ostium primum** [defect in the anteroinferior aspect of the septum, a form of endocardial cushion defect (atrioventricular septal defect)]
- Most small ASDs are asymptomatic

- They cause a left-to-right shunt due to higher pressures on the left side
- Larger shunts can cause exercise intolerance, dyspnoea during exertion, fatigue and atrial arrhythmias, sometimes with palpitations
- Passage of microemboli from the venous circulation across the ASD (paradoxical embolisation), often associated with arrhythmias, may lead to cerebral or systemic thromboembolic disorders
- Rarely, when an ASD is undiagnosed or untreated, Eisenmenger's syndrome develops and the result is a right-to-left shunt with higher pressures on the right side
- A soft midsystolic murmur at the upper left sternal border is common
- Diagnosis is by echocardiography
- Most small ostium secundum ASDs (<3 mm) close spontaneously; about 80% of those between 3 mm and 8 mm close spontaneously by age 18 months. However, ostium primum and sinus venosus ASDs do not close spontaneously
- Treatment is surgical or catheter-based repair
- Patients with moderate to large defects (eg pulmonary to systemic flow ratio >1.5:1) should have the ASD closed, typically between the ages of 2 and 6 years

Ventricular septal defect

- Ventricular septal defect (VSD) can occur alone or with other congenital anomalies (eg tetralogy of Fallot, complete atrioventricular septal defects, transposition of the great arteries)
- VSDs are classified by location: **membranous** (perimembranous), **trabecular muscular**, **outlet** (supracristal or subpulmonary), or **inlet** defects
- Membranous defects (70%-80%) involve varying amounts of muscular tissue adjacent to the membranous septum (thus called perimembranous defects); the most common type occurs immediately below the aortic valve
- Large defects result in a significant left-to-right shunt and produce dyspnoea with feeding and poor growth
- A loud, harsh, pansystolic murmur at the lower left sternal border is common
- Smaller VSDs cause louder murmurs and vice versa
- Recurrent respiratory infections and heart failure may develop
- Diagnosis is by echocardiography
- Small VSDs, particularly muscular septal defects, often close spontaneously during the first few years of life
- A small defect that remains open does not require medical or surgical therapy
- Moderate-sized defects are less likely to close spontaneously

- Diuretics, digoxin and ACE inhibitors are indicated before surgery if heart failure develops
- If infants do not respond to medical treatment or have large shunts (with pulmonary to systemic flow ratio ≥2:1), surgical repair may be done during the first few months of life
- Current surgical mortality rate is 2%-5%
- Surgical complications include residual ventricular shunt, right bundle branch block, complete heart block and ventricular arrhythmias
- Endocarditis prophylaxis is recommended

Patent ductus arteriosus

- Patent ductus arteriosus (PDA) is a persistence of the fetal connection (ductus arteriosus) between the aorta and pulmonary artery after birth, resulting in a left-to-right shunt
- Symptoms may include failure to thrive, poor feeding, tachycardia and tachypnoea
- A continuous machine-like murmur in the upper left sternal border is common
- Diagnosis is by echocardiography
- Administration of indometacin, with or without fluid restriction may be tried in premature infants for duct closure with a significant shunt but not in term infants with PDA
- If the connection persists, surgical or catheter-based correction is indicated
- Endocarditis prophylaxis is recommended before and for 6 to 12 months after correction

Coarctation of the aorta

- Coarctation of the aorta accounts for 8%-10% of congenital heart anomalies
- It occurs in 10%-20% of patients with Turner syndrome
- The male:female ratio is 2:1
- Coarctation of the aorta usually occurs at the proximal thoracic aorta just beyond the left subclavian artery
- It rarely involves the abdominal aorta
- Coarctation can occur alone or with various other congenital anomalies (eg bicuspid aortic valve, VSD, AS, PDA, mitral valve disorders, intracerebral aneurysm)
- It results in upper-extremity hypertension, left ventricular hypertrophy, and malperfusion of the abdominal organs and lower extremities
- Symptoms vary with the anomaly's severity and range from headache, chest pain, cold extremities, fatigue, and leg claudication to fulminant heart failure and shock
- A soft bruit may be heard over the coarctation site and there may be radio-femoral delay along with rib-notching seen on chest X-ray

- Diagnosis is by echocardiography or by CT or MR angiography
- Treatment is balloon angioplasty with stent placement, or surgical correction
- Endocarditis prophylaxis is recommended

Tetralogy of Fallot

- Tetralogy of Fallot consists of four congenital anomalies:
  - A large VSD
  - Right ventricular outflow obstruction (pulmonary stenosis)
  - Right ventricular hypertrophy
  - Overriding of the aorta
- Symptoms include cyanosis, dyspnoea with feeding, poor growth, and tet spells (sudden, potentially lethal episodes of severe cyanosis)
- **Tet spells** may be precipitated by activity and are characterised by paroxysms of hyperpnoea (rapid and deep respirations), irritability and prolonged crying, increasing cyanosis and decreasing intensity of the heart murmur
- The spells occur most often in young infants; peak incidence is age 2–4 months
- A severe spell may lead to limpness, seizures and occasionally death
- During play, some toddlers may intermittently squat, a position that decreases systemic venous return, possibly increases systemic vascular resistance and thus raises arterial O$_2$ saturation
- A harsh systolic murmur at the left upper sternal border with a single S2 is common. Diagnosis is by echocardiography or cardiac catheterisation
- Definitive treatment is surgical repair
- Neonates with severe cyanosis due to ductal constriction are given an infusion of prostaglandin E1 to reopen the ductus arteriosus
- Palliative surgery can be done in patients who are not ideal surgical candidates for complete repair or in some patients with tet spells. In the most popular procedure, a modified Blalock–Taussig shunt, the subclavian artery is connected to the ipsilateral pulmonary artery with a synthetic graft
- Complete repair consists of patch closure of the VSD and widening of the right ventricular outflow tract
- Surgery is usually done electively during the first year of life but, if symptoms are present, it can be done any time after age 3–4 months
- Peri-operative mortality rate is <3% for uncomplicated tetralogy of Fallot
- For untreated patients, survival rates are 55% at 5 years and 30% at 10 years
- Endocarditis prophylaxis is recommended

Transposition of the great arteries

- Transposition of the great arteries occurs when the aorta arises directly from the right ventricle and the pulmonary artery arises from the left ventricle, resulting in independent, parallel pulmonary and systemic circulations
- After returning to the right heart, desaturated systemic venous blood is pumped into the systemic circulation without being oxygenated in the lungs; oxygenated blood entering the left heart goes back to the lungs rather than to the rest of the body
- This anomaly is not compatible with life unless desaturated and oxygenated blood can mix through openings at one or more levels (eg atrial, ventricular, or great artery level)
- Symptoms are primarily cyanosis and those of heart failure
- Heart sounds and murmurs vary depending on the presence of associated congenital anomalies
- Diagnosis is suspected clinically, supported by chest X-ray and ECG, and established by two-dimensional echocardiography with colour flow and Doppler studies
- Initially, prostaglandin E1 is infused to prevent closure of the ductus arteriosus, which allows connection between the two circuits
- Metabolic acidosis is corrected via infusion of sodium bicarbonate
- Pulmonary oedema and respiratory failure may require intubation and mechanical ventilation
- For severely hypoxaemic neonates, cardiac catheterisation and balloon atrial septostomy to cause an atrial septal defect (Rashkind's procedure) can immediately improve systemic arterial saturation
- Definitive repair is the arterial switch operation (Jantene operation), typically done during the first 2 weeks of life. The proximal portions of the great arteries are transected; the coronary arteries are transplanted to the proximal pulmonary artery, and the great arteries are connected to the correct ventricles, correcting the anomaly
- Survival rate after surgery is >90% at 1 year and 5 years
- All patients should be given endocarditis prophylaxis

Atrioventricular septal defect

- Atrioventricular septal defect accounts for about 5% of congenital heart anomalies
- It may be complete or partial
- 30% of patients with the complete form have Down's syndrome
- Atrioventricular septal defect is also common in patients with asplenia or polysplenia syndrome
- Complete atrioventricular septal defect consists of a large ostium primum atrial septal defect, an inlet ventricular septal defect (VSD), and a common AV valve orifice with

regurgitation. A left-to-right shunt occurs at the atrial and ventricular levels

- These defects result from maldevelopment of the endocardial cushions. Defects may be asymptomatic if small
- If large, they may cause heart failure, with dyspnoea with feeding, poor growth, tachypnoea, diaphoresis, or arrhythmias
- A single loud S2 and heart murmur are common
- Diagnosis is by echocardiography or cardiac catheterisation
- Treatment is surgical repair for moderate to severe cases
- Endocarditis prophylaxis is recommended

Hypoplastic left heart syndrome

- Accounts for 1% of congenital heart anomalies
- Consists of hypoplasia of the left ventricle and ascending aorta, maldevelopment of the aortic and mitral valves, an atrial septal defect, and a large PDA
- Unless normal closure of the patent ductus arteriosus is prevented with prostaglandin infusion, cardiogenic shock and death ensue
- A loud single S2 and non-specific systolic murmur are common
- Diagnosis is by emergency echocardiography or cardiac catheterisation
- Definitive treatment is staged surgical correction or heart transplantation
- Endocarditis prophylaxis is recommended

Thoracic surgery

CONTENTS

Thoracic surgery

Thoracic surgery remains an important part of the undergraduate curriculum. The teaching is usually integrated into the 'respiratory module' or firm and students may find difficulty distinguishing respiratory medicine from thoracic surgical disorders. This chapter concentrates on the practice of thoracic surgery at the level required for an undergraduate student. All of the disorders found make up a large fraction of a thoracic surgeon's workload. The only section omitted from here which may be practised by some thoracic surgeons is that of oesophageal disorders, which is covered in Chapter 4.

Revision objectives

You should:
- Be aware of the anatomy of thoracic structures and the differential diagnosis of mediastinal masses arising from these structures
- Know the causes, clinical features and management of pneumothoraces
- Know the causes, clinical features and management of pleural effusions
- Know the aetiology, clinical features and management of lung malignancies and mesotheliomas
- Know briefly about diaphragmatic conditions and their presentations

11.1 THORACIC SURGICAL DISORDERS

Thoracic surgery is the branch of medicine involved in the surgical treatment of diseases affecting organs inside the thorax (the chest) excluding the heart. Generally, thoracic surgeons deal with the treatment of conditions affecting the lungs and pleura, chest wall, oesophagus and diaphragm. This chapter deals with common thoracic surgical disorders with the exception of oesophageal disorders.

11.2 PNEUMOTHORAX

A pneumothorax refers to a collection of air or gas in the pleural space resulting in collapse of the lung on the affected side.

11.2.1 Types of pneumothorax
- **Primary spontaneous pneumothorax** occurs in people without underlying lung disease or trauma to the thorax. Many patients whose condition is labelled as primary spontaneous pneumothorax have an unrecognised lung disease.
- **Secondary spontaneous pneumothorax** occurs in people with underlying parenchymal lung disease.
- **Traumatic pneumothorax** results from injury, often secondary to medical intervention (ie iatrogenic pneumothorax).
- **Tension pneumothorax** occurs when air is trapped in the pleural cavity, resulting in positive pressure. It is a medical emergency!

11.2.2 Aetiology of pneumothorax
Pneumothorax can result from:

- A penetrating chest wound
- Acute infections
- Acupuncture
- Barotrauma to the lungs (ventilation)
- Chronic lung pathologies (including emphysema, asthma)
- Chronic infections, such as tuberculosis
- Cancer
- Catamenial pneumothorax (due to endometriosis in the chest cavity)
- Iatrogenic CVP (line insertion, reflux surgery)
- Spontaneously (most commonly in tall slim young males and in Marfan's syndrome)
- Trauma

11.2.3 Clinical features of pneumothorax
- Sudden shortness of breath, cyanosis and pain felt in the chest and/or back are the main symptoms.
- In penetrating chest wounds, the sound of air flowing through the puncture hole may indicate pneumothorax, hence the term 'sucking' chest wound. The flopping sound of the punctured lung is also occasionally heard.
- If untreated, hypoxia may lead to loss of consciousness and coma.
- In cases of tension pneumothorax, shifting of the mediastinum away from the site of the injury can obstruct the superior and inferior vena cava, resulting in reduced cardiac preload and decreased cardiac output. Untreated, a tension pneumothorax can lead to death within several minutes.
- Spontaneous pneumothoraces are reported in young people with a tall stature. As men are generally taller than women, there is a preponderance among males. The reason

for this association, while unknown, is hypothesised to be the presence of subtle abnormalities in connective tissue.

- Pneumothorax can also occur as part of medical procedures, such as the insertion of a central venous catheter in the subclavian or internal jugular veins. While rare, it is considered a serious complication and needs immediate treatment.

11.2.4 Diagnosis of pneumothorax

The absence of audible breath sounds on auscultation indicates that the lung is collapsed. This, accompanied by hyperresonance (higher pitched sounds than normal) to percussion of the chest wall, is suggestive of the diagnosis. If the signs and symptoms are doubtful, a radiograph of the chest (CXR) can be performed, but in severe hypoxia emergency treatment has to be administered first.

In a supine CXR the deep sulcus sign is diagnostic, which is characterised by a low lateral costophrenic angle on the affected side. Differential diagnosis includes myocardial infarction, oesophageal spasm, pulmonary embolism, pericarditis and pleurodynia.

11.2.5 Treatment of pneumothorax

- Treatment for primary spontaneous pneumothorax includes observation, simple aspiration or chest tube placement.
- Secondary spontaneous pneumothorax and traumatic pneumothorax usually require chest tube placement.
- Iatrogenic pneumothorax is frequently treated with observation or simple aspiration.
- Tension pneumothorax is a medical emergency that requires immediate needle decompression followed by chest tube placement.

Essential note

DO NOT WAIT FOR A CXR when dealing with a tension pneumothorax

---

- Pleurodesis with insufflation of a sclerosing agent or pleural stripping is usually needed for recurrent pneumothorax. A patient treated with this procedure has a recurrence prevention rate greater than 90%. Talc is the preferred agent for pleurodesis. It can be administered by insufflation or as a slurry.
- Video-assisted thoracoscopic surgery (VATS) with resection of large bullous lesions and/or insufflation of talc and thoracotomy are considered the most definitive treatments, with recurrence rates of 2%–14% and 0%–7%,

respectively. While VATS is used to prevent recurrence, not every patient with pneumothorax requires VATS.

- Surgical intervention with VATS or thoracotomy is indicated in the following conditions:
  - Persistent air leak for more than 7 days
  - Recurrent ipsilateral pneumothorax
  - Contralateral pneumothorax
  - Bilateral pneumothorax
  - First-time presentation in a patient with a high-risk occupation (eg diver, pilot)
  - Patients with acquired immunodeficiency syndrome (AIDS) often need this intervention because of extensive underlying necrosis
  - The risk of recurrent pneumothorax may also be unacceptable for patients with plans for extended stays at remote sites.

11.3 PLEURAL EFFUSION

The normal pleural space contains approximately 10–20 ml of fluid, representing the balance between: (1) hydrostatic and oncotic forces in the visceral and parietal pleural vessels and (2) extensive lymphatic drainage. Pleural effusions result from disruption of this balance.

11.3.1 Types of pleural effusion

A pleural effusion can be either a transudate or an exudate. Transudative pleural effusions are caused by systemic factors that alter the balance of the formation and absorption of pleural fluid (eg left ventricular failure, nephrotic syndrome and cirrhosis), while exudative pleural effusions are caused by alterations in local factors that influence the formation and absorption of pleural fluid (eg bacterial pneumonia, cancer, viral infection and pulmonary embolism).

Transudative and exudative pleural effusions are differentiated by comparing chemistries in the pleural fluid with those in the blood. Compared with transudative pleural effusion, exudative pleural effusion has:

- Pleural fluid protein >2.9 g/dl (29 g/l)
- Pleural fluid cholesterol >45 mg/dl (1.16 mmol/l)
- Pleural fluid lactate dehydrogenase (LDH) >60% of upper limit for serum

---

Essential note

It helps in diagnosis to try to classify fluid taken from a pleural tap as either a transudate or an exudate

---

11.3.2 Aetiology of pleural effusion

Transudative pleural effusions are caused by a small, defined group of aetiologies. The following conditions cause transudative pleural effusions:

- Congestive heart failure
- Cirrhosis (hepatic hydrothorax)
- Hypoalbuminaemia
- Nephrotic syndrome
- Peritoneal dialysis
- Myxoedema
- Constrictive pericarditis

Exudative pleural effusions are generally caused by inflammatory and malignant conditions. The more common causes of exudative pleural effusions include the following:

- Pneumonia (parapneumonic)
- Malignancy (carcinoma, lymphoma, mesothelioma)
- Pulmonary embolism
- Collagen-vascular disorders (rheumatoid arthritis, lupus)
- Tuberculous
- Asbestos-related conditions
- Pancreatitis
- Trauma
- Post-cardiac injury syndrome
- Oesophageal perforation
- Radiation pleuritis
- Drugs
- Chylothorax
- Meigs syndrome
- Sarcoidosis
- Yellow nail syndrome

11.3.3 Clinical features of pleural effusion

Pleural effusions may present with:

- No symptoms and are discovered incidentally on physical examination or CXR
- Dyspnoea
- Pleuritic chest pain

Pleuritic chest pain, a vague discomfort or sharp pain that worsens on inspiration indicates inflammation of the parietal pleura.

Physical examination reveals:

- Absent tactile fremitus
- Stony dullness to percussion
- Decreased breath sounds on the side of the effusion

These findings can also be produced by pleural thickening. With large-volume effusions, respiration is usually rapid and shallow. A pleural friction rub, although infrequent, is the classical physical sign.

11.3.4 Diagnosis of pleural effusion

Diagnosis is by physical examination and CXR. Chest aspiration (thoracentesis) and pleural fluid analysis are often required to determine cause. Occasionally a CT or bronchoscopy will help expand on the diagnosis of a lesion found on simple CXR.

11.3.5 Treatment of pleural effusion

The underlying cause is treated. The effusion itself generally does not require treatment if it is asymptomatic, because many resorb spontaneously, especially those due to uncomplicated pneumonias, pulmonary embolism and surgery. Pleuritic pain can usually be managed with oral analgesics, though a short course of oral opioids is sometimes necessary.

Chest aspiration (thoracentesis) or chest drain insertion is sufficient treatment for many symptomatic effusions and can be repeated for effusions that reaccumulate. Removal of >1.5 l of pleural fluid at a time should be avoided, because it can lead to pulmonary oedema due to rapid re-expansion of alveoli previously compressed by fluid.

Effusions that are chronic, recurrent and causing symptoms can be treated with pleurodesis or with an indwelling catheter. Effusions caused by pneumonia and malignancy may require additional specific measures.

11.3.6 Special types of pleural effusion

These include chylothorax, haemothorax and empyema.

Chylothorax

Chylothorax is a milky-white pleural effusion that is high in triglycerides and caused by traumatic or neoplastic (most often lymphomatous) damage to the thoracic duct.

Haemothorax

Haemothorax is the presence of bloody fluid (pleural fluid haematocrit > 50% peripheral haematocrit) in the pleural space due to trauma or, rarely, as a result of coagulopathy or after rupture of a major blood vessel, such as the aorta or pulmonary artery.

Empyema

Empyema is pus in the pleural space. It can occur as a complication of pneumonia, thoracotomy, abscesses (lung, hepatic or subdiaphragmatic), or penetrating trauma. Empyema necessitans is soft-tissue extension of empyema leading to chest wall infection and external drainage.

11.4 PLEURAL MESOTHELIOMA

- Pleural mesothelioma is the only known pleural malignancy and is caused by asbestos exposure in nearly all cases.
- Asbestos workers have up to a 10% lifetime risk of developing the disease, with an average latency of 30 years.
- Risk is independent of smoking.
- Mesothelioma can spread locally or metastasise to the pericardium, diaphragm, peritoneum and, rarely, the tunica vaginalis of the testis.
- Patients most often present with dyspnoea and non-pleuritic chest pain.
- Constitutional symptoms are uncommon at the time of clinical presentation.
- Invasion of the chest wall and other adjacent structures may cause severe pain, hoarseness, dysphagia, Horner's syndrome, brachial plexopathy, or ascites.
- Extrathoracic spread occurs in up to 80% of patients, most commonly including the hilar and mediastinal lymph nodes, liver, adrenals and kidneys.
- Pleural effusions are present in 95% of cases and are typically unilateral, massive effusions.
- Diagnosis is based on pleural fluid cytology or pleural biopsy and, if these are non-diagnostic, biopsy by video-assisted thorascopic surgery (VATS) or thoracotomy.
- Staging is done with chest CT, mediastinoscopy and MRI.
- Mesothelioma remains an incurable cancer.

- Surgery to remove the pleura, ipsilateral lung, phrenic nerve and hemidiaphragm and pericardium (termed pleuropneumonectomy), combined with chemotherapy or radiation therapy may be considered, although it does not substantially change prognosis or survival time, and long-term survival is uncommon. Moreover, complete surgical resection is not feasible in most patients.
- Combination chemotherapy with pemetrexed (an antifolate antimetabolite) and cisplatin is a promising therapeutic option but warrants further study.

11.5 MEDIASTINAL MASSES

Mediastinal masses are caused by a variety of cysts and tumours. The likely causes differ according to the patient's age and to whether the mass occurs in the anterior, middle, or posterior mediastinum (Figure 11.1). The masses may be asymptomatic (in adults) or cause obstructive respiratory symptoms (in children). Diagnosis involves CT scan with biopsy and adjunctive tests as needed. Treatment differs by cause.

11.6 LUNG CANCER

Lung cancer is the number one cause of cancer deaths in men and has surpassed breast cancer as the leading cause of cancer deaths in women. The incidence is rising in women and appears to be levelling off in men. Black men are at especially high risk.

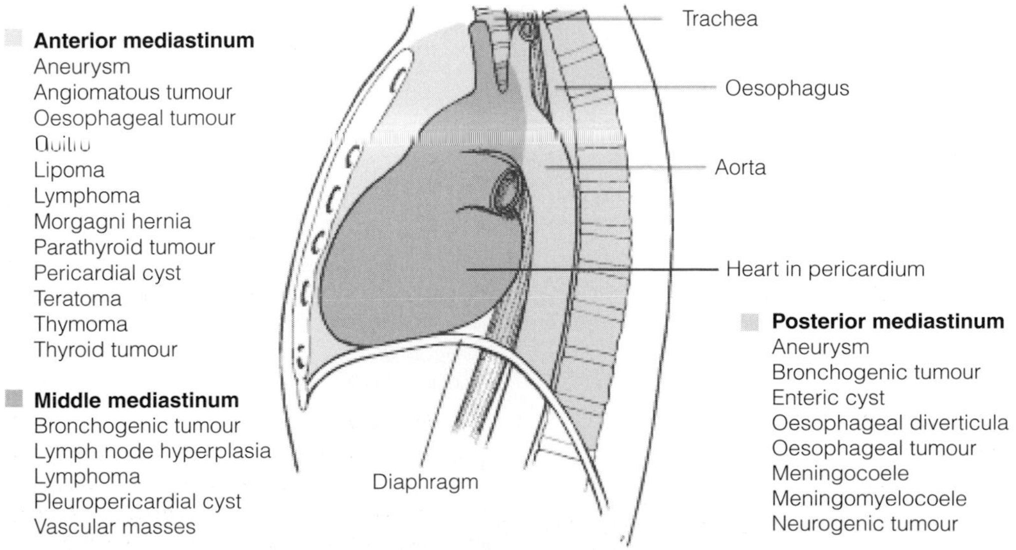

Anterior mediastinum
Aneurysm
Angiomatous tumour
Oesophageal tumour
Goitre
Lipoma
Lymphoma
Morgagni hernia
Parathyroid tumour
Pericardial cyst
Teratoma
Thymoma
Thyroid tumour

Middle mediastinum
Bronchogenic tumour
Lymph node hyperplasia
Lymphoma
Pleuropericardial cyst
Vascular masses

Trachea
Oesophagus
Aorta
Heart in pericardium
Diaphragm

Posterior mediastinum
Aneurysm
Bronchogenic tumour
Enteric cyst
Oesophageal diverticula
Oesophageal tumour
Meningocoele
Meningomyelocoele
Neurogenic tumour

Figure 11.1: Mediastinal masses

11.6.1 Types of lung cancer

Primary lung cancers are usually divided into two groups that account for about 95% of all cases. The division is based on the type of cells that make up the cancer. The two types of lung cancer are classified on the basis of the cell size of the tumour. They are called small-cell lung cancer (SCLC) and non-small-cell lung cancer (NSCLC). NSCLC includes several more types of tumours.

SCLCs are less common, but they grow more quickly and are more likely to metastasise than NSCLCs. Often, SCLCs have already spread to other parts of the body when the disease is diagnosed (Table 11.1).

About 5% of lung cancers are of rare cell types, such as carcinoid tumour and lymphoma. Metastatic (cancers from other parts of the body) cancers also commonly spread to the lungs and make up a large proportion of the lung tumours.

11.6.2 Aetiology of lung cancer

Cigarette smoking is the most significant cause of lung cancer. About 85% of lung cancers occur in a smoker or former smoker.

The risk of developing lung cancer is related to the following factors:

- The number of cigarettes smoked
- The age at which a person started smoking
- How long a person has smoked (or had smoked before quitting)

Other causes of lung cancer:

- Passive smoking, or sidestream smoke, presents another risk for lung cancer. A person living with a smoker has twice the risk of lung cancer of someone not regularly exposed to smoke.
- Air pollution from motor vehicles, factories and other sources may increase the risk for lung cancer, but the degree of increase has not been established accurately.
- Asbestos exposure increases the risk of lung cancer by a factor of 9. A combination of asbestos exposure and cigarette smoking compounds the risk by as much as 50 times.
- Lung diseases, such as tuberculosis and chronic obstructive pulmonary disease (COPD), also create a risk for lung cancer. A person with COPD has a 4–6 times greater risk of

Table 11.1: Characteristics of types of lung cancer				
Feature	Small-cell	Non-small-cell		
		Adenocarcinoma	Squamous cell	Large-cell
Percentage of lung cancers (%)	15%	25%–35%	30%–35%	10%–15%
Location	Submucosa of airways, perihilar mass	Peripheral nodule or mass	Central, endobronchial	Peripheral nodule or mass
Risks	Smoking (100%)	Smoking, occupational exposure (asbestos, radon)		
Treatment	Etoposide or irinotecan or topotecan + carboplatin or cisplatin; concurrent radiation therapy in limited-stage disease; no role for surgery	Stage I and II: surgery with or without adjuvant chemotherapy Stage IIIA: surgery with or without adjuvant therapy or concurrent chemoradiation Stage IIIB: radiation with or without chemotherapy Stage IV: chemotherapy with or without palliative radiation		
Complications	Common cause of SVC syndrome, paraneoplastic syndromes	Haemoptysis, airway obstruction, pneumonia, pleuritic involvement with pain, pleural effusion, SVC syndrome, Pancoast's tumour (shoulder or arm pain), hoarseness (laryngeal nerve involvement), neurological symptoms from brain metastasis, pathological fractures from bone metastasis, jaundice from liver metastasis		
5-year survival with treatment	Limited: 20% Extensive: <5%	Stage I: 57%–67% Stage II: 39%–55% Stage III: 5%–25% Stage IV: <1%		

SVC = superior vena cava

lung cancer, even when the effect of cigarette smoking is excluded.

- Radon exposure poses another risk:
  - Radon is a by-product of naturally occurring radium, which is a product of uranium
  - Radon is present in indoor and outdoor air
  - The risk for lung cancer increases with significant long-term exposure, although no one knows the exact risk.
- Certain occupations where exposure to arsenic, chromium, nickel, aromatic hydrocarbons and ethers occurs may increase the risk of lung cancer.
- A person who has had lung cancer is more likely to develop a second lung cancer than the average person is to develop a first lung cancer.

11.6.3 Clinical features of lung cancer

- About 25% of lung carcinomas are asymptomatic and are detected incidentally with chest imaging.
- Symptoms and signs develop from local tumour, regional spread and metastasis.
- **Symptoms** include:
  - Asymptomatic
  - Dyspnoea
  - Haemoptysis
  - Chest pain
  - Wheezy breathing
  - Hoarseness of voice
  - Dysphagia.
- **Complications** resulting from the tumour may present as:
  - Pleural effusion
  - SVC obstruction
  - Horner's syndrome, especially with Pancoast's apical lung tumour
  - Recurrent laryngeal nerve palsy
  - Metastatic spread to the liver, bones, brain, adrenal glands
  - General symptoms of cachexia, malaise and anorexia.
- **Paraneoplastic syndromes** and constitutional symptoms may occur at any stage. Paraneoplastic syndromes are not caused by cancer directly. Common paraneoplastic syndromes in patients with lung carcinoma include:
  - Hypercalcaemia (caused by tumour production of parathyroid hormone-related protein)
  - Syndrome of inappropriate antidiuretic hormone secretion (SIADH)
  - Finger clubbing, with or without hypertrophic osteoarthropathy
  - Hypercoagulability with migratory superficial thrombophlebitis (Trousseau's syndrome)
  - Myasthenia (Eaton–Lambert syndrome)

- A variety of neurological syndromes, including neuropathies, encephalopathies, encephalitides, myelopathies and cerebellar disease. Mechanisms for neuromuscular syndromes involve tumour expression of autoantigens with production of autoantibodies, but the cause of most others is unknown.

11.6.4 Diagnosis of lung cancer

Diagnosis is suspected by CXR or CT scan and confirmed by biopsy. Bronchoscopy is the procedure most often used for diagnosing lung carcinoma. In theory, the procedure of choice for obtaining tissue is the one that is least invasive. In practice, bronchoscopy is often performed in addition to or instead of less invasive procedures, because diagnostic yields are greater and because bronchoscopy is important for staging. A combination of washings, brushings and fine-needle aspiration of visible endobronchial lesions and of paratracheal, subcarinal, mediastinal and hilar lymph nodes yields a tissue diagnosis in 90%–100% of cases. Mediastinoscopy is a higher-risk procedure and is usually used before surgery to confirm or exclude the presence of tumour in enlarged mediastinal lymph nodes of undetermined significance.

11.6.5 Staging of lung cancer

SCLC is categorised as limited-stage and extensive-stage disease:

- Limited-stage disease is cancer confined to one hemithorax (including ipsilateral lymph nodes) that can be encompassed within one tolerable radiation therapy port, excluding the presence of pleural or pericardial effusion.
- Extensive-stage disease is cancer outside a single hemithorax and the presence of malignant pleural or pericardial effusion.
- About one-third of patients with SCLC have limited-stage disease; the remainder often have extensive distant metastases.

NSCLC staging involves determining tumour size and location (T), lymph node involvement (N) and the presence or absence of distant metastases (M) (Box 11.1).

11.6.6 Treatment of lung cancer

Treatment generally involves assessment of eligibility for surgery followed by choice of surgery, chemotherapy and/or radiation as appropriate, depending on tumour type and stage. Many non-tumour-related factors affect eligibility for surgery and may lead to a decision for palliative over curative treatment or for no treatment at all, even though cure might technically be possible (Box 11.2).

Surgery is reserved for NSCLC (stages I–IIIA) and is performed only on patients who will have adequate pulmonary reserve once a lobe or lung is resected. Patients with pre-operative forced expiratory volume in 1 second (FEV$_1$) >2 litres generally tolerate pneumonectomy. Those with FEV$_1$ <2 I should undergo a quantitative radionuclide perfusion scan to determine the proportion of function the patient can expect to lose from resection.

Multiple **chemotherapy** regimens exist for treatment of lung carcinoma; no one regimen has proved superior. Choice of regimen, therefore, often depends on local practice, contraindications and toxicities.

Radiotherapy also is used as a palliative measure or for treatment of metastases. Radiotherapy carries a risk of radiation pneumonitis when large areas of lung are exposed to high doses of radiation over time.

SCLC of any stage is typically initially responsive to treatment, but responses are usually short-lived. Surgery generally plays no role in treatment of SCLC, although it may be curative in the rare patient who has a small focal tumour without spread (such as a solitary pulmonary nodule). Chemoradiotherapy is the treatment of choice for limited-stage SCLC while extensive-stage disease is treated with chemotherapy alone.

Box 11.1: TNM staging for non-small-cell lung cancer (NSCLC)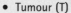

- Tumour (T)
    - TX: Positive malignant cytology results, no lesion seen
    - T1: Diameter smaller than or equal to 3 cm
    - T2: Diameter larger than 3 cm
    - T3: Extension to pleura, chest wall, diaphragm, pericardium, within 2 cm of carina, or total atelectasis
    - T4: Invasion of mediastinal organs (eg oesophagus, trachea, great vessels, heart), malignant pleural effusion, or satellite nodules within the primary lobe
- Regional lymph node involvement (N)
    - N0: No lymph nodes involved
    - N1: Ipsilateral bronchopulmonary or hilar nodes involved
    - N2: Ipsilateral mediastinal or subcarinal nodes
    - N3: Contralateral mediastinal, hilar, any supraclavicular nodes involved
- Metastatic involvement (M)
    - M0: No metastases
    - M1: Metastases present
- Stage groupings
    - IA: T1 N0 M0
    - IB: T2 N0 M0
    - IIA: T1 N1 M0
    - IIB: T2 N1 M0 or T3 N0 M0
    - IIIA: T1–3 N2 M0 or T3 N1 M0
    - IIIB: Any T4 or any N3 M0
    - IV: Any M1

Box 11.2: Indications for palliative surgery in NSCLC

- Poor cardiopulmonary reserve
- Malnutrition
- Frailty or poor physical performance status
- Co-morbidities, including cytopenias
- Psychiatric or cognitive illness

11.6.7 Prognosis of lung cancer

Prognosis is poor, even with newer treatments.

- On average, untreated patients with advanced NSCLC survive 6 months.
- Five-year survival for treated NSCLC patients is about 9 months.
- Patients with extensive-stage SCLC do especially poorly, with a 5-year survival rate <1%.
- The median survival time for limited-stage SCLC disease is 20 months, with a 5-year survival rate of 20%.
- In many patients with SCLC, chemotherapy prolongs life and improves quality of life enough to warrant its use. The 5-year survival rate of patients with NSCLC varies by stage.

11.7 DIAPHRAGMATIC CONDITIONS

Conditions affecting the diaphragm occur infrequently in clinical practice. Trauma, paralysis and hernias are the main conditions that affect the diaphragm clinically. Primary malignancies and primary infections are extremely rare. The two main conditions to remember for finals and at any stage in clinical practice are diaphragmatic paralysis and hernias. Diaphragmatic trauma is dealt with by specialist surgeons.

11.7.2 Diaphragmatic paralysis

- Phrenic nerve (C3,C4,C5) supplies the diaphragm on each side.
- Trauma to this nerve (eg surgery) or even infiltration by a tumour can cause unilateral diaphragmatic paralysis, resulting in a raised hemidiaphragm radiologically.
- Spinal cord lesions above C4 will also result in total diaphragmatic paralysis as the phrenic nerve roots are affected bilaterally. Lifelong breathing is only possible with a ventilator. (Hence the importance of cervical spine protection following any trauma!)

Essential note

Learn how to protect and support the C-spine following trauma. This can save many lives if done properly in the injured patient

11.7.3 Diaphragmatic hernias

- Hernias may be congenital or acquired (rare).
- Diaphragmatic hernias result in the herniation of abdominal contents into the thorax.
- Congenital diaphragmatic hernias occur in between 1 and 5 per 10000 births in the population.
- Survival rate for congenital diaphragmatic hernia is roughly 60%.

- Congenital diaphragmatic hernia may be of the Bochdalek variety (90%) or of the Morgagni type (10%)
- **Bochdalek** hernias occur through **posterolateral** defects of the diaphragm, which results in either failure in the development of the pleuroperitoneal folds or improper or absent migration of the diaphragmatic musculature:
  - Most present in the neonatal period or within the first year of life
  - Mortality rate of 45%–50%
  - Most of the morbidity and mortality of congenital diaphragmatic hernia relates to hypoplasia of the lung and pulmonary hypertension on the affected side
  - Timely diagnosis and proper management remain the key to survival.
- The foramen of **Morgagni** hernia occurs in the **anterior midline** through the sternocostal hiatus of the diaphragm:
  - 90% of cases occur on the right side
  - Treatment is surgical repair and release of the abdominal contents.

Essential note

In remembering diaphragmatic hernias, think **M**idline for **M**orgagni

Vascular surgery

CONTENTS

Vascular surgery

Revision objectives

You should:

- Know how to clinically assess a patient with vascular disease through history and examination of the following:
  - Arterial system examination
  - Venous system examination (lower limbs)
  - Examination of an ulcer (any site)
- Know the epidemiology, causes, clinical features and brief management of arterial vascular disease including:
  - Carotid disease
  - Abdominal aortic aneurysm and peripheral aneurysms
  - Peripheral vascular disease (acute and chronic)
  - Amputations
  - Gangrene
- Know the causes, clinical features and management of venous disease:
  - Venous insufficiency and ulcers
  - Varicose veins
  - Thromboembolic disease
- Know the causes, clinical features and assessment of patients with lymphangitis and lymphoedema

This chapter concentrates on the undergraduate curriculum for vascular surgery, which deals more with clinical assessment, risk factor stratification and epidemiology of vascular disease, with less concentration on management of complex vascular problems. For example, it is more important for the student to know the resuscitation protocol, urgency and mortality rate of a ruptured abdominal aortic aneurysm than to know how and why a repair is performed.

A combination of learning the essential topics covered in this chapter as well as learning the clinical assessment will equip you for most examinations, including the membership exams. Some basic but essential epidemiology is covered below in Section 12.1.1. Please note the learning objectives and concentrate on these important points with regards to learning good basic vascular surgical principles and to answering exam questions with ease.

12.1 INTRODUCTION TO VASCULAR DISEASE

12.1.1 Epidemiology of vascular disease

Arterial disease

- Peripheral arterial disease occurs most commonly due to atherosclerosis and impaired perfusion; basically, when supply < demand
- It affects >30% of people over the age of 70 years
- It affects >30% of people over the age of 50 who smoke or have diabetes
- The incidence increases with age in both sexes
- Risk factors (Figure 12.1) include:
  - Male sex
  - Increasing age
  - Family history
  - Smoking
  - Hypertension
  - Hyperlipidaemia
  - Diabetes mellitus
  - Homocystinaemia
  - Myxoedema
  - Obesity and high-fat diet
- Lower limbs are most commonly affected
- Mortality from arterial disease is most commonly due to myocardial infarction or strokes
- Progression of disease is summarised in Figure 12.2

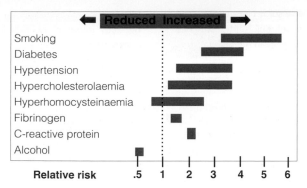

Figure 12.1: Risk factors for peripheral vascular disease (mean follow-up 38 years)

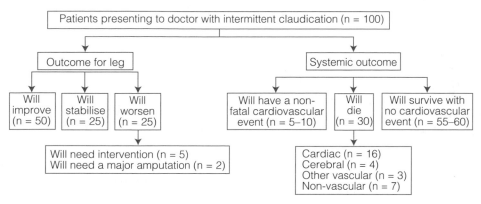

Figure 12.2: Progression of disease

Venous disease

- Venous disease mainly occurs in the lower limbs
- Venous thromboses facts:
  - Most common in hospital patients post-surgery or trauma
  - F>M
  - Numerous risk factors covered later in section
- Varicose veins
  - Affect 4.5% of the population
  - Increasing age, peaking in the sixth decade
  - F>M ratio 4:1
  - There is some association with family history
  - Occupational association with standing for long periods of time
  - Increased in pregnancy and with wearing corsets
  - Can be caused by pelvic pathology compressing venous return

Lymphatic disease

- 80% of lymphoedema affects the lower limbs
- Uncommon disorder in the population
- May be classed into primary (congenital or idiopathic) or secondary (known cause)

12.2.1 Examination of the arterial system

A complete examination includes a full cardiovascular examination, starting with full appropriate exposure of the patient. Although there are variations in examination routines, the general principles of the arterial examination remain the same. Proceed with the examination in a systematic method and get comfortable with whichever you choose to adopt.

General inspection

- Is the patient well or unwell?
- Is there any asymmetry in posture, size, or movements (indicating a previous stroke)?
- Is the patient breathless at rest or in any discomfort?
- Is the patient mobile or immobile (has there been an amputation as a result of vascular disease)?

The hands

- Inspect for discoloration, pallor, peripheral cyanosis
- Do they appear relatively red and well perfused or white/mottled?

- Nail shape and colour might give some clues as well as nicotine staining. Delayed capillary refill is interestingly a common sign of arterial insufficiency in the lower extremity, but it rarely occurs in the arms or hands. Thus, delayed capillary refill in the hands more likely reflects vasospasm or hypovolaemic shock than it does intraluminal arterial obstruction. Severe vasospasm, referred to as Raynaud's phenomenon, occurs most frequently in women after exposure to cool temperatures, causing both hands to become white and painful. The hands then become blue due to stagnant anoxia and subsequently turn red due to reactive hyperaemia.
- Feel for the pulses in the upper limbs as well as checking for radio-radial delays (which indicate a subclavian steal phenomenon).
- Perform a blood pressure check in both arms if you suspect a discrepancy between pulses.

Neck

Palpate for the carotid pulses and listen to them with a stethoscope to identify any bruits. Ask the patient to hold their breath so you don't confuse breath sounds with a bruit.

Abdomen and groin

Proceed to examination of the abdomen unless you feel compelled to examine the heart at this stage. Usually, the cardiac exam can be performed at the end, and in an exam situation do mention that you would perform it for completeness of the assessment. Cardiac examinations are important because certain conditions such as aortic stenosis and cardiac failure render the cardiac pump mechanism inefficient. This results in poor perfusion generally; however, when combined with pre-existing distal vascular disease, the effects can exacerbate the clinical features greatly.

- Inspect and palpate for pulsations that might be caused by an aortic aneurysm.
- The bifurcation of the aorta is generally just below the level of the umbilicus and so aneurysms are generally felt above it.
- Check the groin for pulses as well as for aneurysms.
- Sometimes a saphena varix (swelling over the saphenofemoral junction) can present as a lump on standing. This should be tested by placing a hand over the swelling and tapping the varicose vein lower down the leg to confirm that it is a venous swelling. The lump disappears on lying down.
- Auscultation of the abdomen and groin should be done to listen for bruits or arteriovenous fistulas.

Legs

The legs must be examined for signs of chronic arterial ischaemia:

- **Inspection**
  - Skin colour (pale, red, cyanotic, black)
  - Shiny skin with hair loss
  - Buerger's angle (also known as vascular angle)
  - Dependent rubor (capillary filling time)
  - Venous guttering
  - Trophic skin changes or ulcers
- **Palpation**
  - Capillary refill time
  - Temperature (cold, warm)
  - Pulses (including femoral, popliteal, dorsal pedis, and posterior tibial) Figure 12.3
  - Neuropathy (test muscles and nerves)
  - Auscultation (over main vessels)
  - Doppler pressures should be obtained as well as the ankle–brachial pulse index (ABPI)

Complete the examination with a cardiac examination.

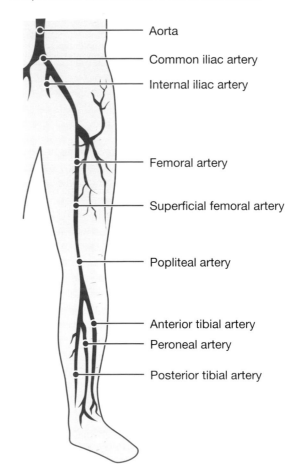

Figure 12.3: Blood supply of the leg

- Aorta
- Common iliac artery
- Internal iliac artery
- Femoral artery
- Superficial femoral artery
- Popliteal artery
- Anterior tibial artery
- Peroneal artery
- Posterior tibial artery

12.2.2 Leg ulcers

An ulcer is defined as a break in the continuity of the epithelial surface. Although there are many causes of leg ulcers, they commonly present to vascular surgeons for treatment.

Causes of leg ulcers
- Venous (post-DVT, varicose veins)
- Arterial (atherosclerotic)
- Neuropathic (diabetes, cerebrovascular accident, spinal lesions)
- Traumatic
- Vasculitic and vasospastic (Raynaud's, polyarteritis nodosa, scleroderma)
- Malignant (basal cell carcinoma, squamous cell carcinoma, melanoma, Marjolin's ulcer, skin metastases)
- Infective (tuberculosis, human immunodeficiency virus)
- Chronic disease (ulcerative colitis, rheumatoid arthritis, systemic lupus erythematosus)
- Malnutrition (scurvy)
- Artefact (self-induced or iatrogenic)
- Lymphatic (infection or trauma)

Examination of leg ulcers
The following should be noted when examining any leg ulcer. This is fairly similar to examining and describing a lump in the body.

- **Site**
  - Describe the precise site of an ulcer using nearby anatomical landmarks
- **Size**
- **Shape** (oval, circular, irregular)
- **Edges**
  - Sloping – healing ulcer (venous stasis ulcers)

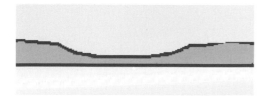

  - Punched out
    - Used to be characteristic of syphilitic ulcers in the pre-antibiotic era
    - Now more commonly neuropathic ulcer in patients with diabetes, or trophic ulcers

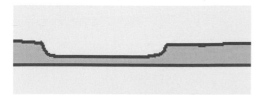

  - Undermined – tuberculosis, decubitus ulcers

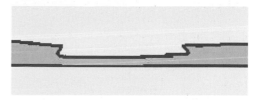

  - Raised – basal cell carcinoma

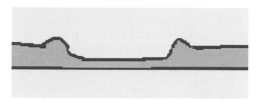

  - Everted – squamous cell carcinoma

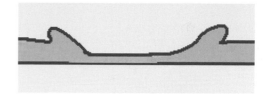

- **Base**
  - Slough/granulation tissue/tendon/bone/depth of base
- **Discharge** (serous, sanguinous, purulent)
- **Colour**
- **Temperature**
- **Tenderness**
- **Odour**
- **Fixation**
- **Surrounding tissues**
  - Varicose veins, lipodermatosclerosis
  - Trophic changes: shiny skin, hair loss, ulcers, loss of subcutaneous tissue, thickened toenails
  - Arterial pulses and ARPI
  - Cutaneous sensation distally (nerves)
  - Bones/joints
- **Regional lymph nodes**
- **General examination**

Diagnostic testing
- Blood tests – FBC, ESR, glucose, autoantibodies
- Microbiological swab of the ulcer
- Duplex Doppler ultrasound
- Ulcer biopsy
- Magnetic resonance angiography (MRA) or CT arteriography (CTA)
- Angiography/venography

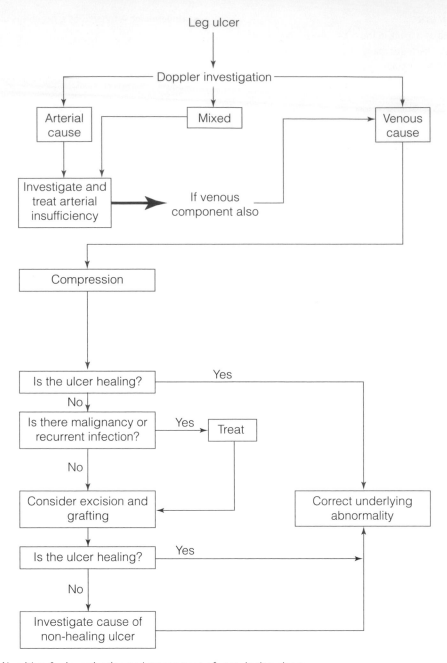

Figure 12.4: Algorithm for investigation and mangement of vascular leg ulcers

Management of leg ulcers (Figure 12.4)

- Treat the underlying cause – this is the most important part of managing any ulcer!
- Treat any infection that may be present.
- Compression bandaging (light compression in arterial disease, 3- or 4-layer compression for venous disease).
- Consider excision and grafting for non-healing ulcers once malignancy and infection are ruled out and any underlying causes have been dealt with appropriately.

12.2.3 Peripheral vascular disease

Peripheral vascular disease affects a significant proportion of elderly patients in the UK. Incidence in both sexes increases with age although it is more commonly found in males. It is predominantly secondary to atherosclerosis causing compromised blood flow, with smoking being the strongest risk factor. Although it can affect any vessel, those of the lower limb are particularly vulnerable. The distal superficial femoral and bifurcation of the common femoral arteries are the most commonly affected sites. The risk factors and epidemiology of peripheral vascular disease are covered in Section 12.1.1. Important terminology and definitions are described below.

Intermittent claudication

Cramping in a muscle which occurs on exertion (walking or running) and is relieved by resting that muscle. This can occur in one or sometimes both legs and although the term is classically used to describe calf pain, it can occur in any muscle including the thigh muscles and buttocks. The pain is due to the muscles having an insufficient blood supply to meet their demands, resulting in ischaemia. This occurs after a variable distance of walking, in some patients after just a few steps and in others after a mile or more. At the shorter distances the pain is usually too severe to allow continued walking but in milder forms it is uncomfortable and a nuisance, making the individual slow down rather than stop. Sometimes the leg also feels 'dead' and sometimes the foot feels numb. All these symptoms almost always improve or disappear within minutes of stopping walking. Patients often find that their quality of life is impaired because of difficulty in continuing normal lifestyle.

Claudication distance

This is used to assess the severity of the disease and is the distance a patient can walk before having to stop due to symptoms of pain. It can be measured in units of length or time.

It is important to rule out a spinal cause (spinal stenosis – pseudoclaudication) – narrowing of the spinal canal due to a prolapsed disc or arthritis of the back causes leg pain when standing and is not relieved by brief resting periods. Relief of pain often occurs by leaning forwards against a stationary object (eg a tree) or sitting.

Other causes of calf pain such as venous claudication, knee arthritis and Baker's cysts need to be clinically ruled out as well.

Critical ischaemia

Collection of symptoms which may occur when blood flow falls below the minimal threshold to maintain limb viability. Rest pain and tissue loss (ulceration) commonly occur. The ABPI is usually less than 0.4 in critically ischaemic limbs.

Rest pain

As atherosclerosis progresses and the blockage becomes more severe, pain may occur in the feet at rest. Classically, the term refers to pain in the foot which occurs on elevation (such as lying in bed) and is relieved by dependency (hanging the feet off the end of the bed or standing). The lack of gravitational assistance caused by elevation of the leg does not help the circulation to the feet and thus rest pain occurs. Rest pain should not be confused with night cramps, which are short and severe muscle cramps of unknown origin. The affected area of rest pain may be very tender and sensitive. Rest pain often implies a state of critical limb ischaemia.

Gangrene

Gangrene is defined as tissue necrosis due to critical ischaemia.

Types of gangrene

- **Dry gangrene**
  - Dry gangrene begins at the distal part of the limb due to ischaemia. Gangrene spreads slowly upwards (proximally) until it reaches the point where the blood supply is adequate to keep the tissue viable.
  - Macroscopically, the affected part is dry, shrunken and dark black, resembling the foot of a mummy. There is usually a clear line of demarcation between the living and the dead tissues. This line of demarcation usually brings about a complete separation, with eventual falling off of the gangrenous tissue if it is not removed surgically.
  - The early signs of dry gangrene are a dull ache and sensation of coldness in the area, along with pallor of the flesh.
  - Dry gangrene occurs in uninfected tissues and this is the main distinction from wet gangrene.
- **Wet gangrene**
  - In wet gangrene, the dead tissue is infected by saprogenic microorganisms and becomes swollen and malodorous. Wet gangrene usually develops rapidly due

to blockage of venous and/or arterial blood flow. The affected part is filled with blood, which favours the rapid growth of bacteria. The toxic products formed by bacteria are absorbed causing the systemic manifestation of septicaemia and finally death.

- Macroscopically the affected part is wet, swollen, soft, putrid, rotten and dark.
- Gangrene is best classified into infected and non-infected rather than wet and dry gangrene, as this often identifies the cause of gangrene and directs appropriate management.
- Wet gangrene should be managed with urgent antibiotic treatment and debridement as necessary.
- **Diabetic gangrene** is due to three factors:
  - Trophic changes resulting from peripheral neuritis
  - Atheroma resulting in ischaemia
  - Lower resistance in tissues to infection due to excess sugar. This type is often associated with gas in the tissues and a foul smell.

12.2.4 Acute arterial insufficiency

Acute arterial insufficiency is loss of perfusion, usually due to a sudden disruption in blood supply of a particular region. **Common causes** include:

- Arterial embolus
- Aortic dissection
- Compression from an external source (eg cervical rib)
- Acute thrombosis of an atheromatous plaque
- Acute thrombosis of an aneurysm
- Trauma
- Intra-arterial injection

Patients with a proximal atherosclerotic lesion usually have a history of intermittent claudication and this acute presentation should be called an 'acute on chronic' event. Cardiac conditions predisposing to emboli include atrial fibrillation (left auricular thrombus), myocardial infarction (mural thrombus), valvular disease and atrial myxoma. Very rarely an embolus originating from the lower legs (DVT) enters the left heart via a septal defect (paradoxical embolus).

The above-mentioned causes can lead to the acute vascular insufficiency of almost any part of the body from the cerebral blood vessels (eg carotid stenosis leading to strokes), to vessels of the gastrointestinal tract (mesenteric ischaemia due to emboli) and to limbs. It should be remembered that emboli can be of air, fat and even amniotic fluid. Presenting signs and symptoms vary according to the end organ affected.

Common obstructions due to emboli

- Brain – the middle cerebral artery or one of its branches; results in hemiplegia

- Retina – passage of a thrombus from an atheromatous plaque into the central retinal artery. Blindness can be caused, known as 'amaurosis fugax'. Patients describe this as a curtain falling over their eyes
- Mesenteric vessels – can cause ischaemia and gangrene of the bowel segment affected
- Spleen – engorgement and local pain
- Kidneys – haematuria and loin pain
- Lungs – pulmonary embolism can be fatal; can cause haemoptysis and dyspnoea

Acute limb ischaemia

Clinical features

The classical six 'Ps': pain, paraesthesia, paralysis, pallor, pulselessness and perishingly cold (Table 12.1). The first three are neurological and the last three vascular in origin. The presence of neurological signs indicates a need for urgent treatment. Sometimes isolated toes/fingers turn blue indicating the segment of occlusion. In the case of acute limb arterial insufficiency, surgery should be performed for acute occlusion within 6 hours for ideal results and avoidance of amputation. With longer ischaemic times, there is a higher chance of amputation and mortality from reperfusion injury and toxins.

Table 12.1: 6 'Ps' for vascular insufficiency	
Neurological	Pain
	Paraesthesia
	Paralysis
Vascular	Pallor
	Pulselessness
	Perishingly cold

Take a history to confirm the exact time of onset as well as a focused vascular and complete general history. In an acutely ischaemic leg caused by a superficial femoral artery embolus (commonest cause), the classic presentation is that of a patient experiencing a sudden onset of pain in their leg. Examination reveals a cold, pale leg which may be tender to touch and has absent pulses. Paraesthesiae and paralysis are late signs.

Investigations
- FBC
- Urea and electrolytes
- Clotting screen
- Glucose
- Cross-match
- ECG
- Urgent arteriography

Treatment

- Resuscitation (IV fluids and oxygen)
- Anticoagulation with 5000 units of IV heparin
- Analgesia
- Consider angiogram/urgent embolectomy/thrombolysis to treat embolus
- Consider fasciotomy if reperfusion injury is suspected

12.2.5 Chronic arterial insufficiency

In the majority of vascular patients arteriosclerosis is the main cause, often due to smoking or diabetes. Multiple recurrent small emboli, Buerger's disease, arteritis and, rarely, Takayasu's arteritis can also compromise vascular flow to the tissues.

It is important from the history to ascertain:

- The severity of the condition
- To what degree is it affecting the patient's lifestyle
- Associated risk factors

The signs and symptoms are relative to the area of occlusion. Common areas of disease are the aortoiliac, iliac and superficial femoral regions. Chronic disease of the upper limb is rare. Common presentations include intermittent claudication, rest pain, ischaemic ulcers and gangrene.

Superficial femoral artery (SFA) disease

Disease affecting the SFA causes intermittent claudication in the calf. In advanced disease, rest pain may occur, implying critical limb ischaemia. These patients may also have many other signs, including ulcers, gangrene and skin changes. Pulses in the SFA are usually absent.

Aortoiliac artery disease

Depending on the severity, any of the above signs and symptoms of SFA occlusion can be observed plus intermittent claudication affecting the buttock or thigh. Disease of the aortoiliac segment can also be associated with impotence (pudendal artery comes off the internal iliac). In men, Leriche's syndrome may be present. Classically, this is a triad of buttock claudication, sexual impotence and absent femoral pulses due to aortoiliac occlusion.

Investigations

- FBC/ESR/U&Es/glucose/HbA$_{1c}$/lipids
- Treadmill test to assess claudication distance
- Doppler studies to assess ABPI (Table 12.2) as well as areas of stenosis
- Arteriography is undertaken when/if surgery or angioplasty is proposed

Table 12.2: Ankle–brachial pulse index (ratio)	
Value	*Interpretation*
0.9–1.2	Normal
0.6–0.8	Mild arterial disease (claudication)
0.4–0.6	Moderate arterial disease (ulcers, claudication, or rest pain)
0.4 or less	Severe disease with rest pain and/or gangrene; requires further investigations/management

Values are an estimate of the degree of claudication.

Note: In diabetic patients a false high ratio is observed due to hardening and calcification of the arterial walls; ABPI >1 common.

Management

It is vital to improve risk factors such as smoking, hypertension and blood lipid profile, and to control diabetes and improve lifestyle factors such as diet, exercise and weight. Advice on foot care should be given.

Medical

- Antiplatelets: aspirin/clopidogrel
- Antihypertensives for aggressive blood pressure control
- Diabetic control (blood sugar)
- Statins for two effects:
  - To lower cholesterol below normal limits
  - To decrease arterial inflammation
- Vasodilators such as prostacyclin and naftidrofuryl, which increase oxygen uptake by muscles and can be used in patients unsuitable for surgical intervention. Cilostazol is a newer agent that is a selective cAMP phosphodiesterase inhibitor and has good antiplatelet and arterial dilator activity

Surgical

- Balloon angioplasty ± stenting (this can be intraluminal or subintimal)
- Arterial bypass with autogenous vein or prosthetic graft
  - For aortoiliac disease, Dacron grafts are usually used
  - For arteries lower down, either vein graft or PTFE graft (polytetrafluoroethylene)
  - For patients with severe aortoiliac disease with poor vessel quality, a prosthetic graft from the axillary arteries can be subcutaneously tunnelled and anastomosed to the femoral(s) – axillary-femoral (ax-fem) bypass graft
- Endarterectomy has largely been superseded by angioplasty, but it is still performed in isolated cases
- Lumbar sympathectomy is used when reconstruction is unfeasible and symptom control is required

12.2.6 Amputation

An amputation is the removal of a body part by surgery or trauma. Surgically, it is performed in cases of gangrene, non-healing ulcers, rest pain not amenable to surgery and malignancies of the limbs. It can also be performed for limbs that have been rendered useless following trauma or nerve damage.

Amputations have been described as early as Hippocrates (c. 460–375 BC) and have an interesting historical development.

General points about amputations

- As the average age of patients is increasing, so is the number of amputations performed, hence prevention is a concern of uttermost importance
- Patients with diabetes are high risk and have a 20 times increased chance of amputation due to a combination of vasculopathy, neuropathy (mainly) and secondary infections

Level of amputation

Main issues influencing decision are as follows:

- Site of higher healing: potential blood supply is richer proximally
- Site where use of limb will be maximised to maintain ambulation as near normal with the least energy expenditure
- Presence or absence of collaterals (ie if SFA is occluded, the decision favours an above-knee over a below-knee amputation)
- Clinical judgement
  - Subjective and objective assessments
  - Clinical judgement is more important, even if it contraindicates laboratory studies

Indications for surgical amputation of limbs

- **Vascular**
  - Severe acute ischaemia due to unreconstructable arterial circulation
  - Chronic arterial insufficiency/inoperable vascular disease (recurrent, failed attempts with endovascular techniques such as angioplasty, stents, grafts)
  - Rest pain, ulceration, gangrenous change with or without infection
- **Infectious:** overwhelming foot sepsis (diabetics), osteomyelitis
- **Trauma:** crush injuries
- **Tumours**
  - Soft tissue, bone (osteogenic sarcoma)
  - Soft tissue sarcomas
  - Melanoma (subungal)

- **Non-functioning limbs**
  - Congenital defects
  - Brachial plexus lesions
  - Poliomyelitis

Levels of amputation (distal to proximal)

- Toes
- Transmetatarsal
- Syme's (heel disarticulation and malleoli excised)
- Below-knee amputation
- Through-knee amputation
- Gritti–Stokes (supracondylar)
- Above-knee amputation
- Hip disarticulation (usually for soft tissue/bony malignancies)

In clinical practice, the commonest amputations are those of the toes, transmetatarsal, below-knee and above-knee.

The other mentioned amputations have very specific indications and are not commonly used.

Complications of amputation

Early complications
- Haemorrhage
- Infection
- Fat embolism
- Haematoma
- Wound dehiscence
- Ischaemic flaps
- Post-operative trauma
- Arterial insufficiency because of inadequate amputation
- Mechanical injury to marginal tissue intraoperatively

Late complications
- Persistent pain
- Sinus formation
- Phantom limb pain
- Ulcers (from constant pressure of prosthesis)
- Osteomyelitis
- Ischaemia of skin flaps

12.2.7 Cerebrovascular insufficiency

Stroke represents one of the most serious causes of mortality and morbidity in the world. Each year 10% of all deaths in the UK occur as a result of a cerebrovascular accident (CVA) and many more patients experience the morbidity of aphasia, blindness, or paralysis. Amongst patients with stroke, extra-cranial carotid disease is the cause in approximately one-half of cases.

Causes of CVA include:

- Thrombosis – 55%
- Emboli – 30%
- Intracranial haemorrhage – 15%

Atherosclerosis is common at the bifurcation of the common carotid artery. Approximately 15% of CVAs are caused by carotid disease.

Clinical features of carotid disease

- Asymptomatic carotid stenosis (bruit audible but no clinical effect)
- Amaurosis fugax: transient total or sectorial monocular loss of vision
- Transient ischaemic attack (TIA) – acute focal neurological loss lasting <24 hours with no persistent defect
- Reversible ischaemic neurological deficit (RIND) – reversible neurological loss lasting >24 hours but less than 30 days
- Ischaemic stroke (CVA) – acute focal neurological loss lasting longer than 24 hours or associated with death
- Clinical presentation of signs and symptoms depends directly on the arterial area affected:
  - Carotid artery – contralateral hemiparesis, dysphasia (dominant hemisphere)
  - Vertebrobasilar diplopia, vertigo, visual blurring, cerebellar signs, facial signs

The risk of stroke increases with the degree of stenosis. Once a stenosis has become symptomatic the risk of a stroke is further increased. The risk of further stroke is ~10% in the first year and ~5% in subsequent years.

Assessment of stenosis

Carotid bruits are an unreliable guide to the severity of stenosis. The correlation between a carotid bruit and a haemodynamically important carotid stenosis is reported to be between 10% and 20%. A cardiac murmur may be transmitted to the neck. Stiff, calcified, or torturous vessels may generate a bruit in the absence of stenosis. Bruits may be absent in cases of severe stenosis.

- Duplex ultrasound
- Carotid angiography
  - Intra-arterial angiography is the traditional method of assessing degree of stenosis but it is associated with complications
    - 4% risk of inducing further neurological event
    - 1% risk of permanent stroke
- Magnetic resonance angiography
- CT brain scan (and carotid vessels with reconstruction)

Magnetic resonance angiography is increasingly used as a non-invasive technique without the complications of traditional angiography. Most surgeons will operate on the basis of non-invasive assessments such as duplex ultrasound in most uncomplicated cases.

Management of carotid disease

Medical management
- Stop smoking
- Pharmacological treatment of hypertension and diabetes
- Prophylactic aspirin/clopidogrel
- Statins

Aspirin prevents around 40 'vascular events' per 1000 patients treated for 3 years. It should be started daily once ischaemic stroke has been confirmed by CT.

Surgery for asymptomatic stenosis
There is evidence to suggest that surgery with a carotid endarterectomy for asymptomatic stenosis of 60% or more may decrease the long-term risk of stroke from 11% to 5%. Most patients in practice are offered surgery once stenosis is greater than 70%. This is currently a controversial topic amongst vascular surgeons.

Surgery for symptomatic stenosis
Surgery for symptomatic stenosis is offered when the stenosis is greater than 70%. The risk of having a subsequent CVA with a carotid stenosis greater than 70% is 20%–30%. Strong evidence suggests that surgery with a carotid endarterectomy reduces the risk of stroke and death due to stroke by more than 50%. This benefit is seen in institutions where there is a low peri-operative stroke and death rate.

Complications of surgery include:
- CVA (1%–2%)
- Transient ischaemic attack (3%–5%)
- Bleeding and haematoma
- Death (1%–2%)
- Nerve injuries
  - Great auricular nerve
  - Hypoglossal nerve
  - Glossopharyngeal nerve
  - Vagus nerve
  - Mandibular branch of the facial nerve

Carotid angioplasty (± stent placement) is being used to dilate stenoses. Recent studies suggest that there is a lower complication rate with stent placement than with carotid endarterectomy although further evidence is still awaited.

12.2.8 Aneurysms

An aneurysm is an abnormal, permanent, dilatation of a segment of an artery to greater than 1.5 times its normal diameter. It is related to a weakness in the wall of the blood vessel. The commonest artery to be affected is the aorta, followed by the popliteal and the femoral artery. An aneurysm of the aorta mandates the examination of the femoral and popliteal arteries to confirm or exclude the presence of an aneurysm. The converse is also true, ie that in the presence of a popliteal or femoral artery aneurysm, there is a 50% chance of an aortic aneurysm being present.

Common classifications

Anatomical (eg infrarenal aortic, suprarenal, iliac, femoral, popliteal)

Most common sites
- Infrarenal aorta
- Iliac
- Popliteal

Pathological
- True: lined by all three layers of arterial wall
- False: formed in the adventitia or completely outside the arterial wall

It is very important to distinguish between true and false aneurysms, as treatment modalities may differ. A false aneurysm is a pulsating haematoma and its cavity is in direct continuation with the lumen of the artery. It is contained by a fibrous capsule and usually results from trauma, eg femoral false aneurysm occurring after a femoral puncture for cardiac catheterisation.

Aetiological
- **Atherosclerotic/degenerative:** 80%
- **Post-traumatic:** 15%
- **Congenital:** 2% in coarctation, berry aneurysm
- **Inflammation:** evidence of peri-adventitial inflammatory and fibrotic response; 10%–15% of abdominal aortic aneurysms have evidence of inflammation, with thick anterior walls which have been known to compress adjacent structures such as the inferior vena cava and the ureters
- **Dissection:** intimal tear due to weakness in the aortic wall. Defect associated with atherosclerosis, hypertension, Marfan's syndrome, trauma
- **Connective tissue disorders:** Marfan's, Ehlers–Danlos, Takayasu's arteritis, tuberous sclerosis
- **Infection:** *Salmonella, Treponema* (syphilis), intravenous drug user (mycotic), infective endocarditis

Many different combinations of the above can be used to describe an aneurysm, eg it may be an inflammatory infrarenal abdominal aortic aneurysm.

Complications of aneurysms

General
- Rupture
- Hypovolaemic shock (due to rupture)
- Arterial embolism
- Insufficient circulation past the aneurysm

Specific to site
- Kidney failure (either direct effect or due to emboli)
- Myocardial infarction
- Stroke
- Aortic dissection
- Fistulation

Abdominal aortic aneurysm (AAA)
- Defined as focal widening > 3 cm
- Commonest in > 60 years; M:F = 6:1
- Mostly infrarenal (95%) with 30% involving iliac arteries
- Risk factors are same as those for peripheral vascular disease
- Plain film: mural calcifications (90%)
- CT: can show size of the aneurysm and peri-aneurysmal fibrosis (10%) which can cause ureteral obstruction
- US: 98% accuracy in width measurement of aneurysm sac but unable to show flow and lumen accurately
- Angiogram: able to show size and lumen calibre accurately. Mural thrombus is present in 80% of cases

Common causes
- Atherosclerosis
- Inflammatory
- Connective tissue disease
- Infection

Prevalence
- Affects 5% of men <65 years
- 6% of men aged 65–74 years
- 9% of men >75 years

Symptoms/signs
- Can be asymptomatic
- Pain in the abdomen
  - Severe, sudden, persistent or constant
  - Not colicky or spasmodic
  - May radiate to back, groin, buttocks, or legs

- Pulsatile abdominal mass
- Rupture
  - Abdominal tenderness and rigidity if ruptured
  - Severe, sudden or persistent pain in the lower back
  - Shock with rapid pulse or heartbeat sensations
- Embolus causing acute limb ischaemia or trash foot

Examination
- Generally unreliable to assess size by examination alone
- Predictability of aneurysm directly proportional to size:
  - 29% accuracy for AAAs of 3.0–3.9 cm
  - 50% accuracy for AAAs of 4.0–4.9 cm
  - 76% accuracy for AAAs of 5.0 cm or greater
- Abdominal obesity decreases the sensitivity of palpation

Investigations
- AXR: calcified wall
- US scan: diameter and relationship to renal arteries – may overestimate the size of an aneurysm compared to intra-operative measurements
- The frequency of scans depends on the size of the aneurysm:
  - For aneurysms between 3 cm and 4 cm, a yearly scan is needed
  - For aneurysms between 4 cm and 5 cm, a 6-monthly scan is needed
  - For aneurysms that are more than 5 cm, a 3-monthly scan is needed

Once the aneurysm is bigger than 5.5 cm an operation should be offered and a CT scan requested to outline the anatomy in greater detail (especially the relationship to the renal arteries).

Surgery
- Indicated if patient is symptomatic or if the size of the abdominal aneurysm is >5.5 cm

Options
- Dacron graft (laparotomy)
- Endovascular repair (stent via femoral arteriotomy)
- Plastic grafts – less than 5% mortality for elective repair
- Elective surgery has a mortality of less than 5%
- Emergency surgery for rupture carries a mortality of 50%–70%

Complications of surgical repair
- Immediate complications
  - Haemorrhage
  - Peripheral embolisation
- Early complications
  - Myocardial infarction
  - Renal failure

- Multiorgan failure
- Disseminated intravascular coagulation
- Acute respiratory distress syndrome
- Colonic ischaemia/spinal cord ischaemia
- Pneumonia
- Stroke
- Deep venous thrombosis/pulmonary embolism
- Late complications
  - Graft infection
  - Spontaneous occlusion of aorta
  - Aortoenteric fistula
  - Anastomotic aneurysm

Popliteal artery aneurysm
- This is the second most common site for atherosclerotic aneurysm
- Accounts for 70% of peripheral aneurysms
- 50% of cases are bilateral
- A third have an associated AAA
- Occasionally, present with a pulsatile mass in the back of the knee but are commonly diagnosed with aneurysm thrombosis or distal emboli leading to peripheral ischaemia
- Rupture is rare
- Aneurysm greater than 2 cm is regarded as significant
- Although most are discovered incidentally, patients may have symptoms of arterial insufficiency
- Investigate with duplex ultrasound/CT or angiogram to assess distal run-off
- Aneurysms of 2.5 cm or greater are usually treated surgically. Smaller ones are screened every 3–6 months
- Most common surgical treatment is ligation of the artery and bypass with a vein graft

Femoral artery aneurysm
- Mostly occur as part of generalised arterial dilatation rather than in isolation (rare)
- Most are false aneurysms following groin puncture
- Rarely rupture or cause symptoms
- Repair by prosthetic graft or reversed vein bypass
- Difficult to treat in IV drug abuse as chronic infections can form in prosthetic grafts

12.3 LYMPHATIC DISORDERS

12.3.1 Lymphoedema
Lymphoedema is the gradual swelling of limb(s) due to progressive failure of the lymphatic system (Box 12.1). It is characterised by painless non-pitting oedema.

Other causes of painless non-pitting oedema include:

- Post-phlebitic limb
- Extrinsic compression of the deep veins
- Deep venous incompetence
- Lymphoedema immobility

Box 12.1: Classification of lymphoedema

Primary lymphoedema
- Congenital (age < 1 year): can be familial or non-familial
- Praecox (age < 35 years): can be familial or non-familial
- Tarda (age > 35 years)

Secondary lymphoedema
- Malignancy/obstruction due to mass effect
- Surgery: axillary surgery or groin dissection
- Radiotherapy
- Infection: parasitic (eg filariasis)

Pathology
- Primary lymphoedema is the result of a spectrum of lymphatic disorders
  - Can be due to aplasia, hypoplasia or hyperplasia of lymphatics
  - In 80%, obliteration of distal lymphatics occurs
  - A proportion of patients have a family history (Milroy's disease)
  - In 10%, proximal occlusion of lymphatics in the abdomen and pelvis is seen
  - In 10%, lymphatic valvular incompetence develops
- Chronic lymphoedema results in subcutaneous fibrosis
- Fibrosis can be worsened by secondary infection

Management
The aims of treatment are to:

- Reduce limb swelling
- Improve limb function
- Prevent infections

Conservative treatment
- Skin care will reduce risk of infection
- Swelling can be reduced by elevation
- Physiotherapy and manual lymph drainage may help
- External pneumatic compression will also help reduce swelling
- Once swelling is reduced, compression stockings should be applied

- Antibiotics should be given at the first sign of infection
- Drugs (eg diuretics) are of no proved benefit

Surgery
- Surgery consists of two approaches
  - Debulking operations
    - Homan's procedure: debulking of subcutaneous tissues with closure
    - Charles' procedure: debulking of subcutaneous tissues with skin grafting
  - Bypass procedures
    - Mesenteric bridge: terminal ileal lymphatics connected to inguinal nodes
- Both aim to produce good functional results, although bypass is rarely successful
- Cosmesis is often poor for debulking procedures

12.3.2 Lymphangitis
Lymphangitis is inflammation of lymphatic channels and is manifested by erythematous streaks. It often accompanies cellulitis and is usually associated with a streptococcal infection. Regional lymphadenopathy is common. The morbidity and mortality associated with lymphangitis are related to the underlying infection. Although no specific data are available for lymphangitis, two-thirds of children with cellulitis are reported to be male and there is no age predilection.

Symptoms and signs
Red tender streaks in the line of lymphatics extending from the area of cellulitis towards local lymph nodes. Overlying skin may be red and it often accompanies cellulitis.

Causes
Group A β-haemolytic *Streptococcus* (GABHS) is most common. Other organisms may include *Staphylococcus aureus* and *Pseudomonas* species.

Treatment
Treat with penicillin if cellulitis is present. Lymphadenitis may follow drainage nodes to the site. Parenteral antibiotics may be required for a patient with signs of systemic illness (eg fever, chills and myalgia, lymphangitis). Analgesia, preferably non-steroidal anti-inflammatory drugs, should be given for pain. Limb elevation helps drainage of the lymphatics and healing with reduction of swelling.

12.4.1 Anatomy of lower limb veins

See Table 12.3 and Figure 12.5a.

Table 12.3: Anatomy of the lower limb
Superficial venous system
Long saphenous vein
1 cm anterior to the medial malleolus → 1 hand's breadth medial to the patella → femoral vein at the saphenofemoral junction (lateral to and 4 cm below the pubic tubercle)
Short saphenous vein
Continuation of the dorsal venous arch behind the lateral malleolus → midline of calf → deep fascia → popliteal vein at the saphenopopliteal junction (popliteal fossa)
Sinusoids
Small blood vessels similar to large capillaries
Deep venous system
Consists of veins and sinusoids
Lies deep within the muscles
Both sinusoids of the deep and superficial system drain into the deep veins through perforating (communicating) veins which traverse the deep fascia. They have valves to prevent backflow into the superficial system

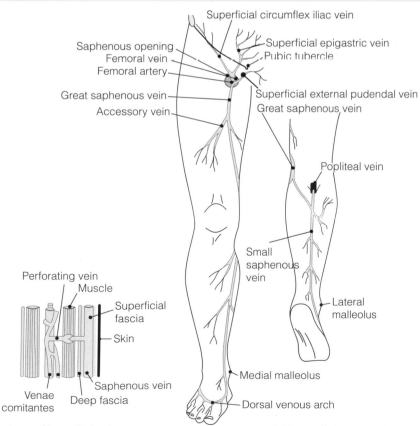

Figure 12.5a: Anatomy of lower limb veins

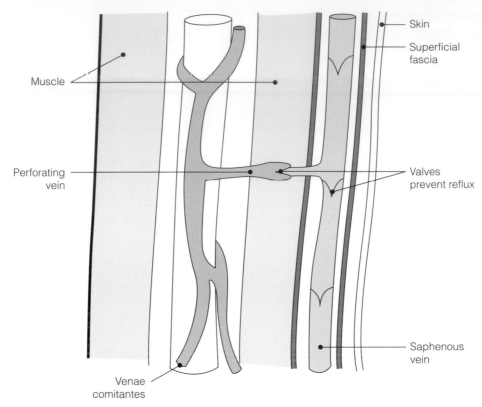

Muscle

Perforating vein

Venae comitantes

Skin

Superficial fascia

Valves prevent reflux

Saphenous vein

Figure 12.5b: Deep and superficial venous systems

Requirements for efficient venous drainage

- Competent heart pump
- Patent venous outflow tracts
- Efficient muscle pump
- Competent valves

Also, venous return is influenced by gravity and venomotor tone.

12.4.2 Examination for varicose veins

- Expose the patient after introducing yourself and obtaining consent to examine
- **Inspection** – start with patient standing
  - Distribution: dilated and tortuous veins in long or short saphenous distribution or other distribution
  - Venous stars: venulectasias – distended bluish vessels that may be palpable
  - Superficial thrombophlebitis: usually shows as inflamed veins which appear firm
  - Haemosiderosis, eczema, ulcers: also check for scarring from previous ulcerations
  - Lipodermatosclerosis: chronic venous hypertension results in fibrin deposition and progressive sclerosis of the skin and subcutaneous fat in the gaiter area
  - Ankle swelling/oedema (pitting): unilateral or bilateral, above/below the knee
  - Erythema: surrounding skin
  - Previous surgery scars: coronary artery bypass grafting usually requires saphenous venous grafts
  - Knee joint swelling, muscle wasting, bony deformity (including obvious disparity in limb length), TEDS
- **Palpation**
  - **Palpate varices:** along the complete length of the veins for any irregularities – notches, lumps (superficial thrombosis), tenderness and hardness (thrombophlebitis), and at the saphenofemoral junction for a saphena varix
  - **Tap test:** prominent veins in the calf are tapped. If there is an incompetent valve, the venous flow is continuous and the tap is felt at the other end
  - **Cough test:** when patient coughs, feel at the saphenofemoral junction for an impulse
- **Tourniquet test/Perthes test** (Box 12.2)
  - Tap, thrill, cough tests have a low sensitivity for detection of incompetent veins
  - Groin lump? Palpate to distinguish between: (1) saphena varix at the saphenofemoral junction, (2) hernia, (3) lymph node

- Compare sides
- Calf tenderness: underlying deep venous thrombosis (Homan's sign not reliable)
- Temperature of both legs
- Distal pulses and sensation (to assess arterial and diabetic disease of the foot)
- Pitting oedema

Box 12.2: Tourniquet and Perthes' tests

Tourniquet test (now outdated as the Doppler probe is used instead)

1 Ask patient to lie down
2 Raise leg and empty veins
3 Tie tourniquet around the mid-thigh – holding it in position, ask patient to stand
4 If veins do not fill, assume that the site of incompetence is above the tourniquet. When you release the tourniquet the veins will fill due to the column of blood flowing down the incompetent valves. Remember: with enough time all veins will fill due to blood passing the arterial system

Perthes' test (assess the deep venous system)
- Tourniquet around the thigh followed by walking/heel raising
- Emptying of surface veins indicates intact deep venous system and incompetence in the saphenous

Full abdominal and pelvic examination should be performed because the patient may have a pelvic mass or a pregnancy causing venous hypertension

Describe as mentioned below:

1 **Inspection findings and whether varicose veins are present:** include ulcers seen, lipodermatosclerosis, venous flares, eczema, swellings
2 **Describe inspection findings** (eg ulcer description, varicose distribution – short or long saphenous or neither)
3 **Where the incompetent valve(s) are:** based on clinical assessment and special tests
4 **Complications:** tenderness/pain, infection
5 **Further assessment findings:** pelvic and abdominal examination as necessary, distal pulses, distal neurology
6 **Plan of further investigation and management plans** (duplex scan, lifestyle changes, compression stocking, potential surgery)

Essential note

It is equally important to assess a patient's deep venous system as it is the superficial system. This can be achieved by a combination of clinical assessment and radiological scans. The reason for this is to inform the clinician of the potential cause of the varicose veins, as well as to give options for the different treatments available. Varicose vein surgery on the superficial system cannot be undertaken in patients with an incompetent or obstructed deep venous system

12.4.3 Varicose veins

Varicose veins are dilated, tortuous and elongated superficial veins. The most commonly affected veins are the long and short saphenous veins. They may be primary or secondary to an obstructed system (eg pelvic mass or deep venous thrombosis).

Demographics
- Affects 4.5% of population
- Peak in the 6th decade
- F:M = 4:1
- Obese
- Positive family history
- Occupations: long standing required (eg surgeons!)
- 20% incidence of recurrence after treatment

Causes
- **Primary or idiopathic (familial):** due to vein-wall laxity resulting in dilatation and valve leakage
- **Secondary:** obstruction/trauma
  - Physical: thrombosis, pelvic tumour
  - Functional: incompetent valves, abnormal communication between the deep and superficial veins
  - High pressure: arteriovenous fistulas, tricuspid incompetence (causing pulsating varicosities)

Signs and symptoms
Varicose veins are generally harmless, with most patients being asymptomatic for many years. Being unsightly is the commonest complaint from patients. Patients may complain of aching legs, itching, ankle swelling, night cramps, superficial thrombophlebitis, haemorrhage due to venous hypertension (eczema and ulceration), skin discoloration due to lipodermatosclerosis, and saphena varix (prominent dilatation at the saphenofemoral junction).

Venous claudication: occurs in severe cases when patients describe acute, bursting pain on walking that is relieved by rest and elevation of the leg.

Note: correlation between signs and symptoms is quite unreliable.

Occasionally patients can present with varicose veins due to a congenital abnormality such as Klippel–Trenaunay syndrome. This consists of:

- Congenital varicose veins
- Port-wine stains
- Bone and soft tissue hypertrophy
- Deep venous abnormalities

Types of veins that may be mistaken for varicose veins

Athletic veins
Normal enlarged veins on muscular legs.

Dilated veins
Known better as thread veins and spider bursts. These are due to a hormonal effect on soft skin. Commonly appear at menarche, during pregnancy and the menopause.

Investigations
- **Hand–held Doppler:** useful to diagnose incompetence at saphenofemoral/saphenopopliteal junctions. Squeezing the calf can augment a signal and a biphasic signal is heard if incompetence is present causing retrograde flow
- **Duplex screening:** investigation of choice as it is accurate and can diagnose valvular and perforator incompetence. It is also non-invasive and quick to perform
- **Venography:** also very accurate but more invasive and rarely required

Management

Conservative measures
- Elastic stockings (graduated compression)
- Weight reduction
- Exercise
- Elevation of legs
- Reassurance

Therapeutic management
The indications for surgery depend primarily on the patient's ability to cope. Any of the signs and symptoms can represent an indication.

Absolute indications would be:

- Lipodermatosclerosis/venous ulcers
- Recurrent superficial thrombophlebitis
- Bleeding from ruptured varix

Therapeutic management modalities:

- Injection sclerotherapy
- Laser therapy
- Surgery

Injection sclerotherapy: sodium tetradecyl sulphate
Sclerotherapy is best applied to small varicosities. Larger veins are unlikely to respond adequately and should be treated by laser or surgery.

A small amount of sclerosant is placed in the lumen of a vein which is then compressed with bandaging. The sclerosant irritates the venous intima, causing inflammation and subsequent fibrosis to obliterate the lumen of the vein. This can also be safely combined with surgery to achieve better results. The sclerosant used is usually a 3% solution of sodium tetradecyl sulphate.

Sclerotherapy rarely gives long-lasting results if the incompetence is either in the groin or at the back of the knee. Surgery is therefore advised in such patients in whom varicosities exist above the knee.

Foam may be used as an alternative to sclerotherapy.

Laser therapy and radiofrequency ablation
Endovenous laser therapy (EVLT) is now standard in most hospitals for treating varicose veins. This has replaced stripping as the results are better, with fewer complications of nerve damage compared with stripping. Equipment is expensive and there is a learning curve to train the surgeons. Most hospitals not offering this form of therapy will continue to use stripping and avulsions (below).

EVLT aims to use laser to coagulate and 'cook' the lumen of the vein along its length. This deliberate inflammation of the vein is to allow healing by fibrosis (damaged endothelium adheres to itself) and subsequent obliteration of the venous lumen. EVLT is naturally followed by compression bandaging during the healing period to allow its purpose to be achieved. EVLT can be combined with avulsions for best results in patients with multiple large varicose veins.

Radiofrequency ablation of the vein follows the exact same procedure and principles as laser therapy, except that it uses radiofrequency energy for coagulation instead of laser. It can be used in theatres not equipped to perform laser surgery.

Surgery

Surgery aims to disconnect the incompetent superficial system from the venous circulation. The commonest procedure is ligation (saphenofemoral or saphenopopliteal junction) and stripping of the long or short saphenous veins, combined with avulsions of the smaller, non-stripped varicosities.

It is essential before performing any surgery on the superficial venous system to ensure that the deep venous system is competent. Removing the superficial system, in the presence of a damaged deep system, can be disastrous to the patient.

Varicose vein complications

Complications arising from varicose veins:

- Superficial thrombophlebitis
- Eczema
- Lipodermatosclerosis – pigmentation due to haemosiderin deposition
- Ulceration
- Haemorrhage
- Marjolin's ulcer (malignant)

Complications of varicose vein surgery:

- Recurrence
- Bleeding and haematoma
- Leg swelling
- Infection
- Pain
- Deep venous thrombosis
- Paraesthesiae and nerve damage
- Scars

12.4.4 Deep venous thrombosis

Deep venous thrombosis (DVT) and pulmonary embolism (PE) are the leading cause of preventable in-hospital mortality in the Western world. Although PE is discussed further in medical textbooks, it must be emphasised that it is primarily a complication of DVT.

Pathophysiology

Virchow's triad, as first formulated, is still the primary mechanism for the development of thrombosis although the importance of each factor is highly debated. The triad consists of:

- Changes in vessel flow (venous stasis)
- Changes in vessel wall (vessel wall injury)
- Changes in blood constituents (hypercoagulable state)

Clinical features

There may be no symptoms relating to the location of the DVT, but the classic symptoms of DVT include pain, swelling and redness of the leg and dilatation of the surface veins. In up to 25% of all hospitalised patients, there may be some form of DVT, which often remains clinically inapparent.

There are several techniques during physical examination to increase the detection of DVT. Measuring the circumference of the affected and the contralateral limb at a fixed point can be helpful. Physical examination is generally unreliable for excluding a diagnosis of DVT.

Homan's sign: discomfort in the calf muscles on forced dorsiflexion of the foot with the knee straight has been a historical sign of DVT presence. This sign is present in fewer than one-third of patients with confirmed DVT and is found in more than 50% of patients without DVT. It is a very non-specific sign and not recommended as it may dislodge the clot.

Risk factors

Many risk factors for DVT have been mentioned in epidemiological studies. Some of the common risk factors are mentioned below. Most patients usually have a combination of a few factors:

- Age over 40
- Obesity
- Previous history of DVT
- Family history of blood clots in veins
- Haematologia: polycythaemia rubra vera, thrombocytosis, inherited disorders of coagulation/fibrinolysis, antithrombin III deficiency, protein C deficiency, protein S deficiency, factor V Leiden, dysfibrinogenaemias and disorders of plasminogen activation
- Malignancy
- Vascular disease or heart failure such as vasculitis, systemic lupus erythematosus (SLE) and the lupus anticoagulant, Behçet's syndrome, homocystinuria
- Immobility: recent surgery or an injury, especially knee or hip surgery, long-haul flights
- Drugs/medications: IV drug abuse, oral contraceptives, oestrogens, heparin-induced thrombocytopenia

The risk of DVT is also increased in women who:

- Take a contraceptive pill that contains oestrogen
- Take hormone replacement therapy (HRT)
- Are pregnant
- Have recently had a baby

It is vital that the clinical assessment also investigates features for a potential pulmonary embolus, as this may warrant further investigation. A careful history has to be taken considering risk factors, including the use of oestrogen-containing methods of hormonal contraception, recent long-haul flying, and a history of miscarriage (which is a feature of several disorders that can also cause thrombosis). A family history can reveal a hereditary factor in the development of DVT.

DVTs can also present in other less common ways. Other presentations of DVT include phlegmasia alba dolens, phlegmasia caerulea dolens and post-thrombotic syndrome. These form a clinical spectrum of the same disorder. All three manifestations result from acute massive venous thrombosis of the larger veins and obstruction of the venous drainage of an extremity.

Phlegmasia alba dolens (white leg)

This thrombosis involves only major deep venous channels of the extremity, therefore sparing collateral veins. The venous drainage is still present; the lack of venous congestion differentiates this entity from caerulea dolens. The leg is pale and swollen secondary to the oedema caused by the DVT.

Phlegmasia caerulea dolens (blue leg)

This is severe thrombophlebitis with extreme pain, oedema, cyanosis and possible ischaemic necrosis. In phlegmasia caerulea dolens, there is an acute and nearly total venous occlusion of the entire extremity outflow, including the iliac and femoral veins. The leg is usually painful, cyanosed and oedematous. Venous gangrene may supervene.

Post-thrombotic syndrome

This happens if DVT damages the valves in the deep veins, so that instead of flowing upwards, the blood pools in the lower leg. This can eventually lead to long-term pain, venous claudication, swelling, lipodermatosclerosis and, in severe cases, ulcers on the leg.

Investigations
- FBC, clotting, thrombophilia screen, duplex ultrasound

Prevention
- General:
  - Leg elevation
  - TED stocking
  - Early post-operative mobilisation
  - Intraoperative pneumatic compressions
  - Risk factor modification (if known, eg stop oral contraceptives)
- Medical:
  - Low-molecular-weight heparin
  - Warfarin
  - Aspirin

Treatment

Initial anticoagulation with heparin if no contraindications exist and then warfarin therapy. The duration of warfarin is dictated by local protocols and influenced by factors such as recurrent or primary DVTs, the presence of pulmonary emboli and other thrombotic risk factors. Prophylactic inferior vena cava filter placement may be performed in patients at extremely high risk (eg quadriplegics, severe closed head injury) or those who have a contraindication to other forms of prophylaxis and/or those who cannot be anticoagulated, but this only prevents pulmonary embolism, not DVT.

Reference

Criqui M H, Fronek A, Barrett-Connor E, Klauber M R, Gabriel S, Goodman D. 1985. The prevalence of peripheral arterial disease in a defined population. Circulation, 71(3), 510–515.

Urology

CONTENTS

Urology

Urology deals with surgical conditions of the urinary system from the kidneys down to the urethra. In males, the penis, scrotum and prostate are also dealt with by urologists and this often makes up a large bulk of any urologist's workload. At the undergraduate level, a sound understanding of the assessment of the urological system in addition to a basic knowledge of the common benign and malignant disorders is required. Congenital urological disorders are dealt with by specialists in paediatric urology and are beyond the scope of this revision text. These conditions, along with a revision of the relevant embryology, should be studied during the paediatric firm.

Revision objectives

You should:

- Know how to perform a urological assessment including history taking, examination and ordering relevant investigations as related to the clinical condition
- Know the different causes of haematuria and how to investigate it further
- Be aware of the classification of renal trauma and its relevance to management
- Know the causes, classification, assessment and management of renal stones
- Know the causes, main clinical features and management of benign urological diseases
- Know the different causes, clinical features and management of scrotal lumps
- Know the causes, epidemiology, clinical and pathological features of renal, bladder, prostate, penile and testicular cancer

13.1 UROLOGICAL ASSESSMENT

13.1.1 Urological history

Urological assessment consists of a general and targeted history in addition to focused examination and investigations. In addition to the standard questions and examination, there are some specific questions and terminology relating to urological conditions. The word 'prostatism' is no longer used by urologists, but it remains a commonly used term; 'lower urinary tract symptoms' (or LUTS) is the preferred term as

these symptoms can occur in men and women and may or may not necessarily be related to the prostate gland.

LUTS

Frequency	How often do you need to void during the day?
Urgency	Do you find it difficult to hold on?
Nocturia	How often do you have to get up in the night?
Dysuria	Do you have pain on passing urine?
Hesitancy	Do you have to wait before you start to void?
Straining	Do you have to strain to void?
Poor stream	How is your flow/stream?
Terminal dribbling	Do you find that you dribble after passing urine?
Intermittency	Do you stop and start during your void?
Incomplete voiding	Do you have the sensation of not emptying your bladder?

LUTS may be best split into two main category of symptoms: obstructive and irritative.

Obstructive symptoms may indicate some degree of obstruction within the urinary tract and include:

- Hesitancy
- Straining
- Poor stream
- Incomplete voiding
- Terminal dribbling

Irritative symptoms may indicate some degree of detrusor instability resulting in involuntary contractions of the distended bladder. These symptoms all may be exacerbated by urinary tract infections (UTIs):

- Frequency
- Urgency
- Nocturia
- Urge incontinence

Other urological symptoms

Loin pain

This may be acute or chronic. Most acute loin pain is thought to be renal colic, but 50% of patients with colic symptoms never pass a stone and also do not have a stone on imaging.

- **Acute pain**
  - Renal or clot colic
  - Pelvi-ureteric junction obstruction (PUJO)
  - Pyelonephritis

- Testicular torsion
- Trauma to the kidney

There are many non-urological causes, the most important of which is a leaking abdominal aortic aneurysm. In the presence of normal imaging, other causes should be investigated.

- **Chronic pain**
  - Tumour
  - Stones
  - Infection
  - PUJO

Urinary incontinence
It is defined as an involuntary leakage of urine. It can be an embarrassing symptom, which needs to be characterised to aid treatment.

Stress incontinence	Leakage of urine with raised abdominal pressure such as cough, sneeze, lifting
Urge incontinence	Leakage of urine preceded by or with a feeling of urgency
Mixed incontinence	A combination of stress and urge incontinence
Nocturnal enuresis	Incontinence while asleep
Continuous incontinence	Overflow incontinence (chronic retention) Permanently wet Implies a fistula or ectopic ureter
Functional incontinence	Incontinence with a normal urinary tract Occurs due to immobility or confusion in the patient

Haematuria (see Section 13.1.3)
- Blood in the urine
- Macroscopic (visible to the naked eye)
- Microscopic (detected on dipstick only)

13.1.2 Urological examination
A urological examination consists of a standard abdominal examination with particular attention to the loin to assess for the presence of a renal mass. The suprapubic region should also be examined by palpation and percussion for an enlarged bladder. Any abdominal examination should include an examination of the regional lymph nodes and external genitalia in males. The examination should be concluded with a digital rectal examination to assess the prostate in males.

- **Scrotum**
  - Number of testes
  - Size of testes
  - Testicular masses
  - Position of testes
  - Peritesticular swellings
  - Transilluminate for hydrocoele
  - Cough impulse for groin hernia
- **Penis**
  - Urethral opening
  - Hypospadias presence
  - Foreskin
- **Digital rectal examination**
  - Size of prostate
  - Texture
  - Nodule presence
  - Pain

13.1.3 Haematuria
This is one of the commonest presenting symptoms in urology. It is macroscopic (gross or frank) if the patient has seen blood. Microscopic or dipstick haematuria is detected by microscopy or dipstick testing and is variably defined as 3–10 red blood cells per high-power field. Microscopic haematuria is often asymptomatic and found incidentally. Dipsticks detect haem with a peroxidase. False positives are possible in the presence of myoglobin, povidone and hypochlorite. Seventy per cent of patients with microscopic haematuria have no significant cause.

Painless macroscopic haematuria should be regarded as being caused by a malignancy until proved otherwise. It is a criterion for being seen within the 2-week rule, as is symptomatic microscopic haematuria in patients >50 years old, although this is a source of much debate among urologists.

The causes of haematuria are listed in Box 13.1.

Investigation of haematuria
Most haematuria referrals are directed to a one-stop haematuria clinic. This aims to minimise repeat appointments for various tests and enables a rapid diagnosis for the patient with faster treatment times. The following investigations are usually available in the one-stop environment:

- Urine culture
- Urine cytology
  - High specificity but low sensitivity for transitional cell carcinoma (TCC)
  - Equivocal results in the presence of infection or instrumentation

Box 13.1: Causes of haematuria

Urological causes
- Cancer
  - Bladder
  - Kidney
  - Prostate
  - Renal pelvis and ureter
- Infection of upper or lower tract
  - Bacterial including TB
  - Parasitic, eg schistosomiasis
  - Fungal
- Stones
  - Renal, ureteric or bladder
- Trauma
  - Renal, bladder, urethra

- Benign prostatic hypertrophy
- Nephrological
  - IgA nephropathy, post-infective glomerulonephritis, etc

Coagulation disorders
- Warfarin
- Congenital

Iatrogenic
- Radiotherapy
- Cyclophosphamide
- Thrombolysis

- Kidney–urinary–bladder (KUB) film
  - May reveal stone disease
- Renal tract ultrasound
  - Renal masses, bladder masses >1 cm. Low pick-up rate for upper tract TCC
- Flexible cystoscopy
  - Bladder tumours, stone disease, colovesical fistula

Flexible cystoscopy is the mainstay of the clinic and allows identification of very small tumours not detected by USS. Further imaging may be required with an intravenous urogram or IVU, if all investigations are normal and there is a high index of suspicion (eg if urine cytology is positive in the absence of a visible bladder tumour).

IVUs are better at initially detecting upper TCCs. CT may be required to further characterise renal masses. Although IVUs are not regarded as diagnostic of upper tract TCC, any filling defect seen needs further investigation with retrograde pyelography and ureteroscopy, which would allow for a tissue diagnosis. If all investigations are normal the patient may be referred back to the GP with a low threshold for re-referral if there should be further bleeding.

13.2 RENAL TRAUMA AND BENIGN UROLOGICAL CONDITIONS

13.2.1 Renal trauma
The majority of renal trauma in the developed world is blunt-force trauma (Europe 97%), with the remainder being penetrating. The reason for this classification is that 95% of blunt injuries can be managed conservatively, whereas 75% of gunshot wounds and 50% of stab wounds require surgery. As

the kidneys are retroperitoneal organs, they are relatively well protected and a significant amount of trauma is required to damage them. Co-existing organ damage is common, especially splenic injuries on the left-hand side. The kidneys are also surrounded by a tough capsule which tamponades the majority of bleeding and allows for conservative treatment.

Renal trauma is graded using the American Association for the Surgery of Trauma organ severity scale (ASST):

Grade I	Contusion or subcapsular haematoma
Grade II	<1 cm deep laceration of cortex, no extravasation of urine
Grade III	>1 cm deep laceration of cortex, no extravasation of urine
Grade IV	Laceration involving cortex, medulla and collecting system, or renal vessel damage with contained bleeding
Grade V	Shattered kidney or avulsion of renal pedicle

Grade I – IV blunt renal injuries are managed conservatively, as are grade V injuries, provided the patient retains haemodynamic stability. Standard trauma management consists of Advanced Trauma Life Support (ATLS) principles with fluid and blood resuscitation, close monitoring and ensuring that the patient remains stable with conservative management. An inability to maintain a stable patient requires aggressive resuscitation and surgery (nephrectomy).

13.2.2 Stone disease
Urological stone disease can be categorised as renal stones and bladder stones. Renal stones make up the majority of stone disease in the UK but bladder stones remain common in Southeast Asia and North Africa.

Stone types (see Box 13.2)

Most stones contain calcium, making them radio-opaque. The amount of calcium within a stone dictates the radiodensity. Up to 20% of uric acid stones contain some calcium oxalate and can be radio-opaque as well at times. Stones form when the concentrations of the constituents rise above the level at which they are metastable and the urine becomes supersaturated. Crystals form around nuclei and aggregate into clumps. Compounds such as magnesium and citrate inhibit aggregation.

Kidney stones

Aetiology

- Commonest between 20 and 50 years old
- Male to female ratio 3:1
- Common in whites (10% by age 70) and Asians, rare in Afro-Caribbeans
- Peak incidence in the summer
- Low fluid intake, <1.2 l a day
- High-protein diet
- Low-calcium diet (calcium in the diet binds to oxalate and phosphate, preventing absorption)

Clinical presentation

Stones either present with symptoms or they are found incidentally on imaging. The commonest symptom is pain, which ranges from an occasional vague discomfort in the loin to classic renal colic.

Renal colic

- Usually loin to groin, but can be groin to loin
- Colicky
- May radiate to testicle
- No position relieves pain
- Nausea and vomiting
- Haematuria, usually microscopic but can be macroscopic
- Not to be confused with a leaking abdominal aortic aneurysm

Stones may act as a nidus for recurrent UTIs and are a cause of micro and macroscopic haematuria.

Management of renal colic

- History and examination (beware abdominal aortic aneurysm)
- Analgesia
- Non-steroidal anti-inflammatory drugs unless contraindicated
- Opiates and antiemetics
- Antibiotics if signs of sepsis (after immediate blood cultures)
- Urine dip and pregnancy test
- FBC and U&E and blood cultures if signs of sepsis are present
- KUB and IVU (CT-KUB if available)
- Further management will depend on the size and position of stone and the presence of sepsis. **The obstructed infected kidney is an emergency, which will require urgent ureteric stenting or nephrostomy**

General investigations for renal stones

- Urine dipstick ± culture
- KUB
  - Good for radio-opaque stones
  - Phleboliths may cause confusion in the pelvis

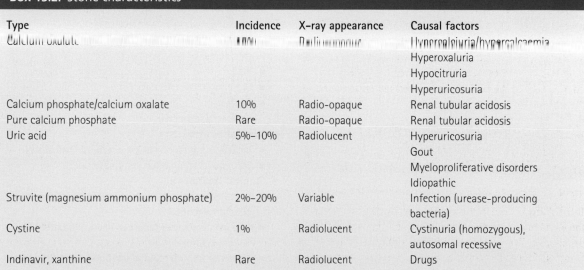

Box 13.2: Stone characteristics

Type	Incidence	X-ray appearance	Causal factors
Calcium oxalate	80%	Radio-opaque	Hypercalciuria/hypercalcaemia Hyperoxaluria Hypocitruria Hyperuricosuria
Calcium phosphate/calcium oxalate	10%	Radio-opaque	Renal tubular acidosis
Pure calcium phosphate	Rare	Radio-opaque	Renal tubular acidosis
Uric acid	5%–10%	Radiolucent	Hyperuricosuria Gout Myeloproliferative disorders Idiopathic
Struvite (magnesium ammonium phosphate)	2%–20%	Variable	Infection (urease-producing bacteria)
Cystine	1%	Radiolucent	Cystinuria (homozygous), autosomal recessive
Indinavir, xanthine	Rare	Radiolucent	Drugs

- USS
  - Up to 95% sensitivity for renal stones
  - Not good for ureteric stones
  - Detects opaque and lucent stones
- IVU (intravenous urogram)
  - Requires injection of intravenous contrast
  - Possible allergic reaction
  - Outlines renal collecting system
  - Helps to detect level of obstruction
  - May require multiple images over a 24-hour period
- CT
  - No contrast needed
  - Detects radiolucent stones

Management options
There are often a number of possible ways to treat any stone. A balance needs to be struck between the number of interventions required and the invasiveness of the procedure. The following options are only a guide.

Asymptomatic stones
- If small and not causing obstruction these may be left
- Annual surveillance may be indicated if large
- Staghorn stones, if treated conservatively, require prophylactic antibiotics

Symptomatic stones
- If <4 mm and in the ureter 95% pass spontaneously
- Large or obstructing stones
  - Endoscopic ureteric stenting
  - Ureteroscopy and extraction
    - Lithoclast
    - Laser
  - Extracorporeal shockwave lithotripsy (ESWL)
    - Depends on machine availability
    - Position of stone if in ureter
- Large stones in the kidney
  - <1 cm
    - Flexible ureteroscopy and laser
    - ESWL
  - >1 cm
    - Percutaneous nephrolithotomy (PCNL)
    - Laparoscopic or open surgery

Bladder stones
In the UK these are usually found in men over the age of 50 with bladder outflow obstruction secondary to benign prostatic hyperplasia. They are also found in the chronically catheterised patient, with no difference in incidence found between urethral or suprapubic catheterisation.

Symptoms include suprapubic pain, haematuria, urgency and incontinence, recurrent UTIs and LUTS. Spinal injury patients may be asymptomatic.

The stones are usually easily visible on KUB or USS.

Most stones can be removed or crushed endoscopically; rarely, a formal cystotomy and extraction is needed.

13.2.3   Benign prostatic and urethral disease
The prostate gland lies inferior to the bladder and surrounds the prostatic urethra. It normally weighs about 20 g, but in prostatic hypertrophy it can enlarge to several times this weight.

Diseases of the prostate and urethral strictures account for the majority of causes of lower urinary tract obstruction. Upper urinary tract obstruction is most commonly caused by stones, malignancy and PUJ obstruction.

Benign prostatic hypertrophy (BPH) (see Figure 13.1)
- Very common condition characterised by an increase in both glandular and stromal components of the prostate gland
- Affects 50% of men over the age of 50, and almost all men by the age of 80
- Unknown aetiology although thought to be due to male hormone imbalance
- Affects the transitional zone of the prostate, with subsequent urethral compression
- Clinical presentations include obstructive LUTS or urinary retention (acute or chronic)
- **Investigate with:**
  - Urinalysis to exclude UTI
  - Renal biochemistry to exclude upper tract obstructive uropathy
  - Prostate-specific antigen (PSA) to check for prostate carcinoma
  - Bladder scan to assess residual volume after voiding
  - Urine flow rate <10 ml/second implies obstruction
  - Urodynamic studies if neurological disease of the bladder is suspected
- **Medical treatments:**
  - Include α_1-antagonists (eg tamsulosin, alfuzosin)
  - 5α-reductase inhibitors (eg finasteride)
- **Surgical treatment:**
  - Indicated in patients with recurrent infections, stones, or acute retention
  - Also indicated after failure of medical treatment to treat symptoms
  - Transurethral resection of the prostate (TURP) is the surgical treatment of choice

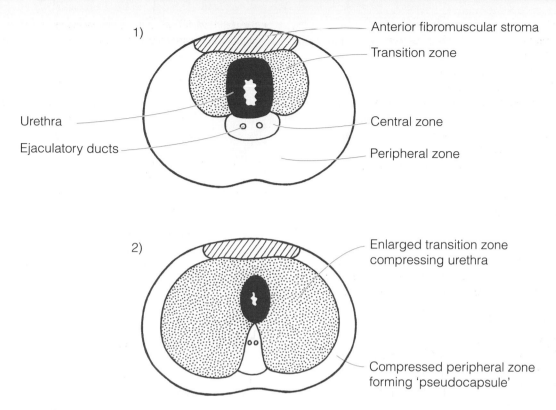

1)

- Anterior fibromuscular stroma
- Transition zone
- Central zone
- Peripheral zone

Urethra

Ejaculatory ducts

2)

- Enlarged transition zone compressing urethra

- Compressed peripheral zone forming 'pseudocapsule'

Figure 13.1: Benign prostatic hypertrophy

TURP complications

- Bleeding
- Infection
- Failure to void
- Incontinence
- Impotence
- Retrograde ejaculation
- Urethral stricture
- **TURP syndrome**
  - Due to absorption of large volumes of irrigation fluid intraoperatively
  - Hypertension, bradycardia, hyponatraemia, nausea, vomiting, cerebral oedema, seizures can all occur
  - Treat with fluid restriction and diuretics, and ITU if necessary

Prostatitis

- Inflammation of the prostate gland, often related to bladder outflow obstruction
- Patient may present with cystitis, fever, purulent discharge, pain on ejaculation, haematospermia
- Investigate with urine culture, blood cultures and transrectal ultrasound of the prostate
- Treat with appropriate antibiotics (usually ciprofloxacin and doxycycline)

Urethral strictures

Urethral stricture is a narrowing of the urethra due to scar tissue. This results in obstructive (LUTS) symptoms as well as recurrent UTIs. Patients can also present with acute urinary retention.

Causes

- Trauma
  - Catheterisation/instrumentation
  - Operative trauma (TURP, bladder neck incision, cystoscopy)
  - Pelvic fractures
  - Straddle injuries
- Infection
  - Gonococcal urethritis
  - Non-gonococcal urethritis
- Neoplasms
  - Penile cancer
  - Prostate cancer
  - Bladder cancer
    - Cystoscopy, TURP, bladder neck incision

Treatment

- Urethral dilation is possible if the stricture is not too tight
- The commonest procedure is optical urethrotomy, where the stricture is divided endoscopically under direct vision. A catheter is left in place for a few days post operatively
  - Repeat surgery is required in about 50% of cases. This can be reduced by intermittent self-dilation
- Long or complicated strictures are best managed with reconstructive surgery such as excision and re-anastomosis or substitution urethroplasty

Urinary retention

Retention of urine may be acute or chronic:

- Acute urinary retention (AUR) – an acute painful condition in which there is an inability to micturate
- Chronic retention – a chronic (usually painless) condition in which there is a post-void residual of more than 300 ml of urine. It may present with renal failure or overflow incontinence

Causes of AUR

- Any cause of lower urinary tract obstruction (bladder outflow obstruction)
  - BPH
  - Prostate carcinoma
  - Urethral stricture
  - Meatal stenosis
  - Congenital posterior urethral valves
  - Bladder or urethral stone
- Neurological disease
  - Detrusor dysfunction
  - Non-coordination between bladder contraction and sphincter relaxation
  - Multiple sclerosis
  - Spinal tumour or cord compression

Predisposing factors

- UTI
- Constipation
- Post-operative (pain, immobility, drugs, anaesthesia)
- Anticholinergic medication

Clinical features

- Painful inability to pass urine (M>F 10:1)
- Tender, distended and palpable bladder

Management

- Urgent urethral or suprapubic catheterisation
- Identify and treat any causes and predisposing factors
- Trial with α_1-blockers and TWOC (trial without catheter) in 48 hours

- Treat BPH with TURP and urethral strictures with dilation or optical urethrotomy
- Long-term catheterisation may be needed in some patients unfit for surgery or those with a neurological cause of retention that does not respond to medications

Management of chronic retention

- Treat with catheterisation until renal function settles
- TURP if BPH is the cause after normalisation of renal function
- Intermittent self-catheterisation or long-term catheterisation for conditions not suitable for surgery or responding to medications

13.2.4 Benign penile conditions

Penile anatomy

The structure of the penis is shown in Figure 13.1.

Circumcision

- Removal of the prepuce (foreskin)
- A simple surgical procedure, though not without potential complications
- Often a full circumcision can be avoided by performing either a frenuloplasty or a preputioplasty

Indications

- Recurrent balanitis, balanoposthitis
- Phimosis that has failed conservative treatment
- HIV prophylaxis
- Religious (not on NHS)

Complications

- Haematoma
- Infection
- Poor cosmetic result
- Necrosis of shaft skin
- Urethrocutaneous fistula

Phimosis

Phimosis is a condition in which the foreskin of the penis is unable to be retracted behind the glans. This is physiologically normal after birth due to preputial adhesions. These break down naturally, and by the age of 5, 90% of boys have a retractile foreskin. By puberty >99% are retractile.

Development of balanitis xerotica obliterans (BXO) can lead to a tight phimosis. If the foreskin is forcibly retracted and becomes stuck, this is known as a paraphimosis. Other complications include, balanitis, chronic inflammation and balanoposthitis, where pus may be retained behind a tight preputial band.

Structure of the Penis

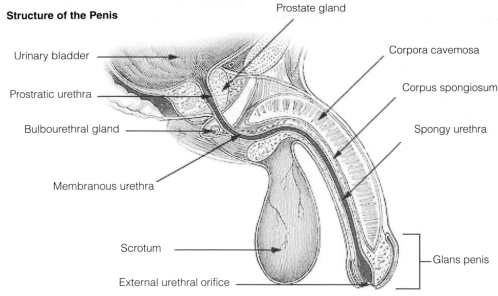

Figure 13.2 Structure of the penis

Treatment is possible with a 6-week course of topical steroid cream. As most phimosis resolves naturally, circumcision should be avoided.

Paraphimosis

This occurs when a tight foreskin has been forcibly retracted and becomes stuck behind the glans. It may also occur iatrogenically if the foreskin is not replaced after catheterisation. If left retracted, it leads to a swollen glans and an oedematous prepuce. The more swollen it becomes the harder it is to reduce. Manual compression is usually enough to reduce the oedema and allow correct positioning; occasionally surgical intervention is required with a dorsal slit. If the prepuce has become necrotic full circumcision may be required.

Balanitis xerotica obliterans

Commonly referred to as BXO and is also called lichen sclerosus et atrophicus.

- Common
- Affects prepuce and glans
- All age groups
- Shiny white appearance
- Can cause meatal stenosis and distal urethral strictures
- Long-standing BXO can be a premalignant condition

Treatment

Treatment is initially with a topical steroid cream. Circumcision may be needed for long-standing BXO. Meatal and urethral lesions may require reconstructive surgery.

Peyronie's disease

Benign condition affecting the penile shaft, leading to curvature in all possible directions.

Men seek treatment due to pain or inability to penetrate during intercourse.

- Up to 1% of men affected
- 40–60 years
- Initial onset may be painful (first 6 months)
- Curvature settles by a year
- Palpable plaque of fibrosis in tunica albuginea
- Thought to be due to micro-trauma
- Linked to Dupuytren's contracture in 10–25% of cases

Treatment

- There is no ideal treatment for this condition
- Medical therapies include vitamin E, tamoxifen and colchicine although results are generally disappointing
- Corrective surgery with Nesbitt's procedure is a last resort to straighten the penis and allow penetration, although shortening always occurs

Priapism

A prolonged and often painful erection lasting more than 4–6 hours without a sexual stimulus.

It was a relatively common occurrence due to the use of intra-cavernosal drugs for erectile dysfunction. With the advent of oral treatments it is far less common.

Low-flow

- Venous occlusion
- Painful, due to ischaemia
- Blood gas from cavernosum, acidotic
- >4 hours requires intervention

Causes

- Drugs
- Intracavernosal prostaglandin PGE_1
- Cocaine, warfarin, heparin, clozapine, antidepressants and α-blockers
- Sickle cell disease, leukaemia, thalassaemia
- Neurogenic
- Malignant invasion

High-flow

- Secondary to an arteriovenous fistula
- Not painful, as not ischaemic
- Fistula caused by penile or perineal trauma

Treatment

If presentation is before 4 hours and secondary to erectile dysfunction medication, try exercise and/or masturbation. If it does not resolve:

- Aspirate corpora, 50 ml at a time
- May require intracavernosal α_1-agonist, eg phenylephrine
- Corporal shunt, large-bore needle through spongiosum into cavernosum
- Sickle cell, treat crisis
- High-flow priapism may respond to cooling, otherwise embolisation is needed

Complications of delayed or failed treatment are fibrosis and impotence.

13.2.5 The scrotum and undescended testis

Scrotal lumps

Scrotal lumps are common in clinical practice and the main causes are listed here. A simple clinical examination should be able to distinguish between the causes, but occasionally an ultrasound examination will be necessary to confirm the diagnosis.

Differential diagnosis

- Inguinal hernia
- Hydrocoele
- Epididymal cyst
- Testicular tumour
- Varicocoele
- Sebaceous cyst
- TB

Inguinal hernia

Inguinal hernia is covered in Section 4.3.2. It suffices to say that if you cannot get above the lump and you are able to reduce it, it is the likely diagnosis.

Hydrocoele

Some fluid between the layers of the tunica vaginalis and tunica albuginea is normal. An abnormal amount constitutes a hydrocoele.

Clinical features

- Smooth, tense
- Painless
- Difficult to feel testis
- Transilluminates
- Primary
  - Idiopathic
  - Slow onset
  - No precipitating factors
  - Classified into
    - Congenital hydrocoele – connects with peritoneal cavity (sac)
    - Vaginal hydrocoele – surrounds testis
    - Infantile hydrocoele – anywhere from testis to deep inguinal ring
    - Hydrocoele of the cord – lies anywhere with the cord (not tunica)
- Secondary
  - Tumour
  - Infection
  - Trauma
    - Haematocoele

Treatment

Treatment is only required if it causes symptoms such as pain or physical inconvenience. Surgery may be performed to either excise the sac (Jaboulay's procedure) or to plicate the sac (Lord's procedure). Haematoma is a common complication due to the lax nature of the scrotum preventing tamponade. Aspiration of the fluid should be restricted to patients who are too unfit for surgery, as it will inevitably recur and may become infected, making surgery more difficult.

Epididymal cysts

These small cysts arise from the collecting tubules:

- Smooth
- Fluctuant
- Separate from testis
- Can get above it
- Usually occurring in men over 40
- Can be single or multiple

- Can be tender although usually slow to enlarge and painless
- Transilluminate if large enough and clear
- Called a spermatocoele if they contain milky-white opalescent fluid
- Aspiration or excision possible
- Caution with surgery in fertile men as can obstruct epididymis

Testicular tumour
See Section 13.3.4 for testicular malignancies.

Varicocoele
Dilatation of the veins surrounding the testis (pampiniform plexus varicosities) and can extend up the cord:

- Occasionally referred to as a varix
- More common on the left side
- Feels like a 'bag of worms'
- Should be examined with the patient standing
- Should disappear on lying
- May cause ache or dragging sensation
- Bilateral varicosities can cause subfertility
- Affected testis may be smaller
- Sudden onset of a left varix may imply a left renal vein obstruction by renal cell cancer

Small varicocoeles are a normal finding and treatment should be reserved for symptoms. A scrotal support may help relieve symptoms. Subfertility or failure of symptoms to resolve are good indications for treatment. Radiological embolisation is popular and a number of surgical approaches exist. All involve ligating the veins at various levels, usually via an inguinal approach. Complications include pain and recurrence.

Sebaceous cyst
A small lump in the scrotal skin no different from a sebaceous cyst anywhere else on the body:

- Fixed to skin
- Smooth
- Punctum

They can be excised if bothersome or they become infected.

Undescended testis
The testes should pass through the inguinal canal after the 24th week of development and descend into the scrotum in the third trimester. Failure to do so results in cryptorchidism.

Incidence
- 5% at birth
- Unilateral > bilateral

- 80% descend by 3 months
- 0.5% have not resolved by 1 year

Aetiology
- Abnormal testis
- Low androgen levels
- Decreased intra-abdominal pressure
  - eg Prune belly syndrome

Risk factors
- Twins
- Pre-term
- Low birth weight

Classification
- Retractile, not true cryptorchidism
- Ectopic (<5%)
  - Perineum
  - Base of penis
  - Femoral region
- Incomplete descent
  - Abdominal
  - Inguinal
  - Superficial inguinal pouch
- Abnormal position after the age of 2 results in histological changes, including:
  - Degeneration of Sertoli cells
  - Abnormal spermatogenesis

Complications
- Relative risk of cancer increase 10-fold
- Reduced fertility
- Increased risk of testicular torsion

Treatment
- Retractile testis is normal and requires parental reassurance
- Otherwise depends on whether the testis is palpable. An orchidopexy can be performed to place the testicle in the scrotum
- If it is not palpable, further imaging (USS or MRI) or laparoscopy may be required. Chromosomal analysis and hormone testing may be required

Testicular torsion
Any acute testicular pain should be regarded as a surgical emergency and torsion until proved otherwise:

- Commonest in adolescence
- Histological damage can occur after 4–6 hours
- Unlikely to survive after 24 hours

- Sudden onset of pain in scrotum with a swollen, painful, high-riding testis
- Can also present with abdominal pain and vomiting
- Pain secondary to testicular ischaemia
- History of intermittent torsion possible

Differential diagnosis
- Trauma
- Infection (epididymo-orchitis)
- Torsion of testicular appendix (hydatid of Morgagni)

Management
If the patient presents within 24 hours, surgical exploration is recommended over imaging, as this may not be conclusive. If the testicle has undergone torsion and does not recover, then orchidectomy is recommended, to reduce the risk of producing anti-sperm antibodies. The contralateral testis should be fixed.

Epididymo-orchitis

Clinical features
- Inflammation of both the epididymis (epididymitis) and testis (orchitis)
- Epididymitis (bacterial) is more common than orchitis (viral – mumps, coxsackievirus)
- Presents with acute-onset testicular pain and swelling, difficult to distinguish from torsion
- Symptoms of UTI and sepsis can be present

Investigations
- Urinalysis
- Ultrasound to exclude an abscess

Pathogenesis
- Usually due to *Chlamydia* or gonorrhoea in young men
- Usually due to *Escherichia coli* in older men

Treatment
- Bedrest
- Scrotal support
- Anti-inflammatory analgesia
- Antibiotics
  - Doxycycline and ciprofloxacin

13.3 UROLOGICAL MALIGNANCY

13.3.1 Bladder cancer
This is the second most common urological malignancy. The majority of cases are curable or controllable.

Aetiology and epidemiology
- Male to female ratio 2.5:1
- Age 60–80
- Risk factors include:
  - Smoking (causes 30%–50% of tumours)
  - Chronic inflammation, eg schistosomiasis, stones, long-term catheters, infections
  - Occupation – rubber, dye, chemical manufacture. Due to β-napthylamine exposure
  - Cyclophosphamide
  - Pelvic radiotherapy

Pathology and staging
In the UK the majority of bladder cancers are transitional cell carcinomas (>90%); worldwide, the commonest are squamous cell carcinomas secondary to schistosomiasis infection. Due to the increase in smoking in the developing world the incidences of the two types are now almost equal. Lymphomas, melanomas and sarcomas are rare. Metastatic deposits may be seen. Direct spread is through the wall of the bladder into local organs. Lymphatic spread is to the iliac and para-aortic nodes haematogenous spread most commonly involves the liver (37%), bone (28%), lung (38%) and adrenal (19%).

Tumour differentiation is graded as well, moderate or poor and is recorded as G1, G2 or G3. Staging is by the TNM system (see Figure 13.2).

The important cut-off in staging is between T1 (superficial), invasion of lamina propria, and T2 (invasive), invasion of the muscle layer. T1 disease can be managed endoscopically, T2 disease requires radical treatment as it carries a 50% 5-year survival. Carcinoma-in-situ is a poorly differentiated tumour

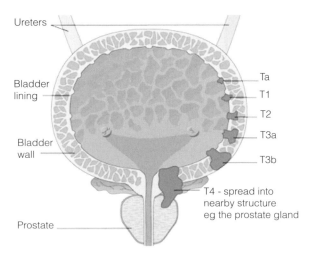

Figure 13.2: Staging of bladder cancer

confined to the epithelial layer. It can be very aggressive with a 40%–80% chance of the tumour becoming invasive.

Presentation

The commonest presenting symptom is painless macroscopic haematuria (85%). Microscopic haematuria is a less reliable symptom, though it requires investigation. Increase in urinary urgency and frequency can be caused by a malignant cystitis or by a tumour mass effect. UTIs can occur secondary to tumour colonisation. Metastatic disease can present with weight loss, lower limb oedema, obstructive renal failure or bone pain.

Diagnosis

The majority of tumours are diagnosed with flexible cystoscopy. This is a quick and easy procedure that forms the backbone of a one-stop haematuria clinic. Urine cytology can be helpful as it is very specific but not highly sensitive, especially in lower grade tumours. Ultrasound can pick up relatively small tumours around 0.5 mm in size, but trabeculated bladders can be misleading. Histology is obtained by transurethral resection (TURBT), and for superficial tumours this is also curative treatment. Staging requires a chest, abdomen and pelvis CT scan.

Treatment

Superficial tumours are managed by TURBT and adjuvant intravesical chemotherapy with mitomycin C, which is instilled into the bladder for 1 hour following resection. This has been shown to reduce recurrence rates. The bladder is followed up for 10 years with regular flexible cystoscopy; any recurrences are treated with TURBT; multiple recurrences may be treated by a course of intravesical chemotherapy over a 6-week period. Intravesical BCG can also be used and is more effective than mitomycin C at preventing recurrences. It works by upregulating the immune response.

Invasive tumours require radical cystectomy, with possible neoadjuvant chemotherapy. Urine is diverted into an ileal conduit or a reconstructed bladder. Patients who are not fit for surgery or who do not wish to have a stoma can have radical radiotherapy.

13.3.2 Prostate cancer

Since the advent of prostate-specific antigen (PSA) testing in 1989, the incidence of prostate cancer has more than doubled. It is the commonest male malignancy and the second commonest cause of cancer deaths in males. There has been little change in the mortality rate over the last 30 years. The majority of prostate cancers do not become clinically significant.

Aetiology and epidemiology

The greatest risk factor for developing adenocarcinoma of the prostate is age: 75% of prostate cancers are diagnosed in men over the age of 65. It is more common in the West: migrants from Asia and Japan are up to 20 times more likely to develop the disease compared with residents in their home nations. This implies an environmental factor, possibly diet. Afro-Caribbean residents in the USA are the highest-risk group. Five to ten per cent of prostate cancers could be hereditary.

Prostate cancer is promoted by testosterone and dihydrotestosterone and removal of testosterone leads to apoptosis of tumour cells. This provides the mechanism for the commonest treatment, chemical castration by hormone manipulation.

Pathology

Adenocarcinomas make up 95% of prostate cancers; they arise from the acinar or ductal epithelium. Some 75% are found in the peripheral zone of the prostate and 20% from the transitional zone (see Figure 13.1). The transitional zone is the area involved in benign hypertrophy. Local spread involves the seminal vesicles and the base of the bladder, which can result in ureteric obstruction. The commonest site for metastases is bone; they are usually sclerotic. Lung, liver and brain metastases are not uncommon. A Gleason grade of 1–5 is given to the two predominant areas in a biopsy, which are combined to give a score of 2–10. In current practice, scores of 6–10 are generally seen. A score of 6 (3+3) is the commonest; the higher the score the more aggressive the tumour.

Presentation

All stages of prostate cancer can present asymptomatically with a raised PSA or abnormal incidental digital rectal examination. Common presenting symptoms include worsening lower urinary tract symptoms (LUTS), haematuria and perineal discomfort, all of which could also result from benign disease. Advanced disease can present with renal failure secondary to ureteric obstruction, lower limb oedema, bone pain or pathological fractures, and neurological signs secondary to cord compression.

Diagnosis

An elevated PSA is the commonest reason for considering a diagnosis of cancer. It is a serine protease detectable in serum. Normal age-specific values are shown in Table 13.1.

Table 13.1: Normal age-specific PSA values

PSA values (ng/ml)	Age (years)
<2.5	40–49
<3.5	50–59
<4.5	60–69
<6.5	70–79

PSA is prostate-specific but not cancer-specific. Other conditions such as BPH, UTI, prostatitis, urinary retention and instrumentation can all elevate readings. Digital rectal examination, though an inexact science, remains an important tool as the majority of tumours are in the peripheral zone, which is posterior and therefore palpable via the rectum. Diagnosis is confirmed by transrectal ultrasound (TRUS) and biopsy. Current guidelines recommend at least ten biopsies. Biopsy should not be performed lightly as it is not without complication; principally, sepsis and deaths have been reported. Tissue for diagnosis may also be obtained following a TURP, although the majority of tissue removed in this procedure is from the transitional zone, not the peripheral zone.

CT, MRI and bone scans are used to help stage the disease, but they are no substitute for histology in making a diagnosis.

Treatment

A multitude of options exist and choosing the best option for the patient can be a lengthy process. Treatments can be separated into curative, palliative and conservative. The appropriateness depends on a number of factors, including PSA, Gleason score, clinical stage, co-morbidity and life expectancy.

Curative surgical treatment with a radical prostatectomy is only a possibility in organ-confined disease. The main complications of surgery are erectile dysfunction and incontinence. Surgical technique is constantly being refined; neurovascular-bundle-sparing surgery has led to improved outcomes. Laparoscopic and robotic techniques are becoming increasingly popular and claim lower complication rates.

Radiotherapy can cause erectile dysfunction especially since it is often combined with hormonal manipulation. Bowel and bladder side-effects are also common; these include haematuria and proctitis.

Brachytherapy, the implantation of radioactive seeds (iodine 125), into the prostate is a newer technique which reduces bowel complications and allows for a higher radiation dose to the prostate. Urinary retention occurs in up to 20% of patients.

High-intensity focused ultrasound (HIFU) and cryotherapy are novel techniques currently undergoing evaluation in clinical trials. Some patients with potentially curable disease choose to go under active surveillance, which consists of regular PSA testing, digital rectal examination and repeat biopsies. This group tends to have low PSAs and Gleason-score tumours, which are slow to progress. They are usually keen to avoid adverse side-effects of radical treatment but can switch to radical treatment if it is felt their disease is progressing.

Symptomatic or high-grade locally advanced and metastatic disease is usually treated by hormonal manipulation, with a luteinising hormone-releasing hormone (LHRH) analogue. In most cases this will bring the PSA back into the normal range for an average of 18 months. Chemical castration leads to a number of side-effects: erectile dysfunction, hot flushes, fatigue, weight gain, mood swings, gynaecomastia and loss of libido. After that the PSA can rise as the tumour ceases to be dependent on testosterone for further growth. This leads to disease progression and worsening local and metastatic symptoms. Asymptomatic patients with PSA values less than 30–40 ng/ml can be managed by PSA surveillance, ie watchful waiting.

- Curative
  - Radical prostatectomy
    - Retropubic, laparoscopic or robotic
  - Radical radiotherapy
    - External-beam, brachytherapy
  - HIFU
  - Cryotherapy
- Palliative
  - Radiotherapy
    - External beam to prostate or metastatic deposits
  - Hormonal manipulation
    - Chemical castration with LHRH analogues
  - Steroids
  - Bisphosphonates
- Conservative
  - Active surveillance
    - Regular PSA checks, low threshold for initiating curative treatment
  - PSA and symptom monitoring, hormonal manipulation if needed

13.3.3 Renal tumours

Renal cell carcinoma

Adenocarcinomas of the kidney may be referred to by many names: renal cell carcinoma (RCC), hypernephroma, Grawitz's tumour and clear cell carcinoma. It makes up 85% of all renal malignancies. Incidence continues to increase due to improvements in and increased access to USS and CT.

Aetiology and risk factors

- Male to female ratio 2:1
- Age 60–80 years
- Risk factors
  - Environmental – smoking, dialysis, asbestos, lead, dmium, polycarbons, phenacetin
  - Polycystic and horseshoe kidneys
  - Gecanetic – von Hippel–Lindau (VHL), autosomal dominant, 50% develop renal tumours

Presentation

- The classical triad of a mass, pain and macroscopic haematuria is now rarely seen (<10%)
- The majority are diagnosed incidentally during imaging for another condition, resulting in a lower stage at diagnosis
- In symptomatic RCC, haematuria (50%) is the commonest symptom
- 25% have symptoms of metastatic disease such as weight loss, night sweats, fever and fatigue
- Lower limb oedema and acute left varicocoele occur secondary to venous obstruction
- 10%–40% of patients suffer from a paraneoplastic syndrome due to the ectopic secretion of hormones such as renin, erythropoietin, or another parahormone

Investigations

- FBC: polycythaemia or anaemia
- U&Es: creatinine (renal failure), hypercalcaemia
- Imaging:
  - USS, staging CT chest, abdomen and pelvis
  - Renogram, DTPA or MAG3 scan to determine split function

Biopsy is rarely indicated due to unreliable results and the risk of haemorrhage and tumour seeding.

Pathology and staging

Renal cell carcinomas are adenocarcinomas arising from the proximal convoluted tubule. They are multifocal in 10%–20% of cases; 25% contain cysts or are cystic in nature. They can spread by direct extension through the renal capsule, into the adrenal or into the renal vein (10%), inferior vena cava and occasionally into the right atrium. Lymphatic spread is to the para-aortic and hilar nodes. Lung, liver, bone and brain are the common sites for haematogenous spread.

Histological subtypes

- **Conventional** (70%–80%) – also known as 'clear cell' due to the histological process that removes the fat from the cells resulting in their characteristic appearance
- **Papillary** (18%) – multifocal in 40%
- **Chromophobe** (5%)

- **Collecting duct** – rare, poor prognosis, young patients
- **Medullary cell** – rare, young, Afro-Caribbean, sickle cell, poor prognosis

Tumours are graded 1–4, 1 being well differentiated and 4 being poor, with the Furhman system.

Staging is via the TNM system. See Box 13.3.

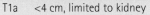

Box 13.3: TNM staging of renal cell carcinoma	
T1a	<4 cm, limited to kidney
T1b	>4 cm, but <7 cm, limited to kidney
T2	>7 cm, limited to kidney
T3	Extension outside the kidney but within Gerota's fascia
T3a	Adrenal or perinephric fat involvement
T3b	Extension into renal vein or IVC below diaphragm
T3c	Extension into IVC above diaphragm
T4	Tumour invades beyond Gerota's fascia
N0	No nodes
N1	Single node
N2	More than one node involved
M0	No distant metastases
M1	Distant metastases present

Treatment

The majority of renal malignancies are treated with surgery. Laproscopic renal surgery is becoming more common, but currently open radical nephrectomy remains the commonest procedure in the UK. Management is dictated by a number of factors including age, co-morbidities, multifocality and the condition of the contralateral kidney. Nephron-sparing surgery with a partial nephrectomy is the preferred option.

Patients with tumours not amenable to partial nephrectomy and who have a normal contralateral kidney may be treated with an open radical nephrectomy or laparoscopic nephrectomy if available. Small tumours may be resected with the kidney in situ. Partial nephrectomy is usually performed open but laparoscopy is used in some centres.

Other options for small and occasionally multiple lesions include cryotherapy and radiofrequency ablation. It should not be forgotten that small incidentally found lesions in the elderly may only require treatment if they become symptomatic. Haematuria can be dealt with by selective embolisation of the tumour.

Metastatic disease is usually managed by oncologists. Single metastases may be resected from the relevant organ if possible and this includes brain metastases. If systemic therapy is planned, oncologists often request the removal of the primary to reduce tumour load.

Immunotherapy with interferon-α and interleukins used to be the commonest treatment. Newer tyrosine kinase inhibitors such as sunitinib and sorafenib are now being used clinically.

Benign renal masses

Renal cysts are present in >50% of the population over the age of 50. This was unknown until the advent of widespread renal tract USS. Simple cysts make up 70% of the benign renal masses and seldom require treatment.

Solid benign masses include oncocytomas and angiomyolipomas. **Oncocytomas** are difficult to distinguish from malignant tumours and are therefore usually removed if found. **Angiomyolipomas** occur sporadically but 20% are associated with tuberous sclerosis. They are composed of blood vessels, smooth muscle and fat. When they become >4 cm, there is a risk of haemorrhage and this requires treatment with embolisation or resection.

13.3.4 Testicular cancer

Primary testicular cancer accounts for 1%–2% of all male cancers, with a lifetime risk of 1 in 500. It is the most curable of all malignancies: in 2001 there were 1990 new cases and only 68 deaths. It rarely occurs before the age of 15 or after the age 60. Bilateral disease occurs in 1%–2% of cases; 95% are germ cell tumours (GCT) and the remaining 5% are stromal tumours or lymphomas.

Epidemiology and aetiology
- Age
  - Teratoma — 20–35 years
  - Seminoma — 35–45 years
  - Lymphoma — >60 years
- **Whites** have four times the incidence compared to the Afro-Caribbean population
- **Undescended testis** (cryptorchidism) increases risk by 10-fold: 10% of tumours occur in undescended testes; risk also increases in a normal contralateral testis. Early orchidopexy, fixation of the testis in the scrotum, does not remove risk but allows for self-examination and earlier detection
- **Intratubular germ cell neoplasia** (ITGCN) is the equivalent of carcinoma-in-situ. Half of all cases develop tumour within 5 years
- **HIV, genetic factors and maternal oestrogen ingestion** also increase risk

Pathology and staging
Testicular tumours are classified by the World Health Organisation (WHO) into germ cell tumours, sex cord tumours and others (see Table 13.2). They are staged by the TNM system. Prognosis for seminomatous tumours is excellent.

The 5-year survival in patients who present without metastases (90%) is 86%; for those with metastases (10%) the 5-year survival is 73%. Prognosis for non-seminomatous germ cell tumours (NSGCT) is also excellent.

Table 13.2: WHO classification of testicular tumours

Germ cell tumours (90%)	Seminoma (48%)	Spermocytic
		Classical
		Anaplastic
	Non-seminomatous GCT (42%)	Teratoma
		Yolk sac tumour
		Choriocarcinoma
		Mixed NSGCT
Other tumours (7%)	Lymphoma (5%)	
	Carcinoid	
	Adenocarcinoma of rete testis	
	Metastatic (1%)	
Sex cord stromal tumours	Leydig cell	
	Sertoli cell	
	Mixed	

Table 13.3: Tumour markers

Alpha-fetoprotein (AFP)	Raised in 70% of teratomas and yolk sac tumours
	Half-life 3–5 days
	Normal <10 ng/ml
Human chorionic gonadotropin (β-hCG)	Choriocarcinoma 100%
	Teratoma 40%, seminoma 10%
	Half-life 24–36 hours
	Normal <5mlU/ml
Lactate dehydrogenase (LDH)	Non-specific
	Used as a guide to tumour burden

Clinical presentation

- Most commonly patients present having found a lump in the testis; there is often a history of minor trauma which initiates the patient's self-examination
- Pain is a rare symptom and occurs in around 5% of cases, usually caused by haemorrhage into the tumour
- Patients may also present with a hydrocoele
- 10% present with metastatic disease, weight loss, lymphadenopathy and chest signs
- 5% of patients present with gynaecomastia due to the production of human chorionic gonadotropin
- Ultrasound is an extension of the physical examination and should be performed. The contralateral testis may feel normal but contain small occult tumours
- Chest X-ray should be performed to exclude metastases
- Blood tests should also be performed to check for and monitor testicular tumour markers

Differential diagnoses

- Epididymo-orchitis
- Epididymal cyst
- Hydrocoele
- Haematoma
- Hernia

Tumour markers

Some germ cell tumours produce measurable proteins (Table 13.3). The presence of these proteins aids in diagnosis, staging and follow-up of the disease.

Treatment

- Radical orchidectomy is the primary treatment in most cases
- If the contralateral testis is abnormal, sperm banking should be offered

- Following surgery the patient is staged with
  - CT of chest, abdomen and pelvis
  - Histology result
  - Tumour marker levels
- Patients who present unwell with metastatic disease can be treated immediately with chemotherapy, without a histological diagnosis
- Radiotherapy can be given to lymph node metastases in seminomatous tumours

13.3.5 Penile cancer

Squamous cell carcinoma of the penis

- This is a rare malignancy with a UK incidence of 1 in 100 000. It is even rarer in countries where circumcision is common (USA) or where levels of personal hygiene are high (Scandinavia)
- Risk factors include advanced age, poor hygiene, BXO and HPV
- The primary usually occurs on the prepuce or glans penis as a painless lesion or ulcer
- If untreated it spreads via the lymphatics to the inguinal lymph nodes
- Patients often present late with metastatic inguinal disease and have a poor prognosis
- Treatment until recently was by partial or complete penile amputation; surgical techniques have been refined, allowing for penis-conserving surgery, in specialist centres
- Prophylactic inguinal node dissection may be required in high-risk cases
- Radiotherapy and chemotherapy (topical 5-fluorouracil) have a very limited role in treatment

Picture permissions

Abdomen

The following figure in this book has been reproduced from Burnand K et al (1992) *The New Aird's Companion in Surgical Studies* (3rd edition) by kind permission of the publisher Elsevier.

Figure 4.13 Goodsall's rule

Endocrine

The following figure in this book has been reproduced from Ellis H (2002) *Clinical Anatomy* (10th edition) by kind permission of the publisher Blackwell Science.

Figure 8.1 The decent of the thyroid

Vascular

The following figure in this book has been reproduced from Snell, R S (2000) *Clinical Anatomy for Medical Students* (6th edition) by kind permission of the publisher Lippincott, Williams and Wilkins.

Figure 12.5a Anatomy of the lower limb veins

Plastic Surgery

The following figure in this book has been adapted from Website Animations, University of Pennsylvania Health System, by kind permission of University of Pennsylvania School of Medicine, Penn Presbyterian Medical Center, Philadelphia.

Figure 9.5 Zones of the hand on the volar surface

Index

Index

315

Index